Sexual and Reproductive Health:
A Growing Concern

Sexual and Reproductive Health: A Growing Concern

Edited by Ross Bell

hayle
medical

New York

Hayle Medical,
750 Third Avenue, 9th Floor,
New York, NY 10017, USA

Visit us on the World Wide Web at:
www.haylemedical.com

ISBN: 978-1-63241-761-9

Cataloging-in-Publication Data

   Sexual and reproductive health : a growing concern / edited by Ross Bell.
      p. cm.
   Includes bibliographical references and index.
   ISBN 978-1-63241-761-9
   1. Sexual health. 2. Reproductive health. 3. Fertility, Human. 4. Human reproduction.
   5. Human biology. 6. Reproduction. I. Bell, Ross.
RG133 .S48 2019
618.178--dc23

Table of Contents

Preface

Every book is a source of knowledge and this one is no exception. The idea that led to the conceptualization of this book was the fact that the world is advancing rapidly; which makes it crucial to document the progress in every field. I am aware that a lot of data is already available, yet, there is a lot more to learn. Hence, I accepted the responsibility of editing this book and contributing my knowledge to the community.

Sexual and reproductive health addresses the reproductive processes, and functions at all stages of life. It focuses on spreading awareness regarding safe, affordable and effective birth control methods. Safe pregnancy and childbirth are intrinsic to reproductive health. Oral pills, condoms, contraceptive patches, vaginal rings, tubectomy, vasectomy and injections for birth control are some of the common methods of birth control. Adolescent sexuality is a major concern, which falls under the scope of sexual and reproductive health. It is a stage of human development concerned with the experience and exploration of sexual feelings in adolescents. This book aims to shed light on some of the unexplored aspects of sexual and reproductive health and the recent researches in this field. It includes some of the vital pieces of work being conducted across the world, on various topics related to sexual and reproductive health. Doctors, researchers and students actively engaged in this field will find this book full of crucial and unexplored concepts.

While editing this book, I had multiple visions for it. Then I finally narrowed down to make every chapter a sole standing text explaining a particular topic, so that they can be used independently. However, the umbrella subject sinews them into a common theme. This makes the book a unique platform of knowledge.

I would like to give the major credit of this book to the experts from every corner of the world, who took the time to share their expertise with us. Also, I owe the completion of this book to the never-ending support of my family, who supported me throughout the project.

Editor

The correlation between raised body mass index and assisted reproductive treatment outcomes

Prasanna Raj Supramaniam[1*], Monica Mittal[1], Enda McVeigh[2] and Lee Nai Lim[1]

Abstract

Background: Public funding for fertility services within the United Kingdom is limited, and therefore, strict guidance exists regarding who can be offered treatment under the National Health Service (NHS). Body mass index (BMI) is a universal criteria adopted by both the public and private sector.

This study addresses an important aspect of the impact of a raised BMI on fertility treatment outcomes. We standardise the analysis of the data by only including studies incorporating the WHO BMI criteria; the current reference point for clinicians and clinical commissioning groups in ascertaining which group of patients should receive treatment. This study is an update of the previous systematic review performed in 2010, with the inclusion of a larger number of cycles from central databases such as the Society for Assisted Reproductive Technology (SART).

Methods: An electronic literature search was conducted through the Cochrane, Medline and Embase libraries. Data extraction for each outcome measure was pooled and expressed as an odds ratio with 95% confidence intervals. Where clinical heterogeneity was evident, the random effects model was used to calculate the risk ratio and a fixed effects model was used for the remaining studies. A p value < 0.05 was considered statistically significant.

Results: A total of 49 studies have been identified and included in this systematic review. Overweight and obese (BMI $\geq$ 25 kg/m^2) women have a statistically significant lower live birth rate (OR 0.81, 95% CI 0.74–0.89, $p < 0.00001$) following Assisted Reproductive Technology (ART) when comparisons are drawn to women with a normal BMI. An increase is also demonstrated in the number of miscarriages experienced by women with a BMI $\geq$ 30 kg/m^2 (OR 1.52, 95% CI 1.28–1.81, $p < 0.00001$).

Conclusion: Although this review concludes that a clear impact of BMI on ART outcomes is demonstrated, there remains questions as to the pathophysiology underlying these differences. This review supports the government's stringent criteria regarding BMI categories under which NHS funding is made available for ART, through a clear description of poor reproductive outcomes in women with a BMI $\geq$ 30 kg/m^2.

Keywords: Body mass index (BMI), Assisted reproductive technology (ART), Overweight, Obese

* Correspondence: prasannaraj@doctors.org.uk
[1]Oxford University Hospitals NHS Foundation Trust, John Radcliffe Hospital, Headley Way, Headington, Oxford OX3 9DU, UK
Full list of author information is available at the end of the article

Plain English summary

This study highlights the impact of an overweight or obese female partner on fertility treatment outcomes, in particular focusing on IVF. Women who are overweight or obese have been shown to be less likely to have a life birth outcome from an IVF cycle. They are also more likely to suffer from early miscarriages whilst undergoing fertility treatments.

Main manuscript

The correlation between raised body mass index and assisted reproductive treatment outcomes: A systematic review and meta-analysis of the evidence.

Background

Obesity is a major challenge for today's clinicians. In 2016, the World Health Organisation (WHO) [1] stated that a staggering 39% of adults aged > 18 years fell into the overweight category, of which 40% were accounted for by women. Furthermore, 13% of the adult population were documented to be obese, with women accounting for 15% (WHO Global Health Observatory Data 2016). A raised body mass index (BMI) has been linked to a number of medical comorbidities, as well as being implicated in having a detrimental impact on the reproductive capacity of women in particular. Women who fall into high BMI categories can present with hypothalamic-pituitary ovarian dysfunction and thus, low fecundity rates. In 2011, Rittenberg et al., [2] concluded that women with a BMI ≥ 25.0 kg/m^2 had a lower live birth rate through assisted reproductive treatments (ART) compared with women of a normal BMI. This has been further supported by multiple large studies evaluating the impact of BMI on ART outcomes.

The WHO classification of BMI is widely referred to, and provides standardisation for comparison of research outcomes. A documented BMI of 18.5–24.9 kg/m^2 is considered normal and healthy and the preferred range. A BMI of 25–29.9 kg/m^2 refers to overweight and a BMI ≥ 30 kg/m^2 is considered obese. The latter range is further subdivided into Class 1 (30.0–34.9 kg/m^2), Class 2 (35.0–39.9 kg/m^2) and Class 3 (≥ 40.0 kg/m^2).

This paper, considers the current evidence regarding the impact of raised BMI on outcomes following ART treatment. A systematic review and meta-analysis of the available evidence will help provide or refute the current recommendations from the government regarding the allocation of resources for fertility treatment.

Methods

Search strategy

Literature searches were conducted through the Cochrane, Embase and Medline libraries (1966–2017). The medical subject headings (MeSH) were generated for two categories: 1. Body mass index (BMI, overweight, obesity); 2. in vitro fertilisation (IVF)/ intracytoplasmic sperm injection (ICSI) (embryo, embryo transfer, ART). All identified papers were reviewed by two authors (PRS and MM) independently. All discrepancies, regarding inclusion or exclusion of the data were discussed with a final decision mutually agreed upon.

Study inclusion and exclusion criteria

All relevant published studies reporting on the effects of BMI on IVF and ICSI pregnancy outcomes were included. Studies that reported donor cycles, conception by natural cycles, intrauterine insemination, waist hip ratio, and non-WHO classification of BMI were excluded. In addition, studies reporting on the effects of paternal body mass index on IVF/ ICSI outcomes were also excluded.

Outcome measures

The primary outcome measure assessed was live birth rate following an IVF/ ICSI cycle. Secondary outcome measures included: clinical pregnancy rate; and, miscarriage rate. The presence of a gestational sac on an ultrasound scan at least four weeks following on from an embryo transfer was used as confirmation for a clinical pregnancy. The clinical pregnancy rate was calculated per IVF/ ICSI cycle. For the purpose of this review, miscarriage was defined as pregnancy loss ≤ 20 weeks gestation. The miscarriage rate was calculated per clinical pregnancy.

Statistical analysis

Data extraction for each outcome measure was pooled and expressed as an odds ratio (OR) with a 95% confidence interval (CI). Clinical heterogeneity (I^2) [3] was considered significant when the I^2 value was < 50%. Where clinical heterogeneity was evident, the random effects model (DerSimonian and Laird, 1986) was used to calculate the risk ratio, and clinical heterogeneity was explored by comparing the variation in studies, such as, study design, study quality and interventions. Particular care was taken to further evaluate studies with similar first authors to avoid heterogeneity in the study population. For the remaining pooled data, the fixed effect model [4] was used to calculate the risk ratio. Statistical analysis was performed using the RevMan 5.3 software. A p value < 0.05 was considered statistically significant.

Results

The search strategy yielded 7458 electronic citations (Fig. 1). Of this, 2830 were removed secondary to duplications. Titles and abstracts were reviewed for the remaining 4628 publications. After screening of the titles and abstracts, 4508 publications were further excluded.

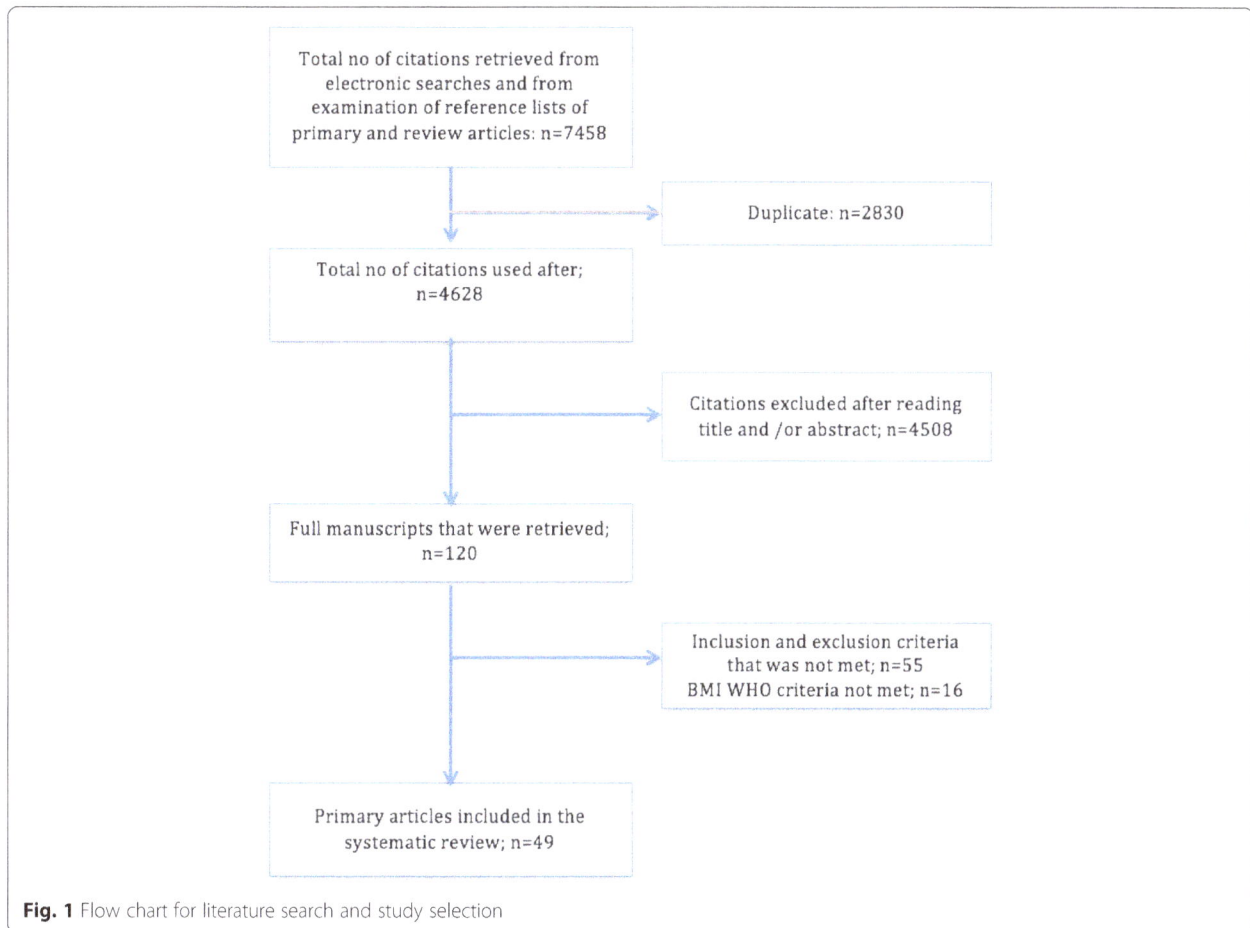

Fig. 1 Flow chart for literature search and study selection

Full manuscripts were obtained for the remaining 120 articles. A further 16 articles were excluded as they did not use the WHO classification for BMI categories. A further 55 articles were excluded as per the inclusion exclusion criteria. The remaining 49 articles met all requirements and were included in this systematic review and meta-analysis (Table 1).

Primary outcome measure
Life birth rate per IVF/ ICSI cycle
In women with a BMI $\geq$25 kg/m^2 versus BMI < 25 kg/m^2, a total of 14 studies were pooled and a statistically significant reduction in the live birth rate (OR 0.81, 95% CI 0.74–0.89, $p < 0.00001$; Fig. 2a) was seen. There was significant heterogeneity between the included studies ($I^2 = 65\%$).

A total of 11 studies compared women with a normal BMI against those who were overweight (BMI 25–29.9 kg/m^2). An analysis of the pooled data showed a statistically significant reduction in the live birth rate in women with a BMI 25–29.9 (OR 0.92, 95% CI 0.86–0.97, $p = 0.005$; Fig. 2b). No significant heterogeneity ($I^2 = 18\%$) was documented.

Data for women with a normal BMI versus BMI $\geq$ 30 kg/m^2 came from the pooling of 10 studies. The live birth rate for women with a BMI $\geq$30 kg/m^2 was statistically significantly lower than for women with a normal BMI (OR 0.81, 95% CI 0.79–0.82, $p < 0.00001$; Fig. 2c). No significant heterogeneity ($I^2 = 0\%$) was detected in the data source.

Secondary outcome measures
Clinical pregnancy rate
A total of 37 studies were pooled for BMI < 25 kg/m^2 versus BMI $\geq$25 kg/m^2. A statistically significant reduction in the clinical pregnancy rate was demonstrated for women with a BMI $\geq$25 kg/m^2 (OR 0.82, 95% CI 0.77–0.88, $p < 0.00001$; Fig. 3a). However, there was significant heterogeneity ($I^2 = 58\%$, $p < 0.00001$) between the studies analysed.

A statistically significant reduction in the clinical pregnancy rate was demonstrated for women with a BMI between 25 and 29.9 kg/m^2 when compared to women with a normal BMI (19 studies pooled, OR 0.89, 95% CI 0.84–0.94, $p < 0.00001$; Fig. 3b). No significant heterogeneity ($I^2 = 31\%$) was seen between the studies.

Table 1 Details of included studies

Study	Methodology (population size)	Intervention	Exclusion Criteria	BMI Categories (kg/m^2) and numbers	Outcome Measures
Fedorcsak et al. 2000 [8] (1996–1998)	Retrospective Cohort study (383 women)	IVF/ICSI	12 patients excluded as incomplete data	< 25.0 (304 women) ≥25.0 (79 women)	Live birth rate Fertilization rate No of oocytes retrieved Abortion rate
Wittemer et al. 2000 [9] (1997–1998)	Retrospective study (398 women)	IVF/ICSI	None stated	< 20.0 (87 women) 20.0–25.0 (222 women) ≥ 25.0 (89 women)	Pregnancy rate Delivery rate Miscarriage rate
Wang et al. 2000 [10] (1987–1998)	Retrospective study (3586 women)	IVF/ICSI and GIFT	None stated	< 20.0 (441 women) 20.0–24.9 (1910 women) 25.0–29.9 (814 women) 30.0–34.9 (304 women) ≥35.0 (117 women)	Probability of achieving at least one pregnancy
Loveland et al. 2001 [11] (1997–1999)	Retrospective study (139 women / 180 cycles)	IVF	Women > 40 years of age, blastocyst or frozen embryo transfer, donor cycles	≤25 (70 women / 87 cycles) > 25 (69 women / 93 cycles)	Number of oocytes Clinical pregnancy rate Spontaneous abortion Ongoing pregnancy rate
Wang et al. 2001 [12] (1987–1999)	Cohort study (1018 women)	IVF/ICSI/ GIFT	Women whose BMI or PCOS status was not assessed	< 20.0 (112 women) 20.0–24.9 (509 women) 25.0–29.9 (231 women) 30.0–34.9 (116 women) ≥35.0 (50 women)	Spontaneous abortion
Wang et al. 2002 [13] (1987–1999)	Retrospective analysis (2349 women)	IVF/ICSI/ GIFT	Ectopic pregnancy, late pregnancy, women whose BMI was measured >/= 1 year before pregnancy	< 18.5 (70 women) 18.5–24.9 (1508 women) 25–29.9 (503 women) 30–34.9 (198 women) ≥35 (70 women)	Spontaneous miscarriage
Winter et al. 2002 [14] (1994–1999)	Cohort (1123 women / 1196 cycles)	IVF/ICSI/ GIFT		< 18.5 (26 women) 18.5–25.0 (701 women) 25.1–30.0 (243 women) 30.1–35.0 (107 women) > 35.0 (46 women)	Early pregnancy loss
Doody et al. 2003 [15] (2000–2003)	Retrospective analysis (822 retrievals)	IVF/ICSI	Donor cycles, age > 40 years	< 25 (460 women) 25–29.9 (194 women) 30–34.9 (89 women) > 35 (79 women)	Pregnancy rate Implantation rate No of oocytes No of embryos transferred Ongoing pregnancy rate
Fedorscak et al. 2004 [16] (1996–2002)	Retrospective Study (2660 women / 5019 cycles)	IVF/ICSI	None stated	< 18.5 (76 women/136 cycles) 18.5–24.9 (1839 women/ 3457 cycles) 25.0–29.9 (504 women/ 963 cycles) ≥30.0 (241 women/ 463 cycles)	No of oocytes collected No of embryo transferred No of embryo transfers No of biochemical pregnancies Early pregnancy loss Miscarriage (6–12 weeks), (> 12 weeks) Ectopic pregnancy Stillbirth Live birth rate Dose of FSH Duration of FSH
Ryley et al. 2004 [17]	Retrospective study (6827 cycles)	IVF	Women with BMI > 40	< 20.0 (466 cycles) 20.0–24.9 (3605 cycles) 25.0–29.9 (1632 cycles) 30.0–34.9 (724 cycles) =35 (400 cycles)	Clinical pregnancy rate No of oocytes
Van Swieten et al. 2005 [18]	Observational (162 women/ 288 cycle)	IVF/ICSI	None stated	< 25 (101 women) 25–30 (32 women) > 30 (29 women)	Fertilisation rate No oocytes retrieved Clinical pregnancy rate Abortion rate

Table 1 Details of included studies (Continued)

Study	Methodology (population size)	Intervention	Exclusion Criteria	BMI Categories (kg/m^2) and numbers	Outcome Measures
Hammadeh et al. 2005 [19]	Prospective (52 women)	IVF	None stated	≤25.0 (28 women) > 25.0 (24 women)	Pregnancy rate
Dechaud et al. 2006 [20]	Prospective study (573 women/ 789 cycles)	IVF/ICSI	Women with a history of uterine surgery, hydrosalpinges evidenced by ultrasonography, three or more failed attempts at IVF, frozen-thawed cycles, women undergoing pre-implantation diagnosis and those using a protocol other than the long protocol	< 20 (186 women/ 264 cycles) 20–25 (283 women/ 394 cycles) 25–30 (68 women/ 83 cycles) ≥30 (36 women/ 48 cycles)	Duration of ovarian stimulation Dose of FSH Implantation rate No of oocytes Fertilization rate Clinical pregnancy rate Miscarriage rate
Dokras et al. 2006 [21] (1995–2005)	Retrospective Study (1293 women)	IVF/IVF with ICSI	Women > 38 years of age, day 2 transfer cycles, cryopreserved embryo transfers, donor oocyte cycle, gamete intrafallopian transfer and zygote intrafallopian transfer cycles	< 25 (683 women) 25–29.9 (295 women) 30.0–39.9 (236 women) ≥40 (79 women)	No of follicles aspirated Fertilization rate No of embryo(s) transferred Clinical pregnancy rate Miscarriage rate Delivery rate Days of stimulation
Mitwally et al. 2006 [22]	Cohort (183 cycles)	IVF	None stated	< 25.0 (102 cycles) ≥25.0 (81 cycles)	Clinical pregnancy rate
Metwally 2007 [23] (2001–2006)	Retrospective analysis (426 women)	IVF/ICSI	Cycles on women whose BMI was unrecorded	19–24.9 (241 women) 25–29.9 (113 women) ≥30 (72 women)	Fertilization rate Clinical pregnancy rate Dose of FSH Duration of FSH No of oocytes collected
Esinler et al. 2008 [24]	Retrospective Study (775 women/ 1113 cycles)	ICSI	Freeze-thaw cycles, female age > 40, presence of PCOS, history of irregular menstrual cycle and suspected poor ovarian response	18.5–24.9 (451 women/ 627 cycles) 25.0–29.9 (222 women/ 339 cycles) ≥30.0 (102 women/ 147 cycles)	Clinical pregnancy rate Fertilization rate No of miscarriages No of oocytes Dose of FSH Duration of FSH
Martinuzzi et al. 2008 [25] (2004–2006)	Retrospective study (417 women)	IVF	Women > 36 years of age, cycle day-3	< 18.5 (21 women) 18.5–24.9 (267 women) 25.0–29.9 (77 women) ≥30 (52 women)	No of oocytes Fertilization rate Implantation rate Clinical pregnancy rate Ongoing pregnancy rate
Moini et al. 2008 [26] (2002–2003)	Cross-sectional study (287 women)	IVF/ICSI	Women who did not have polycystic ovary syndrome, age > 40 years, BMI < 20, women with hypo/ hyperthyroidism, hyperprolactinemia and diabetes type 1	20–25 (133 women) 25.1–30 (117 women) > 30 (37 women)	No of oocytes No of transferred embryos Clinical pregnancy rate Miscarriage rate
Sneed et al. 2008 [27] (2005–2006)	Retrospective analysis (1273 women)	IVF	Frozen cycles, donor oocyte or gestational surrogacy cycles, age > 44 years	< 18.5 (28 women) > 18.5–24.9 (613 women) > 25–29.9 (325 women) > 30 (307 women)	No of oocytes No of embryo transfers Fertilization rate Implantation rate Spontaneous abortion Clinical pregnancies Live birth rate
Ozgun et al. 2009 [28] (2006–2007)	Prospective study (604 women)	ICSI	Women > 42 years old, medical co-morbidities such as diabetes mellitus, hyper or hypothyroidism, basal FSH > 15 IU/L, thawed embryo transfer cycles, history of prior ovarian surgery, poor responders, couples with more than one etiology for their infertility	< 18.5 (10 women) 18.5–24.9 (232 women) 25–29.9 (229 women) 30–35.9 (111 women) ≥36 (22 women)	No of Pregnancy Total FSH dosage

Table 1 Details of included studies *(Continued)*

Study	Methodology (population size)	Intervention	Exclusion Criteria	BMI Categories (kg/m^2) and numbers	Outcome Measures
Sathya et al. 2010 [29]	Retrospective study (308 women)	IVF	Women > 40 years of age, FSH > 10 mIU/ml	< 25 (88 women) 25–30 (147 women) > 30 (73 women)	No of embryos transferred Clinical pregnancy rate Missed abortion rate Multiple pregnancy rate Ectopic pregnancy rate Implantation rate Gonadotrophin dosage
Zhang et al. 2010 [30] (2002–2008)	Retrospective study (2628 women)	IVF/ICSI	Patients with severe endometriosis (III and IV stage) diagnosed by laparoscopy, more than two failed previous attempts, preimplantation diagnosis cycles, frozen thawed cycles, protocols other than the long protocol	18.5–24.9 (2222 women) 25.0–29.9 (379 women) ≥30.0 (27 women)	No of oocytes Fertilization rate Pregnancy rate Early pregnancy loss rate Ectopic pregnancy Miscarriage rate Live birth rate Days of FSH stimulation Dosage of FSH stimulation Ongoing pregnancy rate
Bellver et al. 2010 [31] (2001–2007)	Retrospective study (6500 cycles)	IVF/ICSI	None stated	< 20 (669 women / 1070 cycles) 20–24.9 (2620 women/ 3930 cycles) 25–29.9 (676 women/ 1081 cycles) ≥ 30 (262 cycles/ 419 cycles)	Total dose of gonadotrophin No of oocytes Fertilization rate No of embryos transferred Implantation rate Pregnancy rate Clinical pregnancy rate Clinical and global miscarriage rate Live birth rate
Vilarino et al. 2010 [32] (2008)	Retrospective (208 cycles/ 191 women)	IVF/ICSI	Frozen and donor oocyte-derived cycles	< 25 (137 cycles) ≥25 (71 cycles)	Fertilisation rate No of transferred embryos Pregnancy rate Early pregnancy loss Clinical miscarriage rate Ectopic pregnancy Live birth rate Dosage of FSH
Farhi et al. 2010 [33] (2006–2007)	Retrospective study (233 women/ 233 cycles)	IVF	Women ≥38 years of age, other than 2 high-quality embryos, ≥3 previous IVF attempts, women with hydrosalpinx, fibroid uterus, congenital uterine anomaly and chronic illness	≤25.0 (160 women) > 25.0 (73 women)	Live birth rate Pregnancy rate No of oocytes Fertilization rate
Davies et al. 2010 [34] (2008–2009)	232 cycles	IVF	Donor egg, gestational carrier and pre-implantation genetic diagnosis cycles	< 25.0 (176 cycles) > 25.0 (56 cycles)	Fetal heartbeat rates
Funabiki et al. 2011 [35] (2006–2010)	Retrospective study (859 women)	IVF	None stated	< 18.5 (152 women) 18.5–25.0 (648 women) ≥25.0 (59 women)	Pregnancy rate Ongoing pregnancy rate Miscarriage rate No of oocytes
Hill et al. 2011 [36]	Prospective study (117 women)	IVF	Women > 42 years of age, patients with elevated FSH levels (≥12 mIU/mL)	< 25.0 (58 women) ≥25.0 (59 women) < 30.0 (96 women) ≥30.0 (21 women)	Live birth rate Pregnancy rate Implantation rate No of oocytes No of embryo transferred Days of stimulation

Table 1 Details of included studies (Continued)

Study	Methodology (population size)	Intervention	Exclusion Criteria	BMI Categories (kg/m^2) and numbers	Outcome Measures
Pinborg et al. 2011 [37] (2005–2006)	Cohort study (487 women/ 1417 cycles)	IVF/ ICSI/ FET	Patients undergoing intrauterine insemination cycles, patients with an existing child from fertility treatment, couples who had adopted a child in the 12th month follow-up period and couples who had no treatment during the first 12 months of follow up	< 18.5 (20 women) 18.5–24.9 (305 women) 25.0–29.9 (103 women) ≥30.0 (59 women)	Fertilization rate No of oocytes Biochemical pregnancy rate Ectopic pregnancy rate Ongoing pregnancy rate Miscarriage rate Live birth rate Dose of gonadotrophin stimulation
Parker et al. 2011 [38] (2010–2011)	Retrospective study (995 patients)	IVF/ICSI	None stated	< 18.5 (18 women) 18.5–24.9 (475 women) 25–29.9 (241 women) > 30 (221 women)	No of oocytes Clinical pregnancy rate Implantation rate Ongoing pregnancy rate Total FSH dosage No of embryo transferred
Rittenberg et al. 2011 [39] (2006–2010)	Cohort Study (413 women)	IVF/ICSI	Women > 40 years, BMI < 18.5, BMI > 35, pre-implantation genetic diagnosis, donor oocyte or embryos frozen for fertility preservation prior to cancer therapy cycles, mullerian duct anomalies, monozygotic twin gestations	18.5–24.9 (192 women) ≥25 (133 women)	Oocyte fertilisation rate No of oocytes Clinical pregnancy rate Live birth rate Miscarriage rate Duration of stimulation
Singh et al. 2011 [40] (2008–2010)	Retrospective Study (328 women/ 342 cycles)	IVF/ICSI	Women with confounding factors for poor response, endometrial pathologies, hydrosalpinx, ≥3 previous failed attempts, frozen thawed cycles	< 18.5 (26 women) 18.5–24.9 (141 women) 25–29.9 (131 women) > 30 (18 women)	Fertilisation rate Pregnancy rate Total dose of FSH Total days of stimulation No of oocytes retrieved Fertilization rate Clinical pregnancy rate
Luke et al. 2011 [41] (2007–2008)	Historical cohort study (152,500 cycles)	IVF	Women whose height and weight were not recorded, gestational carrier cycles, research or embryo banking with no outcome reported	< 18.5 (4254 cycles) 18.5–24.9 (86,860 cycles) 25–29.9 (35,452 cycles) 30.0–34.9 (15,406 cycles) 35.0–39.9 (6920 cycles) 40.0–44.9 (2513 cycles) 45.0–49.9 (805 cycles)	Pregnancy rate Fetal death or stillborn
Chavarro et al. 2012 [42] (2004–2011)	Prospective study (170 women/ 233 cycles)	IVF/ICSI	Women < 18 and > 45 years of age	< 20 (22 women) 20–22.4 (47 women) 22.5–24.9 (42 women) 25–29.9 (35 women) ≥30 (24 women)	Clinical pregnancy rate Total gonadotrophin dose Fertilization rate Clinical pregnancy rate Live birth rate
Galal et al. 2012 [43]	Prospective cohort (220 women)	ICSI	None stated	< 25.0 (110 women) > 25.0 (110 women)	No of oocytes Fertilization rate Clinical pregnancy rate No of embryos transferred
Werner et al. 2012 [44] (2008–2012)	Retrospective study (355 women)	IVF	None stated	< 18.5 (13 women) 18.5–24.9 (209 women) 25.0–29.9 (88 women) > 30.0 (45 women)	Pregnancy rate Clinical implantation rate Sustained implantation rate
Zander-Fox et al. 2012 [45] (2006–2007)	Retrospective study (2089 cycles)	IVF/ICSI	Women > 38 years of age, natural and donor cycles	18.5–24.9 (1065 cycles) 25.0–29.9 (486 cycles) 30.0–34.9 (244 cycles) 35.0–39.9 (144 cycles) ≥40.0 (118 cycles)	No of oocytes Fertilisation rate Live delivery Clinical pregnancy No of oocytes
Ozgun et al. 2012 [46] (2005–2010)	Retrospective cohort (935 women)	ICSI	No exclusion criteria	< 18.5 (18 women) 18.5–24.9 (398 women) 25–29.9 (355 women) ≥30 (164 women)	Clinical pregnancy rateNo of oocytes Miscarriage rate Total gonadotrophin dose

Table 1 Details of included studies *(Continued)*

Study	Methodology (population size)	Intervention	Exclusion Criteria	BMI Categories (kg/m^2) and numbers	Outcome Measures
Ramezanzadeh et al. 2012 [47] (2010–2011)	Prospective study (236 women)	IVF	Male factor infertility according to the WHO criteria, presence of systemic disease, age < 18 years or > 40 years and donor oocytes	< 25 (93 women) 25–30 (94 women) > 30 (49 women)	No of oocytes Fertilization rate No of embryo transferred Biochemical pregnancies Clinical pregnancy rate Implantation rate
Moragianni et al. 2012 [48] (2007–2008)	Retrospective cohort study (4609 women)	IVF/ IVF-ICSI	Women < 20 years and > 47 years of age, donor oocytes, gestational surrogacy, cryopreserved embryos or those that lacked BMI documentation	< 18.5 (92 women) 18.5–24.99 (2605 women) 25.0–29.99 (1027 women) 30.00–34.99 (477 women) 35.00–39.99 (275 women) > 40.0 (133 women)	No of oocytes retrieved Duration of stimulation Total dosage of gonadotrophin No of embryo transferred Implantation Clinical pregnancy Biochemical pregnancy Global miscarriage Ectopic pregnancy Live birth Multiple birth
Bailey et al. 2014 [49] (2001–2010)	Retrospective Cohort Study (79 women / 101 cycles)	IVF/ICSI	Women < 40 years of age, height and weight measurements > 3 months from the start of cycle, in-vitro maturation, FSH > 10 mIU/mL, uncontrolled thyroid disease, history of chemotherapy or radiation exposure, recurrent pregnancy loss, uterine factor, balanced translocation in either partner, surgically documented endometriosis or pelvic adhesions, history of pelvic inflammatory disease, adenomyosis and submucosal myoma	18.7–24.9 (51 cycles) 25.0–29.9 (19 cycles) ≥30.0 (31 cycles)	Chemical pregnancy Miscarriage Clinical Pregnancy Live Birth rate Duration of stimulation of gonadotrophin Dosage of gonadotrophin No of oocytes retrieved
Schliep et al. 2014 [50] (2005–2010)	Prospective Cohort Study (721 women)	IVF/ICSI	Men with non-obstructive azoospermia	< 18.5 (32 women) 18.5–24.9 (407 women) 25–29.9 (147 women) 30–34.9 (72 women) ≥35 (63 women)	Fertilization rate Pregnancy rate Live birth rate
Cai et al. 2017 [51] (2013–2014)	Retrospective Cohort Study (4401 women / 4798 fresh transfer cycles)	IVF/ICSI	Mild stimulation cycles, natural cycles and luteal-phase stimulation cycle, patients with diabetes, glucose intolerance and thyroid abnormality	< 18.5 (886 cycles) 18.5–24.9 (3642 cycles) ≥25 (670 cycles)	Fertilization rate Live birth rate Miscarriage rate Dosage of gonadotrophin
Ozekinci et al. 2015 [52] (2008–2013)	Retrospective Cohort Study (298 women)	IVF-ICSI	Underweight women, women > 38 years of age, transfer of > 2 embryos, frozen cycles	18.5–24.9 (164 cycles) 25–29.9 (70 cycles) ≥30 (64 cycles)	Dosage of gonadotrophin Duration of stimulation
Caillon et al. 2015 [53] (2006–2009)	Retrospective study (582 women)	IVF-ICSI	Underweight women	18.5–24.9 (409 women) ≥25 (149 women)	Dosage of gonadotrophin Implantation rate Miscarriage rate Live birth rate
Provost et al. 2016 [54] 2008–2010	Retrospective Cohort Study (239,127 cycles)	IVF	Women with a height < 48 in. and weight < 70 pounds	< 18.5 (7149 cycles) 18.5–24.9 (134,588 cycles) 25–29.9 (54,822 cycles) 30–34.9 (24,922 cycles) 35–39.9 (11,747 cycles) 40–44.9 (4084 cycles) 45–49.9 (1292 cycles) > 50 (463 cycles)	Implantation rate Clinical pregnancy rate Miscarriage rate Live birth rate
Russo et al. 2017 [55] 2010–2014	Retrospective Cohort Study (520 women)	Not specified	Congenital uterine anomalies, endometrial polyps, intrauterine synechiae, adenomyosis, intra-cavity fibroids, hydrosalpinges, donor cycles, poor quality embryos, cleavage stage embryos, and women > 40 years	< 20 (51 women) 20–24.9 (294 women) 25–29.9 (64 women) 30–39.9 (58 women) ≥40 (54 women)	Miscarriage rate Clinical pregnancy rate Live birth rate Dosage of gonadotrophin

Table 1 Details of included studies *(Continued)*

Study	Methodology (population size)	Intervention	Exclusion Criteria	BMI Categories (kg/m^2) and numbers	Outcome Measures
Christensen et al. 2016 [56] (1999–2009)	Retrospective Cohort Study (5342 cycles)	IVF/ICSI	Missing information on BMI or treatment type, premature ovulation before oocyte retrieval, intrauterine insemination cycles	< 18.5 (158 cycles) 18.5–24.9 (3539 cycles) 25–29.9 (1171 cycles) ≥30 (474 cycles)	Dosage of gonadotrophin Clinical pregnancy rate

BMI Body Mass Index, *IVF* in vitro fertilization, *ICSI* intracytoplasmic sperm injection, *OHSS* ovarian hyperstimulation syndrome, *GIFT* gamete intra-Fallopian transfer, *HCG* human chorionic gonadotrophin, *FSH* follicle stimulation hormone

Pooled analysis from 18 studies demonstrated a statistically significant reduction in the clinical pregnancy rate for women with a BMI ≥30 kg/m^2 when compared to women with a normal BMI (OR 0.80, 95% CI 0.74–0.87, $p < 0.00001$; Fig. 3c). There was no significant heterogeneity ($I^2 = 32\%$) present between the studies.

Miscarriage rate

An increased risk of miscarriage is demonstrated in women with a BMI ≥25 kg/m^2 when compared to women with a BMI < 25 kg/m^2 (26 studies pooled, OR 1.30, 95% CI 1.15–1.48, $p < 0.0001$; Fig. 4a). However, significant heterogeneity ($I^2 = 53\%$, $p = 0.0001$) was seen between the studies.

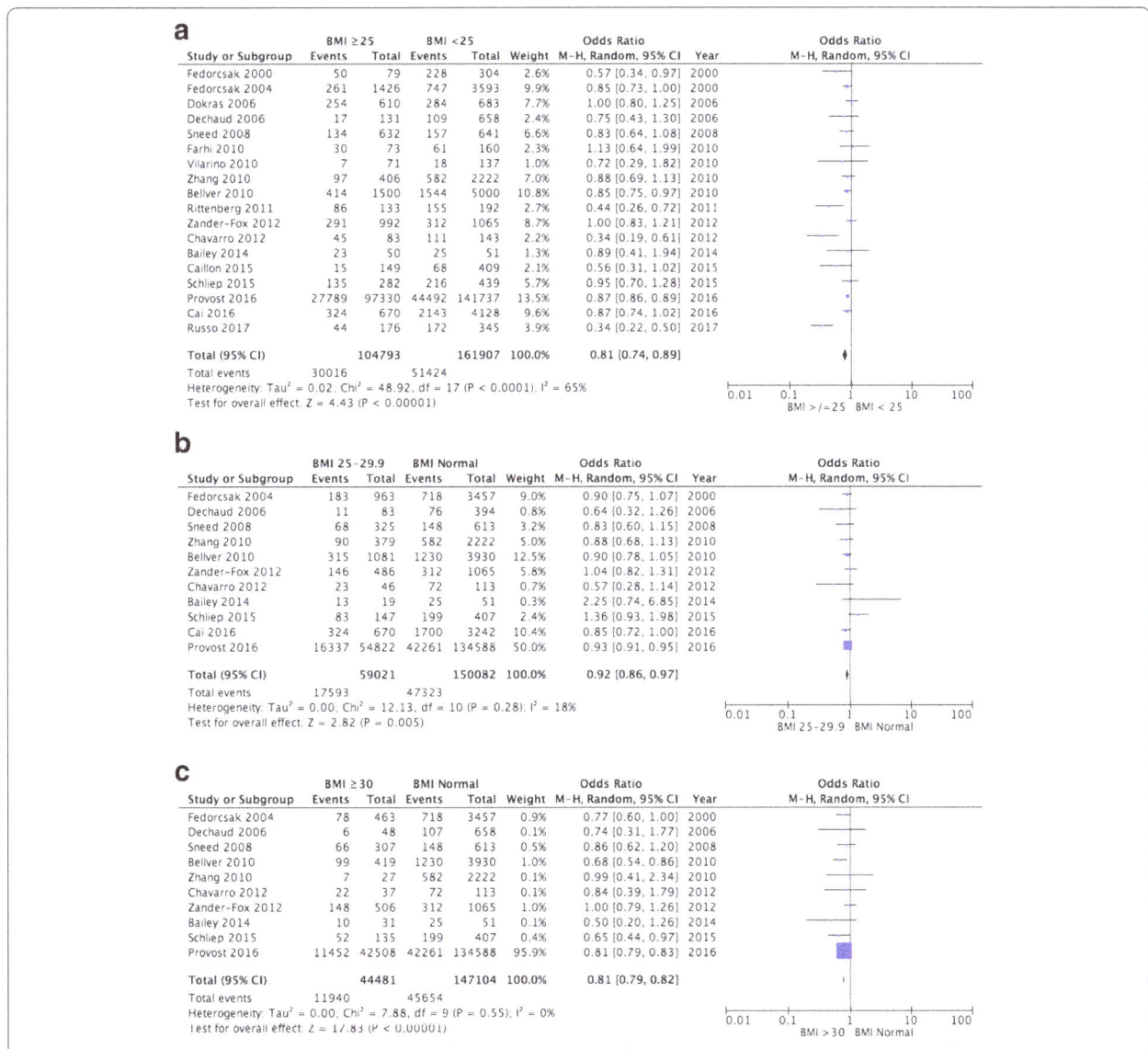

Fig. 2 Meta-analysis of live-birth rate: (**a**) BMI ≥25 kg/m^2 versus BMI < 25 kg/m^2; (**b**) Normal BMI versus BMI 25–29.9 kg/m^2; (**c**) Normal BMI versus BMI ≥30 kg/m^2

a

Study or Subgroup	BMI ≥25 Events	Total	BMI <25 Events	Total	Weight	Odds Ratio M–H, Random, 95% CI	Year
Wang 2000	499	1232	1116	2351	6.2%	0.75 [0.66, 0.87]	2000
Wittemer 2000	20	70	60	255	1.1%	1.30 [0.72, 2.35]	2000
Loveland 2001	24	93	42	87	1.0%	0.37 [0.20, 0.70]	2001
Doody 2003	127	362	195	460	3.3%	0.73 [0.55, 0.98]	2003
Ryley 2004	739	2756	1283	4071	7.0%	0.80 [0.72, 0.89]	2004
Hammadeh 2005	8	24	13	28	0.3%	0.58 [0.19, 1.78]	2005
Van Swieten 2005	20	61	46	101	0.9%	0.58 [0.30, 1.13]	2005
Mitwally 2006	28	81	52	102	1.1%	0.51 [0.28, 0.93]	2006
Metwally 2007	51	185	73	241	1.9%	0.88 [0.57, 1.34]	2006
Dokras 2006	295	610	320	683	4.5%	1.06 [0.85, 1.32]	2006
Dechaud 2006	17	131	109	658	1.3%	0.75 [0.43, 1.30]	2006
Sneed 2008	166	632	185	641	4.0%	0.88 [0.69, 1.12]	2008
Moini 2008	30	154	39	133	1.3%	0.58 [0.34, 1.01]	2008
Davies 2010	21	56	101	176	1.0%	0.45 [0.24, 0.83]	2010
Vilarino 2010	16	71	36	137	0.9%	0.82 [0.42, 1.60]	2010
Zhang 2010	134	406	754	2222	4.3%	0.96 [0.77, 1.20]	2010
Farhi 2010	16	73	29	160	0.8%	1.27 [0.64, 2.52]	2010
Bellver 2010	616	1500	2243	5000	6.8%	0.86 [0.76, 0.96]	2010
Sathya 2010	90	220	38	88	1.5%	0.91 [0.55, 1.50]	2010
Rittenberg 2011	124	133	181	192	0.5%	0.84 [0.34, 2.08]	2011
Funabiki 2011	11	34	117	332	0.7%	0.88 [0.41, 1.87]	2011
Parker 2011	222	462	234	493	3.8%	1.02 [0.79, 1.32]	2011
Pinborg 2011	105	435	213	746	3.5%	0.80 [0.61, 1.04]	2011
Hill 2011	31	59	28	58	0.8%	1.19 [0.57, 2.45]	2011
Werner 2012	93	133	149	222	1.7%	1.14 [0.72, 1.81]	2012
Ramezanzadeh 2012	47	190	30	93	1.3%	0.69 [0.40, 1.19]	2012
Chavarro 2012	63	83	124	143	0.8%	0.48 [0.24, 0.97]	2012
Ozgun 2012	124	519	128	416	3.3%	0.71 [0.53, 0.94]	2012
Galai 2012	58	110	75	110	1.3%	0.52 [0.30, 0.90]	2012
Zander-Fox 2012	354	992	385	1065	5.3%	0.98 [0.82, 1.17]	2012
Bailey 2014	25	50	29	51	0.7%	0.76 [0.35, 1.66]	2014
Schliep 2015	149	282	242	439	3.1%	0.92 [0.68, 1.23]	2015
Ozekinci 2015	49	134	52	164	1.5%	0.92 [0.56, 1.50]	2015
Provost 2016	34872	97330	53704	141737	8.6%	0.92 [0.90, 0.93]	2016
Cai 2016	376	670	2451	4128	5.6%	0.88 [0.74, 1.03]	2016
Christensen 2016	353	1645	949	3697	6.3%	0.79 [0.69, 0.91]	2016
Russo 2017	44	176	172	345	2.1%	0.34 [0.22, 0.50]	2017
Total (95% CI)		112154		172025	100.0%	0.82 [0.77, 0.88]	
Total events	40008		65997				

Heterogeneity: Tau² = 0.01; Chi² = 85.35, df = 36 (P < 0.00001); I² = 58%
Test for overall effect: Z = 5.82 (P < 0.00001)

b

Study or Subgroup	BMI 25–29.9 Events	Total	BMI Normal Events	Total	Weight	Odds Ratio M–H, Random, 95% CI	Year
Wang 2000	342	814	917	1910	8.1%	0.78 [0.66, 0.93]	2000
Ryley 2004	450	1632	1130	3605	11.0%	0.83 [0.73, 0.95]	2004
Dechaud 2006	11	83	76	394	0.7%	0.64 [0.32, 1.26]	2006
Metwally 2007	34	113	73	241	1.3%	0.99 [0.61, 1.61]	2006
Moini 2008	25	117	39	133	0.9%	0.65 [0.37, 1.17]	2008
Sneed 2008	106	325	221	613	3.5%	0.86 [0.65, 1.14]	2008
Bellver 2010	457	1081	1761	3930	10.4%	0.90 [0.79, 1.03]	2010
Zhang 2010	125	379	754	2222	4.9%	0.96 [0.76, 1.21]	2010
Pinborg 2011	68	257	199	702	2.8%	0.91 [0.66, 1.26]	2011
Parker 2011	121	241	219	475	3.0%	1.18 [0.86, 1.61]	2011
Chavarro 2012	34	46	83	113	0.5%	1.02 [0.47, 2.23]	2012
Zander-Fox 2012	385	1065	182	486	5.3%	0.95 [0.76, 1.18]	2012
Ozgun 2012	87	355	123	398	2.8%	0.73 [0.53, 1.00]	2012
Werner 2012	58	88	142	209	1.1%	0.91 [0.54, 1.55]	2012
Schliep 2015	89	147	225	407	2.1%	1.24 [0.85, 1.82]	2015
Ozekinci 2015	22	70	52	164	0.9%	0.99 [0.54, 1.80]	2015
Christensen 2016	247	1171	905	3539	8.5%	0.78 [0.66, 0.91]	2016
Cai 2016	376	670	1928	3242	8.0%	0.87 [0.74, 1.03]	2016
Provost 2016	20175	54822	51009	134588	24.1%	0.95 [0.93, 0.97]	2016
Total (95% CI)		63476		157371	100.0%	0.89 [0.84, 0.94]	
Total events	23212		60038				

Heterogeneity: Tau² = 0.00; Chi² = 26.16, df = 18 (P = 0.10); I² = 31%
Test for overall effect: Z = 3.92 (P < 0.0001)

c

Study or Subgroup	BMI ≥30 Events	Total	BMI Normal Events	Total	Weight	Odds Ratio M–H, Random, 95% CI	Year
Wang 2000	157	421	917	1910	8.7%	0.64 [0.52, 0.80]	2000
Ryley 2004	289	1124	1130	3605	13.2%	0.76 [0.65, 0.88]	2004
Metwally 2007	17	72	73	241	1.6%	0.71 [0.39, 1.31]	2006
Dechaud 2006	6	48	76	394	0.8%	0.60 [0.25, 1.46]	2006
Moini 2008	5	37	39	133	0.6%	0.38 [0.14, 1.04]	2008
Sneed 2008	80	307	175	618	5.2%	0.89 [0.65, 1.22]	2008
Zhang 2010	9	27	754	2222	0.9%	0.97 [0.44, 2.18]	2010
Bellver 2010	159	419	1761	3930	9.2%	0.75 [0.61, 0.93]	2010
Parker 2011	101	221	219	475	4.9%	0.98 [0.71, 1.36]	2011
Pinborg 2011	37	178	199	702	3.4%	0.66 [0.45, 0.99]	2011
Chavarro 2012	29	37	83	113	0.8%	1.31 [0.54, 3.18]	2012
Werner 2012	35	45	142	209	1.0%	1.65 [0.77, 3.53]	2012
Ozgun 2012	37	164	123	398	3.0%	0.65 [0.43, 0.99]	2012
Zander-Fox 2012	172	506	385	1065	8.4%	0.91 [0.73, 1.14]	2012
Schliep 2015	60	135	225	407	3.5%	0.65 [0.44, 0.96]	2015
Ozekinci 2015	18	64	52	164	1.4%	0.84 [0.45, 1.59]	2015
Christensen 2016	106	474	905	3539	8.1%	0.84 [0.67, 1.05]	2016
Provost 2016	14697	42508	51009	134588	25.3%	0.87 [0.85, 0.89]	2016
Total (95% CI)		46787		154713	100.0%	0.80 [0.74, 0.87]	
Total events	16014		58267				

Heterogeneity: Tau² = 0.01; Chi² = 25.08, df = 17 (P = 0.09); I² = 32%
Test for overall effect: Z = 5.47 (P < 0.00001)

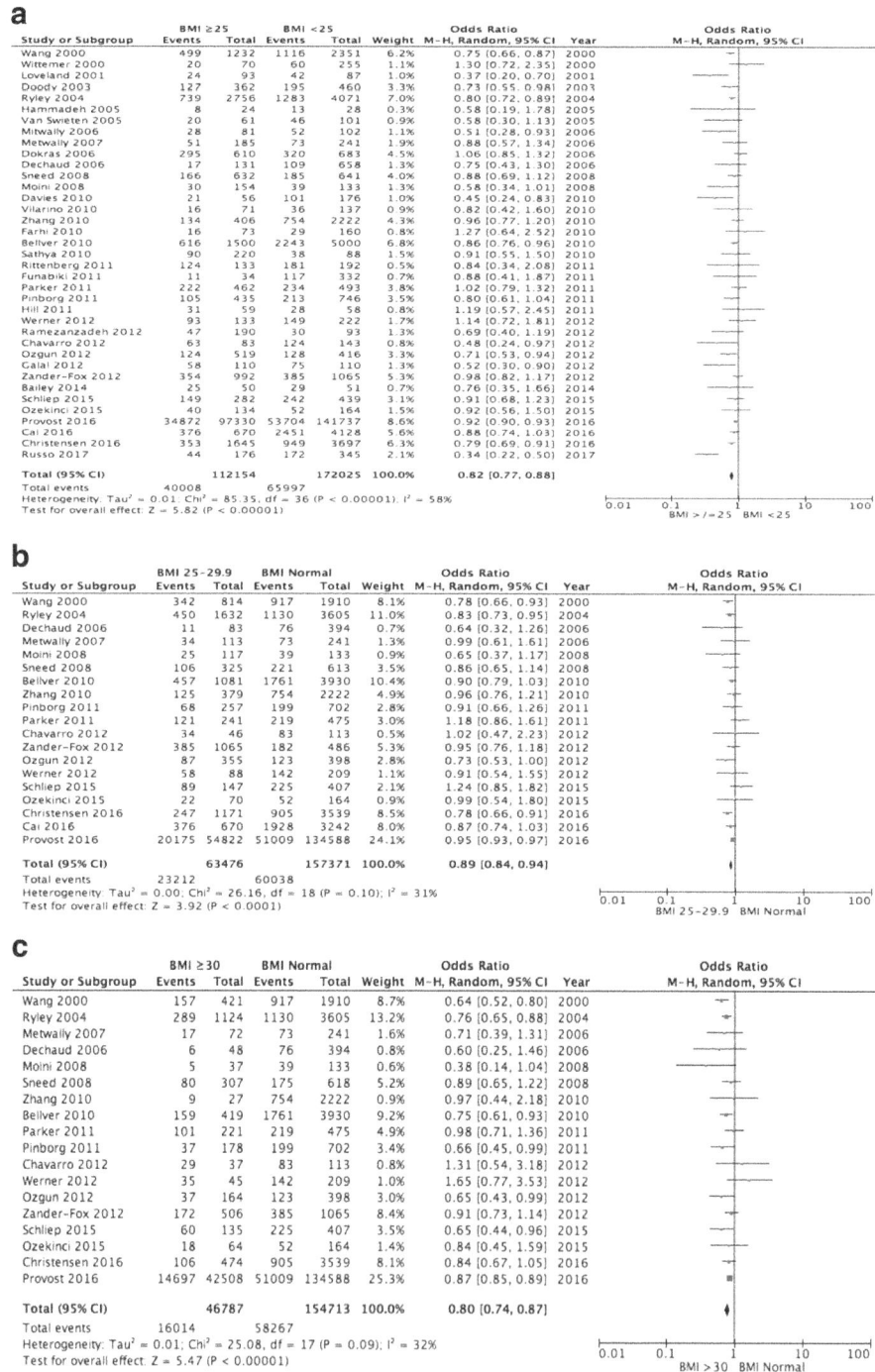

Fig. 3 Meta-analysis of clinical pregnancy rate: (**a**) BMI ≥25 kg/m² versus BMI < 25 kg/m²; (**b**) Normal BMI versus BMI 25–29.9 kg/m²; (**c**) Normal BMI versus BMI ≥30 kg/m²

Women with a BMI 25–29.9 kg/m² were also more likely to have a miscarriage when compared to women with a normal BMI (18 studies pooled, OR 1.15 95% CI 1.05–1.26, $p = 0.002$; Fig. 4b). There was no significant clinical heterogeneity ($I^2 = 16\%$) in this group.

The risk of miscarriage is further increased in women with a BMI ≥30 kg/m² when compared to women who fall into a normal BMI category (17 studies pooled, OR 1.52, 95% CI 1.28–1.81, $p < 0.00001$; Fig. 4c). No significant heterogeneity ($I^2 = 46\%$) was demonstrated between the studies.

a

Study or Subgroup	BMI ≥25 Events	Total	BMI <25 Events	Total	Weight	Odds Ratio M-H, Random, 95% CI	Year
Fedorcsak 2004	153	430	289	1073	8.8%	1.50 [1.18, 1.90]	2000
Fedorcsak 2000	28	79	68	304	3.9%	1.91 [1.12, 3.25]	2000
Wittemer 2000	7	20	14	60	1.2%	1.77 [0.59, 5.30]	2000
Wang 2001	103	397	108	621	7.4%	1.66 [1.23, 2.26]	2001
Loveland 2001	5	24	3	42	0.7%	3.42 [0.74, 15.84]	2001
Wang 2002	186	771	283	1578	9.5%	1.45 [1.18, 1.79]	2002
Winter 2002	55	396	133	727	6.7%	0.72 [0.51, 1.01]	2002
Van Swieten 2005	4	20	12	46	0.9%	0.71 [0.20, 2.54]	2005
Dechaud 2006	4	28	14	159	1.0%	1.73 [0.52, 5.69]	2006
Dokras 2006	40	295	35	320	4.5%	1.28 [0.79, 2.07]	2006
Moini 2008	17	30	12	39	1.5%	2.94 [1.09, 7.93]	2008
Esinler 2008	28	181	34	252	3.9%	1.17 [0.68, 2.02]	2008
Sneed 2008	25	196	39	231	3.8%	0.72 [0.42, 1.24]	2008
Vilarino 2010	2	16	6	36	0.5%	0.71 [0.13, 3.99]	2010
Zhang 2010	18	134	63	754	3.7%	1.70 [0.97, 2.98]	2010
Farhi 2010	8	38	21	82	1.6%	0.77 [0.31, 1.95]	2010
Sathya 2010	20	90	2	38	0.7%	5.14 [1.14, 23.24]	2010
Bellver 2010	73	616	256	2242	8.0%	1.04 [0.79, 1.38]	2010
Pinborg 2011	17	118	235	235	2.9%	1.41 [0.73, 2.74]	2011
Funabiki 2011	5	11	18	117	0.9%	4.58 [1.26, 16.63]	2011
Rittenberg 2011	47	124	377	181	4.2%	2.38 [1.42, 3.96]	2011
Ozgun 2012	14	124	23	128	2.5%	0.58 [0.28, 1.19]	2012
Bailey 2014	1	25	2	29	0.3%	0.56 [0.05, 6.60]	2014
Ozekinci 2015	6	134	6	164	1.1%	1.23 [0.39, 3.92]	2015
Provost 2016	13323	97330	16023	141737	12.8%	1.24 [1.21, 1.28]	2016
Cai 2016	49	376	278	2451	7.0%	1.17 [0.85, 1.62]	2016
Total (95% CI)		102003		153646	100.0%	1.30 [1.15, 1.48]	
Total events	14238		17804				

Heterogeneity: Tau² = 0.03, Chi² = 52.78, df = 25 (P = 0.0010), I² = 53%
Test for overall effect: Z = 4.08 (P < 0.0001)

b

Study or Subgroup	BMI 25-29.9 Events	Total	BMI Normal Events	Total	Weight	Odds Ratio M-H, Random, 95% CI	Year
Fedorcsak 2004	98	292	279	1033	8.5%	1.37 [1.03, 1.80]	2000
Wang 2001	53	231	97	509	5.1%	1.26 [0.87, 1.85]	2001
Wang 2002	111	503	271	1508	10.2%	1.29 [1.01, 1.66]	2002
Winter 2002	29	243	124	701	4.0%	0.63 [0.41, 0.97]	2002
Van Swieten 2005	0	8	6	46	0.1%	0.37 [0.02, 7.14]	2005
Dokras 2006	14	141	35	320	1.9%	0.90 [0.47, 1.73]	2006
Dechaud 2006	3	20	8	105	0.4%	2.14 [0.52, 8.88]	2006
Sneed 2008	16	106	39	221	2.0%	0.83 [0.44, 1.56]	2008
Moini 2008	14	25	12	39	0.7%	2.86 [1.01, 8.12]	2008
Esinler 2008	17	124	34	252	2.0%	1.02 [0.54, 1.91]	2008
Bellver 2010	189	457	680	1761	13.1%	1.12 [0.91, 1.38]	2010
Zhang 2010	17	125	63	754	2.4%	1.73 [0.97, 3.06]	2010
Pinborg 2011	8	75	24	221	1.1%	0.98 [0.42, 2.29]	2011
Ozgun 2012	11	87	21	123	1.3%	0.70 [0.32, 1.55]	2012
Bailey 2014	0	14	2	29	0.1%	0.38 [0.02, 8.44]	2014
Ozekinci 2015	3	70	6	164	0.4%	1.18 [0.29, 4.85]	2015
Provost 2016	6962	54822	15208	134588	40.4%	1.14 [1.11, 1.18]	2016
Cai 2016	49	376	206	1928	6.3%	1.25 [0.90, 1.75]	2016
Total (95% CI)		57719		144302	100.0%	1.15 [1.05, 1.26]	
Total events	7594		17115				

Heterogeneity: Tau² = 0.01, Chi² = 20.32, df = 17 (P = 0.26), I² = 16%
Test for overall effect: Z = 3.05 (P = 0.002)

c

Study or Subgroup	BMI ≥30 Events	Total	BMI Normal Events	Total	Weight	Odds Ratio M-H, Random, 95% CI	Year
Fedorcsak 2004	55	138	279	1033	10.8%	1.79 [1.24, 2.59]	2000
Wang 2001	50	166	97	509	9.9%	1.83 [1.23, 2.73]	2001
Winter 2002	26	153	124	701	8.4%	0.95 [0.60, 1.52]	2002
Wang 2002	75	268	271	1508	13.0%	1.77 [1.32, 2.39]	2002
Van Swieten 2005	2	12	6	46	0.9%	1.33 [0.23, 7.63]	2005
Dechaud 2006	1	8	8	105	0.6%	1.73 [0.19, 15.88]	2006
Dokras 2006	26	154	35	320	6.8%	1.65 [0.96, 2.86]	2006
Moini 2008	3	5	12	39	0.8%	3.38 [0.50, 22.88]	2008
Sneed 2008	9	90	39	221	4.1%	0.52 [0.24, 1.12]	2008
Esinler 2008	11	58	34	252	4.3%	1.50 [0.71, 3.17]	2008
Zhang 2010	1	9	63	754	0.7%	1.37 [0.17, 11.14]	2010
Bellver 2010	94	159	680	1761	11.9%	2.30 [1.65, 3.20]	2010
Pinborg 2011	9	43	24	221	3.5%	2.17 [0.93, 5.07]	2011
Ozgun 2012	3	37	21	123	1.7%	0.43 [0.12, 1.53]	2012
Bailey 2014	1	11	2	29	0.5%	1.35 [0.11, 16.57]	2014
Ozekinci 2015	3	64	6	164	1.4%	1.30 [0.31, 5.34]	2015
Provost 2016	6361	42508	15208	134588	20.8%	1.38 [1.34, 1.43]	2016
Total (95% CI)		43883		142374	100.0%	1.52 [1.28, 1.81]	
Total events	6730		16909				

Heterogeneity: Tau² = 0.04, Chi² = 29.78, df = 16 (P = 0.02), I² = 46%
Test for overall effect: Z = 4.74 (P < 0.00001)

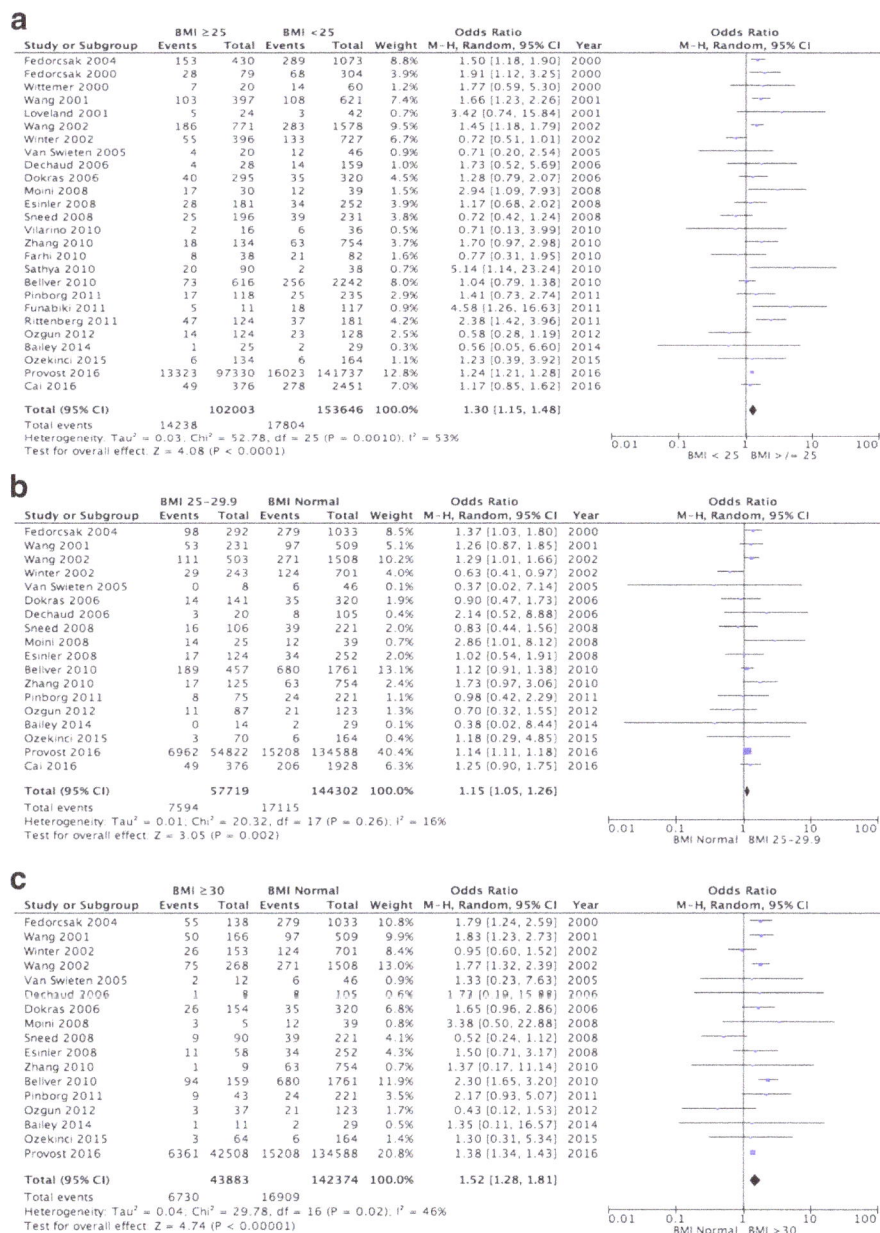

Fig. 4 Meta-analysis of miscarriage rate: (**a**) BMI ≥25 kg/m² versus BMI < 25 kg/m²; (**b**) Normal BMI versus BMI 25–29.9 kg/m²; (**c**) Normal BMI versus BMI ≥30 kg/m²

Dosage of gonadotrophin stimulation

Women with a BMI ≥25 kg/m² required significantly larger total gonadotrophin dosages than women with a BMI < 25 kg/m² (15 studies pooled, weighted mean difference [WMD] 196.03iu, 95% CI 131.91–260.16, $p < 0.00001$; Fig. 5a). However, significant heterogeneity (I² = 75%, $p < 0.00001$) was present between the studies.

Women with a BMI 25–29.9 kg/m² were demonstrated to require significantly higher total gonadotrophin dosages than women with a normal BMI (12 studies pooled, WMD 83.67iu, 95% CI 24.54–142.80, $p = 0.006$; Fig. 5b). However, significant heterogeneity (I² = 80%, $p < 0.00001$) existed between the studies.

Furthermore, increased total dosages of gonadotrophin was documented for women with a BMI ≥30 kg/m² when compared to women whose BMI fell into the normal category (13 studies pooled, WMD 363.58iu, 95% CI 252.99–474.17, p < 0.00001; Fig. 5c). However, significant heterogeneity (I² = 81%, $p < 0.00001$) was present between the studies.

a

Study or Subgroup	BMI ≥25 Mean	SD	Total	BMI <25 Mean	SD	Total	Weight	Mean Difference IV, Random, 95% CI	Year
Dechaud 2006	2,344	897	131	2,046	879	658	6.4%	298.00 [130.35, 465.65]	2006
Metwally 2007	1,986	200	185	1,797	227	241	10.9%	189.00 [148.36, 229.64]	2006
Esinler 2008	2,921	1,199	486	2,517	1,057	627	7.6%	404.00 [269.06, 538.94]	2008
Ozgun 2009	2,765	1,158	519	2,342	1,038	416	7.4%	423.00 [282.02, 563.98]	2009
Zhang 2010	2,727	1,049	406	2,587	933	2222	8.6%	140.00 [30.84, 249.16]	2010
Sathya 2010	2,680	996	220	2,491	1,058	88	4.0%	189.00 [-68.27, 446.27]	2010
Bellver 2010	2,265	874	1500	2,178	918	5000	10.7%	87.00 [35.97, 138.03]	2010
Farhi 2010	2,462	1,219	73	2,085	1,032	160	2.9%	377.00 [54.87, 699.13]	2010
Vilarino 2010	1,494	489	71	1,545	481	137	7.4%	-51.00 [-190.37, 88.37]	2010
Luke 2011	3,467.1	2,279.5	61386	3,446.7	20,538	91114	7.6%	20.40 [-114.17, 154.97]	2011
Singh 2011	2,892	962	149	2,577	1,053	167	4.8%	315.00 [92.82, 537.18]	2012
Moragianni 2012	2,989	1,834	1912	2,835	1,921	2697	8.6%	154.00 [44.39, 263.61]	2012
Chavarro 2012	1,987	896	59	1,701	989	111	3.4%	286.00 [-7.46, 579.46]	2012
Bailey 2014	2,049	1,176	50	1,755	1,008	51	1.9%	294.00 [-133.53, 721.53]	2014
Caillon 2015	2,314	703.6	149	2,146	659.8	409	7.8%	168.00 [38.18, 297.82]	2015
Total (95% CI)			67296			104098	100.0%	196.03 [131.91, 260.16]	

Heterogeneity: Tau² = 9358.56; Chi² = 56.00, df = 14 (P < 0.00001), I² = 75%
Test for overall effect: Z = 5.99 (P < 0.00001)

BMI <25 BMI >/=25

b

Study or Subgroup	BMI 25-29.9 Mean	SD	Total	BMI Normal Mean	SD	Total	Weight	Mean Difference IV, Random, 95% CI
Bailey 2014	1,305	545.5	19	1,755	1,008	51	2.2%	-450.00 [-819.72, -80.28]
Bellver 2010	2,215.4	859.2	1081	2,176.9	919.9	3930	13.8%	38.50 [-20.24, 97.24]
Chavarro 2012	1,867	913	35	1,746.3	993.8	89	2.2%	120.70 [-245.52, 486.92]
Dechaud 2006	2,281	967	83	2,047	888	394	4.8%	234.00 [8.24, 459.76]
Esinler 2008	2,779.1	1,160.1	339	2,516.5	1,057.2	627	7.9%	262.60 [113.95, 411.25]
Luke 2011	3,434	2,517	35452	3,458	21,031	86860	8.3%	-24.00 [-166.29, 118.29]
Metwally 2007	1,970.8	239.6	113	1,979.1	227.3	241	14.1%	-8.30 [-60.98, 44.38]
Moragianni 2012	3,014	2,044.5	1027	2,844.9	1,918.8	2605	8.1%	169.10 [23.96, 314.24]
Ozekinci 2015	2,015	968	70	1,859	1,065	164	3.5%	156.00 [-123.27, 435.27]
Ozgun 2012	2,661	1,136	355	2,344	1,918.8	2605	8.5%	317.00 [177.74, 456.26]
Singh 2011	9.92	1.66	131	10.25	1.79	141	15.9%	-0.33 [-0.74, 0.08]
Zhang 2010	2,688	966	379	2,587	933	2222	10.6%	101.00 [-3.71, 205.71]
Total (95% CI)			39084			99929	100.0%	83.67 [24.54, 142.80]

Heterogeneity: Tau² = 5713.28; Chi² = 54.11, df = 11 (P < 0.00001); I² = 80%
Test for overall effect: Z = 2.77 (P = 0.006)

BMI 25-29.9 BMI Normal

c

Study or Subgroup	BMI ≥30 Mean	SD	Total	BMI Normal Mean	SD	Total	Weight	Mean Difference IV, Random, 95% CI	Year
Dechaud 2006	2,454	757	48	2,047	888	394	8.2%	407.00 [175.59, 638.41]	2006
Metwally 2007	2,009	109	72	1,797	227	241	12.5%	212.00 [173.85, 250.15]	2006
Esinler 2008	3,248	1,255	147	2,517	1,057	627	8.5%	731.00 [511.90, 950.10]	2008
Sathya 2010	2,658	887	73	2,490	1,058	88	6.6%	168.00 [-132.44, 468.44]	2010
Bellver 2010	2,395	899	419	2,177	920	3930	11.7%	218.00 [127.24, 308.76]	2010
Zhang 2010	3,272	1,798	27	2,587	933	2222	2.2%	685.00 [5.69, 1364.31]	2010
Luke 2011	3,507.7	1,907.6	25644	3,458	21,031	86860	10.5%	49.70 [-92.10, 191.50]	2011
Moragianni 2012	2,959	1,554	885	2,845	1,919	2605	10.9%	114.00 [-12.15, 240.15]	2012
Chavarro 2012	2,163	860	24	1,746	994	89	4.8%	417.00 [15.72, 818.28]	2012
Singh 2011	3,150	520	18	2,567	1,088	141	6.6%	583.00 [283.07, 882.93]	2012
Ozgun 2012	2,991	1,175	164	2,344	1,022	398	8.8%	647.00 [441.04, 852.96]	2012
Bailey 2014	2,505	1,230	31	1,755	1,008	51	3.4%	750.00 [236.18, 1263.82]	2014
Ozekinci 2015	2,455	1,343	64	1,859	1,065	164	5.3%	596.00 [228.81, 963.19]	2015
Total (95% CI)			27616			97810	100.0%	363.58 [252.99, 474.17]	

Heterogeneity: Tau² = 25006.12; Chi² = 64.21, df = 12 (P < 0.00001); I² = 81%
Test for overall effect: Z = 6.44 (P < 0.00001)

BMI Normal BMI >30

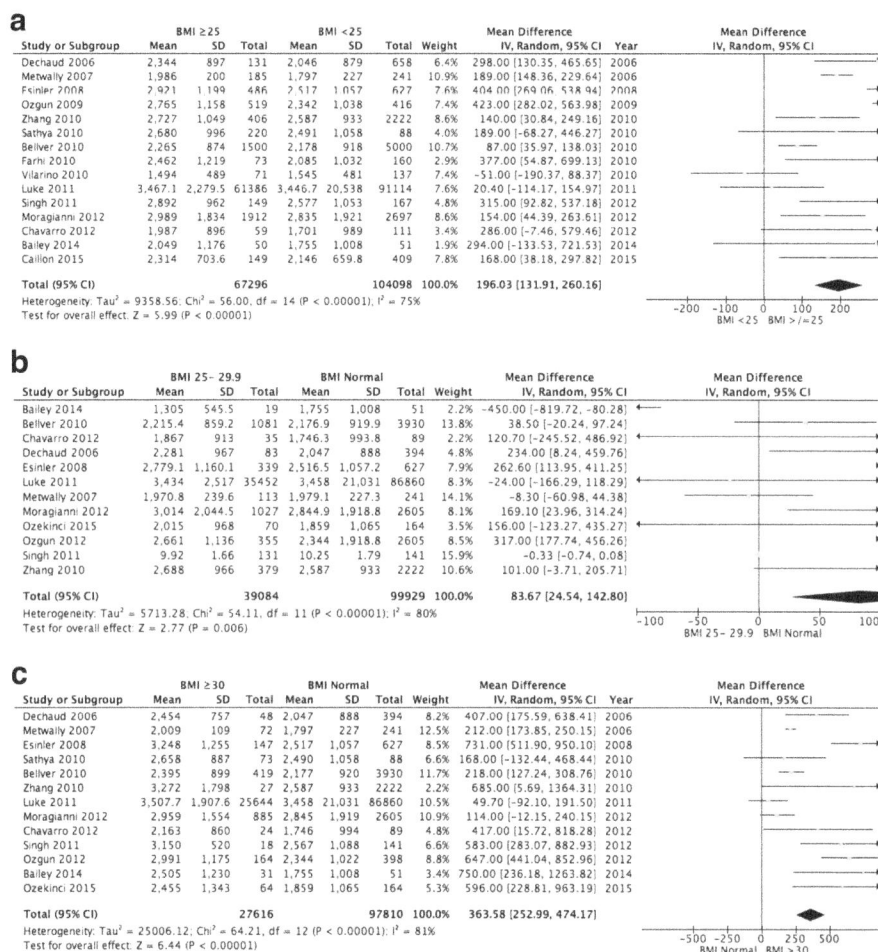

Fig. 5 Meta-analysis of total gonadotrophin dose: (**a**) BMI ≥25 kg/m² versus BMI < 25 kg/m²; (**b**) Normal BMI versus BMI 25–29.9 kg/m²; (**c**) Normal BMI versus BMI ≥30 kg/m²

Duration of gonadotrophin stimulation

No significant difference in duration of stimulation therapy was documented between women with a BMI < 25 kg/m² or ≥25 kg/m² (13 studies pooled, WMD 0.10, 95% CI -0.10-0.31, $p = 0.32$; Fig. 6a), however significant heterogeneity ($I^2 = 95\%$, $p < 0.00001$) existed between the included studies.

Furthermore, no significant difference was seen for duration of gonadotrophin stimulation between women with a BMI 25–29.9 kg/m² versus a normal BMI (8 pooled studies, WMD 0.02, 95% CI -0.10-0.13, $p = 0.79$, $I^2 = 48\%$; Fig. 6b) or for women with a BMI ≥30 kg/m² versus a normal BMI (12 pooled studies, WMD 0.12 95% CI -0.24-0.47, $p = 0.52$; Fig. 6c), however significant heterogeneity ($I^2 = 96\%$, $p < 0.00001$) was noted between the studies for the latter comparison.

Discussion

Public funding for fertility services within the United Kingdom is limited, and therefore, strict guidance exists regarding who can be offered treatment under the National Health Service (NHS). Body mass index (BMI) is a universal criteria adopted by both the public and private sector. This study addresses an important aspect of the impact of a raised BMI on fertility treatment outcomes.

We standardise the analysis of the data by only including studies incorporating the WHO BMI criteria; the current reference point for clinicians and clinical commissioning groups in ascertaining which group of patients should receive treatment. This study is an update of the previous systematic review performed in 2010, with the inclusion of a larger number of cycles from central databases such as the Society for Assisted Reproductive Technology (SART).

This systematic review and meta-analysis has clearly highlighted the negative impact of a raised BMI on the outcomes following ART treatment, with documented lower success rates and higher rates of miscarriages as well as higher total dosage of gonadotrophin usage with

a

Study or Subgroup	BMI ≥25 Mean	SD	Total	BMI <25 Mean	SD	Total	Weight	Mean Difference IV, Random, 95% CI	Year
Van Swieten 2005	12.4	2.6	61	12.4	2.08	101	4.6%	0.00 [-0.77, 0.77]	2005
Metwally 2007	11.12	0.36	185	11.23	0.24	241	12.5%	-0.11 [-0.17, -0.05]	2006
Dechaud 2006	10.9	1.7	131	10.5	1.9	658	9.6%	0.40 [0.07, 0.73]	2006
Dokras 2006	10.1	0.3	610	9.8	0.06	683	12.6%	0.30 [0.28, 0.32]	2006
Esinler 2008	10.4	2.7	486	10.1	1.7	627	10.3%	0.30 [0.03, 0.57]	2008
Farhi 2010	10.9	5.9	73	10.3	2.5	160	1.8%	0.60 [-0.81, 2.01]	2010
Zhang 2010	10.7	2.4	406	10.4	2.03	2222	10.7%	0.30 [0.05, 0.55]	2010
Rittenberg 2011	11.2	2.2	133	10.5	1.7	192	8.0%	0.70 [0.26, 1.14]	2011
Hill 2011	9.7	1.3	59	10.4	12.2	58	0.4%	-0.70 [-3.86, 2.46]	2011
Ramezanzadeh 2012	12.6	2.4	143	12.7	1.7	93	7.0%	-0.10 [-0.62, 0.42]	2012
Moragianni 2012	9.1	2.1	1912	9.4	2.1	2697	12.1%	-0.30 [-0.42, -0.18]	2012
Singh 2011	10	1.7	149	10.25	1.79	141	8.5%	-0.25 [-0.65, 0.15]	2012
Bailey 2014	10.7	2.8	50	11.7	3.9	51	2.0%	-1.00 [-2.32, 0.32]	2014
Total (95% CI)			**4398**			**7924**	**100.0%**	**0.10 [-0.10, 0.31]**	

Heterogeneity: Tau² = 0.09; Chi² = 243.38, df = 12 (P < 0.00001); I² = 95%
Test for overall effect: Z = 0.99 (P = 0.32)

BMI <25   BMI >/=25

b

Study or Subgroup	BMI 25 - 29.9 Mean	SD	Total	BMI Normal Mean	SD	Total	Weight	Mean Difference IV, Random, 95% CI
Bailey 2014	10.3	2	19	11.7	3.9	51	0.7%	-1.40 [-2.80, -0.00]
Dechaud 2006	10.9	1.9	83	10.7	2	394	5.7%	0.20 [-0.25, 0.65]
Esinler 2008	10.3	2.7	339	10.1	1.7	627	10.1%	0.20 [-0.12, 0.52]
Metwally 2007	11.2	0.37	113	11.23	0.24	241	32.7%	-0.03 [-0.10, 0.04]
Moragianni 2012	9.34	1.91	1027	9.38	2.13	2605	24.3%	-0.04 [-0.18, 0.10]
Ozekinci 2015	8.9	1.9	70	8.7	1.8	164	4.5%	0.20 [-0.32, 0.72]
Singh 2011	9.92	1.66	131	10.25	1.79	141	6.8%	-0.33 [-0.74, 0.08]
Zhang 2010	10.6	2.16	379	10.42	2.03	2222	15.2%	0.18 [-0.05, 0.41]
Total (95% CI)			**2161**			**6445**	**100.0%**	**0.02 [-0.10, 0.13]**

Heterogeneity: Tau² = 0.01; Chi² = 12.26, df = 7 (P = 0.09); I² = 43%
Test for overall effect: Z = 0.27 (P = 0.79)

BMI 25 - 29.9   BMI Normal

c

Study or Subgroup	BMI ≥30 Mean	SD	Total	BMI Normal Mean	SD	Total	Weight	Mean Difference IV, Random, 95% CI	Year
Van Swieten 2005	12.5	3.3	29	12.4	2.1	101	4.7%	0.10 [-1.17, 1.37]	2005
Dokras 2006	10.3	0.4	315	9.8	0.1	683	11.8%	0.50 [0.46, 0.54]	2006
Metwally 2007	11	0.3	40	11.2	0.2	165	11.7%	-0.20 [-0.30, -0.10]	2006
Dechaud 2006	10.9	1.4	48	10.7	2	394	10.0%	0.20 [-0.24, 0.64]	2006
Esinler 2008	10.6	2.6	147	10.1	1.7	627	10.0%	0.50 [0.06, 0.94]	2008
Zhang 2010	11.89	4.57	27	10.42	2.03	2222	3.1%	1.47 [-0.26, 3.20]	2010
Hill 2011	10	1	21	10.4	1.2	58	9.4%	-0.40 [-0.93, 0.13]	2011
Singh 2011	10.22	1.78	18	10.25	1.79	141	6.9%	-0.03 [-0.90, 0.84]	2012
Ramezanzadeh 2012	12.7	1.8	49	12.7	1.7	93	8.8%	0.00 [-0.61, 0.61]	2012
Moragianni 2012	8.8	2.3	885	9.38	2.13	2605	11.5%	-0.58 [-0.75, -0.41]	2012
Bailey 2014	11	3.2	31	11.7	3.9	51	3.6%	-0.70 [-2.25, 0.85]	2014
Ozekinci 2015	9.8	2.4	64	8.7	1.8	164	8.5%	1.10 [0.45, 1.75]	2015
Total (95% CI)			**1674**			**7304**	**100.0%**	**0.12 [-0.24, 0.47]**	

Heterogeneity: Tau² = 0.28; Chi² = 294.14, df = 11 (P < 0.00001); I² = 96%
Test for overall effect: Z = 0.65 (P = 0.52)

BMI Normal   BMI >30

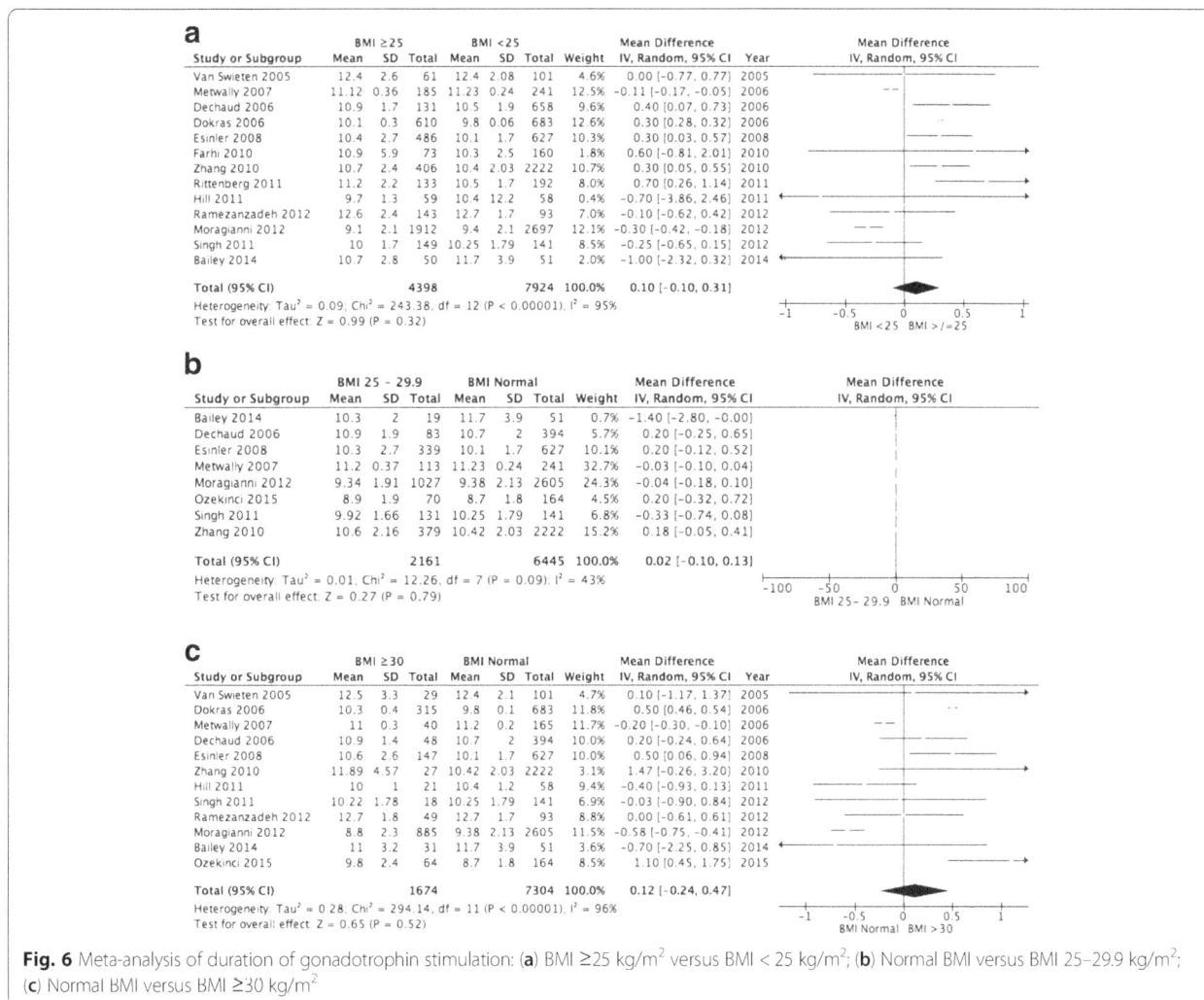

Fig. 6 Meta-analysis of duration of gonadotrophin stimulation: (**a**) BMI ≥25 kg/m² versus BMI < 25 kg/m²; (**b**) Normal BMI versus BMI 25–29.9 kg/m²; (**c**) Normal BMI versus BMI ≥30 kg/m²

no effect on the duration of stimulation. The latter may have been balanced by higher dosages of treatment which can also have a cost implication. However, as most studies have included a BMI category of < 25 kg/m², which would also include underweight women with a BMI < 18 kg/m², the detrimental effects of which have been addressed in a number of previous studies, a risk of bias cannot be confidently excluded. This has been addressed through the inclusion of studies allowing for a sub-group analysis of women with a normal BMI with overweight and obese women.

The presented data is able to demonstrate statistical significance with low clinical heterogeneity for a number of factors reflective of success through ART treatment. Despite this, caution is advised for interpretation of the presented information as only a few of the included studies controlled for confounding factors such as age, smoking and duration of infertility. In order to reduce further clinical heterogeneity, studies not incorporating the WHO classification for BMI and paternal BMI were excluded.

The included studies were considered relevant if they conformed to the WHO classification of BMI, despite this, a considerable amount of methodological and clinical heterogeneity existed. The level of statistical heterogeneity for the primary outcome measure live birth rate and secondary outcome measures clinical pregnancy rate and miscarriage rate were limited. However, despite a significant increase in total gonadotrophin dosage requirements with increasing BMI categories, the studies demonstrated significant statistical heterogeneity, limiting their value.

The presented data can act as an aid in the counselling of subjects secondary to a clear impact on ART outcomes being demonstrated across all BMI categories. The evidence supports the government's stringent allocation of funding when resources are significantly limited.

A raised BMI impacts reproductive health at the pre and post embryological stage of development, affecting oocyte quality and the endometrial environment [2].

A recent meta-analysis and systematic review by Best et al., [5] has demonstrated that weight loss can improve pregnancy rate and ovulatory status with a trend favouring spontaneous conception. However, these effects have not been seen through ART. Of note, miscarriage rates were unaltered with a change in weight.

Besides the reproductive health effects of a raised BMI, clinicians should also be aware of the increased rate of pregnancy complications such as pregnancy induced hypertension, pre-eclampsia and gestational diabetes in women with a raised BMI. Women are also at an increased risk of an emergency caesarean section with increasing BMI [6, 7].

A holistic approach should be used when counselling patients seeking ART treatments using an open discussion method to inform patients of the effects of raised BMI on ART and obstetric care. This will allow couples to make an informed decision and to take ownership of their well-being.

Conclusion

This systematic review and meta-analysis further emphasises the negative impact of a raised BMI on ART outcomes. However, the underlying pathophysiology is beyond the scope of this systematic review and will need to be evaluated in future studies. The quality of this systematic review would be further improved if future study designs included the WHO classification of BMI and controlled for confounding variables.

Abbreviations
ART: Assisted reproductive technology; BMI: Body Mass Index; FSH: Follicle stimulation hormone; GIFT: Gamete intra-Fallopian transfer; HCG: Human chorionic gonadotrophin; ICSI: Intracytoplasmic sperm injection; IVF: In vitro fertilization; MeSH: Medical subject headings; NHS: National Health Service; OHSS: Ovarian hyperstimulation syndrome; SART: Society for Assisted Reproductive Technology

Acknowledgements
Not applicable.

Funding
Not applicable.

Authors' contributions
PRS and MM analyzed and interpreted the data. LNL developed the initial idea. EM and LNL oversaw the progress of the manuscript. All authors read and approved the final manuscript.

Competing interests
The authors declare that they have no competing interests.

Author details
[1]Oxford University Hospitals NHS Foundation Trust, John Radcliffe Hospital, Headley Way, Headington, Oxford OX3 9DU, UK. [2]Nuffield Department of Women's and Reproductive Health, University of Oxford, Level 3, Women's Centre, John Radcliffe Hospital, Oxford OX3 9DU, UK.

References
1. WHO. Obesity and overweight. Geneva: World Health Organization. Fact Sheet 311. Available from http://www.who.int/mediacentre/factsheets/fs311/en/.
2. Rittenberg V, Seshadri S, Sunkara SK, Sobaleva S, Oteng-Ntim E, El-Toukhy T. Effect of body mass index on IVF treatment outcome: an updated systematic review and meta-analysis. Reprod BioMed Online. 2011;23(4): 421–39.
3. Higgins JPT, Thompson SG. Quantifying heterogeneity in a meta-analysis. Stat Med. 2002;21(11):1539–58.
4. Mantel N, Haenszel W. Statistical aspects of the analysis of data from retrospective studies of disease. J Natl Cancer Inst. 1959;22:719–48.
5. Best D, Avenell A, Bhattacharya S. How effective are weight-loss interventions for improving fertility in women and men who are overweight or obese? A systematic review and meta-analysis of the evidence. Hum Reprod Update. 2017;23(6):681–705.
6. Aly H, Hammad T, Nada A, Mohamed M, Bathgate S, El-Mohandes A. Maternal obesity, associated complications and risk of prematurity. J Perinatol. 2010;30(7):447–51.
7. Bhattacharya S, Campbell DM, Liston WA, Bhattacharya S. Effect of body mass index on pregnancy outcomes in nulliparous women delivering singleton babies. BMC Public Health. 2007;7:168.
8. Fedorcsak P, et al. Obesity is a risk factor for early pregnancy loss after IVF or ICSI. Acta Obstet Gynecol Scand. 2000;79(1):43–8.
9. Wittemer C, et al. Does body mass index of infertile women have an impact on IVF procedure and outcome? J Assist Reprod Genet. 2000;17(10):547–52.
10. Wang JX, Davies M, Norman RJ. Body mass and probability of pregnancy during assisted reproduction treatment: retrospective study. Br Med J. 2000; 321(7272):1320–1.
11. Loveland JB, et al. Increased body mass index has a deleterious effect on in vitro fertilization outcome. J Assist Reprod Genet. 2001;18(7):382–6.
12. Wang JX, Davies MJ, Norman RJ. Polycystic ovarian syndrome and the risk of spontaneous abortion following assisted reproductive technology treatment. Hum Reprod. 2001;16(12):2606–9.
13. Wang X, Davies J, Norman J. Obesity increases the risk of spontaneous abortion during infertility treatment. Obes Res. 2002;10(6):551–4.
14. Winter E, Wang J, Davies MJ, Norman RJ. Early pregnancy loss following assisted reproductive technology treatment. Hum Reprod. 2002;12:3220–3.
15. Doody KM, Langley MT, Marek DE, Nackley AC, Doody KJ. Morbid obesity adversely impacts outcomes with IVF. Fertility Sterility. 2003;80:S160.
16. Fedorcsák P, Dale PO, Storeng R, Ertzeid G, Bjercke S, Oldereid N, Omland AK, Abyholm T, Tanbo T. Impact of overweight and underweight on assisted reproduction treatment. Hum Reprod. 2004;19(11):2523–8.
17. Ryley DA, Bayer SR, Eaton J, Zimon A, Klipstein S, Reindollar. Influence of body mass index (BMI) on the outcome of 6,827 IVF cycles. Fertil Steril. 2004;82(Supplement 2):S38–9.
18. Van ECAM, et al. Obesity and clomiphene challenge test as predictors of outcome of in vitro fertilization and intracytoplasmic sperm injection. Gynecol Obstet Investig. 2005;59(4):220–4.
19. Hammadeh ME, Sykoutris A, Amer AS, Schmidt. Relationship between body mass index (BMI) and plasma lipid concentration and their effect on IVF/ICSI outcome. Fertil Steril. 2005;84(Supplement 1):S422.
20. Dechaud H, et al. Obesity does not adversely affect results in patients who are undergoing in vitro fertilization and embryo transfer. European Journal of Obstetrics Gynecology and Reproductive Biology. 2006;127(1):88–93.
21. Dokras A, et al. Obstetric outcomes after in vitro fertilization in obese and morbidly obese women. Obstet Gynecol. 2006;108(1):61–9.
22. Mitwally MF, Leduc MM, Ogunleye O, Albuarki H, Diamond MP, Abuzeid M. The effect of body mass index (BMI) on the outcome of IVF and embryo transfer in women of different ethnic backgrounds. Fertility Sterility. 2006;86:S68–9.
23. Metwally M, Cutting R, Tipton A, Skull J, Ledger WL, Li TC. Effect of increased body mass index on oocyte and embryo quality in IVF patients. Reprod BioMed Online. 2007;15:532–8.
24. Esinler I, Bozdag G, Yarali H. Impact of isolated obesity on ICSI outcome. Reprod BioMed Online. 2008;17(4):583–7.
25. Martinuzzi K, et al. Elevated body mass index (BMI) does not adversely affect in vitro fertilization outcome in young women. J Assist Reprod Genet. 2008; 25(5):169–75.
26. Moini A, et al. The effect of body mass index on the outcome of IVF/ICSI cycles in non polycystic ovary syndrome women. International Journal of Fertility and Sterility. 2008;2(2):82–5.

27. Sneed ML, et al. Body mass index: impact on IVF success appears age-related. Hum Reprod. 2008;23(8):1835–9.
28. Ozgun MT, et al. The influence of body mass index on FSH dose and pregnancy rate in women undergoing ICSI-embryo transfer. Journal of the Turkish German Gynecology Association. 2009;10(1):1–5.
29. Sathya A, et al. Effect of body mass index on in vitro fertilization outcomes in women. Journal of Human Reproductive Sciences. 2010;3(3):135–8.
30. Zhang D, et al. Overweight and obesity negatively affect the outcomes of ovarian stimulation and in vitro fertilisation: a cohort study of 2628 Chinese women. Gynecol Endocrinol. 2010;26(5):325–32.
31. Bellver J, et al. Female obesity impairs in vitro fertilization outcome without affecting embryo quality. Fertil Steril. 2010;93(2):447–54.
32. Vilarino Lima F, et al. Body mass index and fertility: is there a correlation with human reproduction outcomes? Gynecol Endocrinol. 2011;27(4):232–6.
33. Farhi J, et al. High-quality embryos retain their implantation capability in overweight women. Reprod BioMed Online. 2010;21(5):706–11.
34. Davies D, et al. Are the negative effects of being overweight on reproductive potential evident in FET cycles? Reprod BioMed Online. 2010;20(Supplement S2):S58.
35. Funabiki M, et al. The influence of body mass index (BMI) on pregnancy outcomes among Japanese infertile women. Fertil Steril. 2011;96(3 Supplement 1):S115.
36. Hill MJ, Hong S, Frattarelli JL. Body mass index impacts in vitro fertilization stimulation. ISRN Obstetrics and Gynecology. 2011;2010:1–5.
37. Pinborg A, et al. Influence of female bodyweight on IVF outcome: a longitudinal multicentre cohort study of 487 infertile couples. Reprod BioMed Online. 2011;23(4):490–9.
38. Parker K, et al. Does body mass index (BMI) affect IVF outcomes? Fertil Steril. 2011;96(3 Supplement 1):S124.
39. Rittenberg V, Sobaleva S, et al. Influence of BMI on risk of miscarriage after single blastocyst transfer. Hum Reprod. 2011;26(10):2642–50.
40. Singh N, et al. Correlation of body mass index with outcome of in vitro fertilization in a developing country. Arch Gynecol Obstet. 2012;285(1):259–63.
41. Luke B, et al. Female obesity adversely affects assisted reproductive technology (ART) pregnancy and live birth rates. Hum Reprod. 2011;26(1):245–52.
42. Chavarro JE, et al. Body mass index and short-term weight change in relation to treatment outcomes in women undergoing assisted reproduction. Fertil Steril. 2012;98(1):109–16.
43. Galal AF, Elhelaly DN. Higher body mass index significantly affects intracytoplasmic sperm injection success rate. Fertil Steril. 2012;97(3 Supplement 1).S9–S10.
44. Werner M, et al. Body mass index (BMI) does not impact endometrial receptivity in fresh IVF cycles: evaluation of implantation rates (IR) and ongoing pregnancy rates (PR) following the transfer of euploid blastocysts. Fertil Steril. 2012;98(3 Supplement 1):S286–7.
45. Zander-Fox DL, et al. Does obesity really matter? The impact of BMI on embryo quality and pregnancy outcomes after IVF in women aged <38 years. Aust N Z J Obstet Gynaecol. 2012;52(3):270–6.
46. Ozgun MT, et al. Effect of body mass index on the risk of miscarriage after ICSI. Int J Gynecol Obstet. 2012;119:S535.
47. Ramezanzadeh F, et al. Impact of body mass index versus physical activity and calorie intake on assisted reproduction outcomes. European Journal of Obstetrics Gynecology and Reproductive Biology. 2012;163(1):52–6.
48. Moragianni VA, Jones SML, Ryley DA. The effect of body mass index on the outcomes of first assisted reproductive technology cycles. Fertil Steril. 2012;98(1):102–8.
49. Bailey AP, et al. Effect of body mass index on in vitro fertilization outcomes in women with polycystic ovary syndrome. Am J Obstet Gynecol. 2014;211(2):163.e1–6.
50. Schliep KC, et al. Effect of male and female body mass index on pregnancy and live birth success after in vitro fertilization. Fertil Steril. 2015;103(2):388–95.
51. Cai J, Liu L, Zhang J, Qiu H, Jiang X, Li P, Sha A, Ren J. Low body mass index compromises live birth rate in fresh transfer in vitro fertilization cycles: a retrospective study in a Chinese population. Fertility Sterility. 2017;107(2):422–9.
52. Ozekinci M, Seven A, Olgan S, Sakinci M, Keskin U, Akar ME, Ceyhan ST, Ergun A. Does obesity have detrimental effects on IVF treatment outcomes? BMC Womens Health. 2015;15:61. https://doi.org/10.1186/s12905-015-0223-0.
53. Caillon H, Fréour T, Bach-Ngohou K, Colombel A, Denis MG, Barrière P, Masson D. Effects of female increased body mass index on in vitro fertilization cycles outcome. Obesity Research & Clinical Practice. 2015;9:382–8.
54. Provost MP, Acharya KS, Acharya CR, Yeh JS, Steward JG, Eaton JL, Goldfarb JM, Muasher SJ. Pregnancy outcomes decline with increasing body mass index: analysis of 239,127 fresh autologous in vitro fertilization cycles from the 2008-2010 Society for Assisted Reproductive Technology registry. Fertil Steril. 2016;105(3):663–9.
55. Russo M, Ates S, Shaulov T, Dahan MH. Morbid obesity and pregnancy outcomes after single blastocyst transfer: a retrospective, north American study. J Assist Reprod Genet. 2017; https://doi.org/10.1007/s10815-017-0883-9.
56. Christensen MW, Ingerslev HJ, Degn B, Kesmodel US. Effect of female body mass index on oocyte quantity in fertility treatments (IVF): treatment cycle number is a possible effect modifier. A Register-Based Cohort Study PLoS ONE. 2016;11(9):e0163393. https://doi.org/10.1371/journal.

2

Ugandan providers' views on the acceptability of contraceptive self-injection for adolescents

Jane Cover[1][*] (iD), Allen Namagembe[2], Justine Tumusiime[2], Jeanette Lim[1] and Carie Muntifering Cox[3]

Abstract

Background: Self-injection of subcutaneous depot medroxyprogesterone acetate may offer greater discretion and increase access to injectable contraception, particularly for those who face challenges accessing clinic services. In particular, unmarried adolescents often encounter stigma when seeking services, and may also lack the financial means to travel to clinics on the quarterly basis that injectable contraception requires. Whether self-injection is offered to women on a wide scale basis, and to adolescents specifically, will depend in part upon the willingness of providers to train clients of diverse ages and educational backgrounds. This study explores the views of providers with regard to self-injection as an option for women and adolescents in Uganda.

Methods: In-depth qualitative interviews were conducted with family planning providers in Gulu district, to understand their views on injectable self-injection for women, with a specific focus on unmarried adolescents ages 15 to 19 years. The in-depth interviews, which lasted up to 60 min were audio-recorded, translated and transcribed simultaneously, and analyzed using Atlas.ti software to identify key themes and common perspectives.

Results: A total of 40 health care providers were interviewed with equal numbers of each type (public, NGO, and private clinics, pharmacies, and community-based health workers). While most providers were receptive to self-injection for adult women, fewer than half were supportive of adolescent self-injection. Their reservations focused on age, marital status and parity concerns around adolescent use of the injectable more broadly, and concerns about the ability of adolescents to self-inject safely.

Conclusions: Self-injection presents an opportunity to reduce the enormous burden on the public sector health system in Uganda, which is particularly compounded by the heavy reliance on injectable contraception requiring quarterly clinic visits. The results of this study reveal a level of cautious support for self-injection among providers when it comes to self-injection by adult women. With respect to adolescent clients, family planning policymakers and program implementers should design, implement, and evaluate self-injection interventions with the needs of adolescent clients uppermost in mind, recognizing that extra attention will likely be needed to reduce provider-imposed restrictions on adolescent access to this injectable delivery modality.

Keywords: Self-injection, Injectable contraception, DMPA-SC, Depot medroxyprogesterone acetate, Adolescents, Family planning

* Correspondence: jcover@path.org
[1]PATH, PO Box 900922, Seattle, WA 98109, USA
Full list of author information is available at the end of the article

Ugandan providers' views on the acceptability of contraceptive self-injection...

17

Plain English summary

Self-administration of contraception may offer greater privacy and increase access to injectable contraception, particularly for those who face challenges accessing clinic services. In particular, unmarried adolescents often encounter negative stigma when seeking services, and may also lack the financial means to travel to clinics for regular reinjection. Whether self-injection is offered to adolescent women will depend on the willingness of providers to train clients of diverse ages and backgrounds. This study explores the views of providers with regard to self-injection as an option for women and adolescents in Uganda.

In-depth qualitative interviews were conducted with family planning providers in Gulu district, to understand their views on injectable self-injection for women, with a specific focus on unmarried adolescents.

A total of 40 health care providers were interviewed from public, NGO, and private clinics, pharmacies, and community-based settings. While most providers were receptive to self-injection for adult women, fewer than half were supportive of adolescent self-injection. Their reservations focused on whether young women, women who are unmarried, and women without children should use the injectable, in addition to concerns about the ability of adolescents to self-inject safely.

Self-injection presents an opportunity to reduce the enormous burden on the public health system imposed by quarterly reinjection clinic visits. These results reveal cautious support for self-injection among providers when it comes to self-injection by adult women. With respect to adolescent clients, extra attention will likely be needed to reduce provider-imposed restrictions on adolescent access to this mode of delivery for injectable contraception.

Background

The introduction of subcutaneous depot medroxyprogesterone acetate (DMPA-SC) in a number of African countries in 2014 has opened the door to the possibility of self-injection of injectable contraception [1]. Self-injection may offer greater discretion and increase access to the injectable, particularly for those who face challenges accessing clinic services. Many women could benefit in terms of reduced travel and opportunity costs if they could manage their injectable use independently of the health system. In particular, unmarried adolescents often encounter stigma when seeking contraceptives at public sector clinics, and may lack the financial and physical independence to travel to clinics on the periodic basis that injectable contraception requires. Whether self-injection is offered to women on a wide scale basis, and to adolescents specifically, will depend on the willingness of providers as gatekeepers to DMPA-SC. This qualitative study explores the views of providers – public, NGO, private and community-based – with regard to

self-injection as an option for women and adolescents in Uganda.

Like the intramuscular version, DMPA-SC is a three-month, progestin-only product that is stable at room temperature. The subcutaneous version now available in a number of African countries has a lower dose of DMPA (104 mg. vs. 150 mg.), but with comparable safety and efficacy [2]. DMPA-SC is packaged in the Uniject™ injection system – a small, prefilled, auto-disable device designed for easy administration after minimal training. The easy-to-use injection system provides opportunities for women to administer themselves through self-injection. DMPA-SC (brand name Sayana Press) was registered for administration by providers by the Ugandan National Drug Authority (NDA) in 2014.

While the total fertility rate in Uganda is declining – from 6.2 children per woman in 2011 to 5.4 in 2016 – it remains among the highest in the world [3, 4]. Unmet need for contraception is also high, at 28% among currently married women and 32% among sexually active unmarried women, suggesting that a substantial share of women are not using a method though they would like to wait an additional 2 years before their next birth or to limit childbearing altogether [5]. Adolescents aged 15–19 years represent about 11% of the population in Uganda, and one quarter of them have already begun childbearing [5]. The modern contraceptive prevalence rate is 36% among married women ages 15 to 49 years, and the injectable is the most popular method (for married and unmarried women alike), representing nearly half (46%) of the modern method mix [6].Studies of the appeal of DMPA-SC in Uganda found that more than four out of five women preferred it to the intramuscular version (DMPA-IM) [7]. The the country is now undergoing rapid scale up to offer DMPA-SC nationwide, and as of 2018, DMPA-SC represents 11% of the contraceptive method mix among married women [6].

The popularity of injectable contraception, and the growing appeal of DMPA-SC in Uganda creates potentially fertile ground for self-administration. Self-injection of DMPA-SC could overcome barriers for many women, and particularly for adolescents. While women may initially need training from a clinic- or community-based health worker, subsequent self-injection at home will eliminate the need to see a provider every 3 months. Self-injection reduces the financial burden and opportunity costs associated with travelling to the clinic and waiting for services. The ability to store the product at home will make women less vulnerable to stock outs. For women wishing to use the injectable discreetly, self-injection may enhance confidentiality. In short, self-injection may improve injectable continuation by reducing clinic access challenges while simultaneously enhancing women's autonomy and control over contraceptive use [8–11].

Self-injection may offer solutions to the particular access challenges often faced by unmarried adolescents, including concerns about privacy and confidentiality stemming from the stigma of contraceptive use and premarital sex; the cost of travel and distance to health facilities for adolescents who lack financial autonomy and face challenges travelling independently; and inconvenient clinic hours, which can be particularly difficult for school-attending adolescents [12, 13]. Despite efforts to improve services for adolescents, there continues to be a pronounced lack of youth-friendly services, of which non-judgmental, supportive front line health care providers are the critical component [14, 15].

Numerous studies have found that health care workers sometimes refuse to provide contraception to unmarried adolescents because of deeply held negative opinions about premarital sex, or limit their contraceptive options due to misperceptions about who can use certain methods safely and effectively [13]. Misplaced fears that some forms of contraception impair fertility lead to parity and/or age restrictions [16, 17]. Recent research from Nigeria found that the most common restriction imposed on contraceptive provision was an age requirement [18]. In Tanzania, more than one in three providers impose age restrictions on injectable use, more than one in four impose parity restrictions and one in five impose marriage restrictions [19]. More specific to Uganda, a simulated client survey found that two thirds of providers chose a method on behalf of their clients. The authors observed that 'younger clients seemed to be treated differently than older clients', with more discussion focused on method side effects when the simulated client was younger and unmarried [20]. Another study from Uganda found that one in five providers indicated they would not offer injectable contraception to adolescents, with the authors concluding that most providers had misunderstandings about contraceptives, negative attitudes toward providing contraceptives to young women, and imposed age restrictions and consent requirements on adolescents [21]. While self-injection does not eliminate the challenge of provider bias, it improves the autonomy of clients and may enable unmarried adolescents to minimize the stigma they experience when seeking contraceptives in clinic settings.

Research suggests that self-injection is a feasible mode of administration, including for women in low resource settings as well as for adolescent women. Among adult research participants in Uganda, 88% self-injected proficiently three-months after being trained by a nurse [22]. Studies from high resource settings have similarly shown that self-injection of DMPA-SC is feasible [23–25]. One study in the United States specifically assessed adolescent competency and acceptability in self-administering DMPA-SC, finding moderate proficiency (63%) after a single training session. Though the study was small, the authors concluded that self-injection was feasible for

adolescents with training and support [26]. A qualitative study of Ugandan adolescent interest in self-injection found that approximately half were personally interested in taking up self-injection if that option were available to them [27].

With respect to self-injection in Uganda, the NDA granted approval for self-injection in 2017, and subsequently that year, a pilot self-injection program was launched in four districts – the first offer of self-injection in sub-Saharan Africa outside of a research setting. However, successful implementation and scale up of self-injection as a delivery strategy in Uganda will require buy-in from family planning providers who are the gatekeepers to self-injection training. To the extent that providers doubt women's ability to self-inject safely and effectively, or feel that self-injection will encourage promiscuity among unmarried adolescents, they will limit the availability of training, or provide training only to particular types of women, such as more educated or married adult women.

This qualitative study is designed to better understand Ugandan providers' willingness to endorse and train women, including adolescents, for self-injection. To that end, we first explore providers' views of appropriate contraceptive methods for adolescents, including injectable contraceptive use, as a necessary precondition to self-injection. The study then examines their views regarding self-injection for all women of reproductive age. Lastly it solicits their opinions regarding key program characteristics—such as the training approach and appropriate follow-up—that might facilitate self-injection, and how the program design requirements may be varied to better serve adolescent clients.

Methods

Study sites and participants

The study was conducted between October – December 2015 in the district of Gulu in Northern Uganda, in collaboration with the Ugandan Ministry of Health. Facilities and establishments from which participants were drawn were identified from a full list of potential sites in the district, and those selected were based on the willingness of facility administrators to have their staff participate, and with consideration for the accessibility of the site. Health care personnel were recruited purposively from private clinics, NGO clinics, public sector clinics, public sector village health teams (VHTs), and pharmacies. Clinic-based family planning providers and community health workers were eligible if they were providing family planning counseling and services as part of their main responsibilities, while pharmacy staff were eligible if their pharmacy was selling injectable contraceptives. Participants were recruited through face to face interaction at facilities and interviews conducted either at the facility or at a location convenient to the provider. Participants were required to speak English or

Acholi—the major local language, to provide voluntary informed consent and to agree to being audio-recorded.

Study design and procedures

We conducted qualitative in-depth interviews with family planning providers to understand their views on injectable self-injection for women, with a specific focus on unmarried adolescents ages 15 to 19 years. Participants included a mix of individuals who had previously been trained to administer DMPA- SC, and others who were unfamiliar with DMPA-SC. Health workers who had not been trained to administer DMPA-SC were given basic information, received a demonstration during the interview, and had an opportunity to administer DMPA-SC on a prosthetic. No injections or self-injections were performed during this study.

Semi-structured interview guides were developed to facilitate the interviews. Different interview guides were prepared for family planning providers who had previously been trained to administer DMPA-SC, family planning providers not familiar with DMPA-SC, and with pharmacy staff.

The data collection team was comprised of both male (2) and female (2) research assistants from Gulu district. They participated in a 5-day training covering recruiting and screening procedures, research ethics and administering informed consent, qualitative interviewing techniques and conducting in-depth interviews, translating and transcribing audio recordings, and data quality assurance.

The in-depth interviews lasted up to 60 min and were conducted in English or Acholi, as preferred by the participant. Interviews were audio-recorded, and translated and transcribed simultaneously.

Interviews were designed to move from the general to specific, beginning with views on contraceptive use and recommended methods for women in general, and for adolescents specifically, and progressing to views about injectable contraception and self-injection as a delivery modality for adult as well as adolescent women. Interviewers also solicited ideas for program design to facilitate self-injection—such as training, supervision, and reminders – with an eye toward what additional support, if any, might be necessary for adolescent populations.

Data analysis

Data analysis was conducted using the qualitative software program Atlas.ti. The coding scheme was developed and transcripts were coded through an iterative process by two coders, with any discrepancies reviewed and resolved. Coded text was reviewed for each main code and, subsequently, memos were developed to summarize key patterns and themes. Where appropriate, findings were compared by the type of provider (private clinic/public clinic/commercial provider/community based).

Ethical conduct of the study

All research study team members involved in data collection, management, or analysis were trained on research ethics, including confidentiality. This study was approved by the Mulago Hospital institutional review board, the Uganda National Council for Science and Technology, and the PATH Research Ethics Committee.

Results

Participant characteristics

To capture the views from various types of providers, we interviewed 40 providers in total, 29 of whom were women. The median number of years worked as a health care provider was 6, with a range of one to 30 years. The median age was 32, with a range of 24 to 75 years. To maximize the diversity of experience, providers were drawn equally from public sector health centers, NGO facilities, for profit clinics, pharmacies and the public sector community-based distribution program. Participant characteristics are shown in Table 1.

Below we present summaries of themes that emerged from interviews, along with illustrative comments from these 40 health care providers.

Informed choice for adult women, less so for adolescents

When asked what family planning methods they recommend to a client, about three fourths of providers ($n = 28$) stated that they do not recommend specific methods, but rather, counsel the woman about available family planning methods and allow her to choose.

"I do not decide for the mothers any methods. But when they come, I counsel them and then they choose for themselves." – VHT provider

The remaining providers who stated that they recommend particular methods were evenly split between those who recommend injectables and those who promote long acting reversible methods and sterilization (intrauterine devices or IUDs, implants and tubal ligation). No one offered that they recommend condoms or oral contraceptives.

With regard to unmarried adolescents under age 20 however, far fewer providers ($n = 14$) expressed that all (non-permanent) methods are potentially appropriate for adolescent women. The most common method actively promoted to adolescents was the condom ($n = 18$). Two thirds of providers recommending condoms ($n = 12$) were concerned about exposure to sexually transmitted infections (STIs), and the remaining one third ($n = 6$) expressed reservations about premarital adolescent sexual activity,

Table 1 Participant characteristics

	N (Total = 40)	%
Median age (and range)	32 (24–75)	
Gender		
Male	11	27.5
Female	29	72.5
Religion		
Catholic	22	55.0
Protestant	12	30.0
Pentacostal	4	10.0
Seventh Day Adventist	2	5.0
Facility		
Private clinic	9	22.5
Pharmacy	8	20.0
Public Community Health Worker	8	20.0
Public clinic	8	20.0
NGO clinic	7	17.5
Title/Background		
Clinical officer	5	12.5
Midwife	7	17.5
Nurse/Nursing officer	14	35.0
Nursing assistant	4	10.0
VHT (Community Health Worker)	8	20.0
Pharmacist	1	2.5
Business manager	1	2.5
Median number of years as health worker (and range)	6 (1–30)	

recommending the 'ABCs' – Abstain, Be faithful but if not, use Condoms.

> *"The method that I feel is appropriate for an adolescent according to me is only condom. Because like for the female adolescent there are side effects of these contraceptives and it can become problematic especially to those who are school going. So condom is okay since it doesn't only prevent them from pregnancy but also from other diseases like the STDs (sexually transmitted diseases), for instance HIV/AIDs (Human immunodeficiency Virus/Acquired Immune Deficiency Syndrome)."* - Pharmacy provider

> *"But you know when we talking about adolescents, we are not only looking at preventing pregnancy in them but also other STDs and STIs. Like adolescents who have not yet given birth in their life, as long as they know they are free from getting pregnant, they are very vulnerable and they would forget about HIVs. That*

> *would also be my fear that much as we are trying to prevent pregnancy in especially adolescents, we should always not forget to encourage them to use condom on top of preventing pregnancy. Remind them that HIV is still there, so they should protect themselves."* - NGO provider

> *"Being an adolescent is really not something easy because we always advocate for abstinence, you see that. And whoever cannot really do that should use condom."* (Public provider)

Consistent with this tendency to prescribe specific methods to adolescent clients, a substantial share of providers ($n = 15$) volunteered specific methods they would advise adolescents NOT to use. In particular, they singled out the IUD ($n = 4$), hormonal methods generally ($n = 2$), injectable contraception ($n = 3$), cycle or moon beads ($n = 2$), long term methods of any type ($n = 1$), oral contraceptives ($n = 1$), implants ($n = 1$) and condoms ($n = 1$). Their rationales for restricting adolescent choice included concerns about low efficacy (condoms and cycle or moon beads), concerns about possible infertility or cervical cancer due to STI exposure during IUD use, and more commonly, concerns about the impact of hormonal contraception on fertility.

Providers divided on injectable use by adolescents

When asked specifically about injectable contraception, just over half of providers ($n = 22$) expressed support for adolescent use of this method, with many citing the importance of injectable contraception in preventing unwanted pregnancy and reducing the incidence of school drop due to pregnancy. Other stated benefits of the injectable included the short duration, manageable side effects, and accessibility of the method.

> *"I would [offer injectable contraceptive to adolescents] because first of all I know it has no other future dangerous effect to the youth. Secondly it's going to protect them from having unwanted pregnancy. And they will also continue with their studies at school. That is the reason I recommend the injectables to the youth. It's very safe and it has no future effect."* - Public provider

> *"My own opinion is generally that it's actually good for adolescents to use injectable contraception because the injectable is a short term method, and the side effects are easily manageable and it can easily be accessed and administered."* - NGO provider

The remaining providers ($n = 18$) expressed reservations about adolescent use of the injectable. Their reservations were sometimes tied to marital status, rooted either in the perceived immorality of premarital sexual activity or in the risk of exposure to STIs through multiple sexual partners.

"Assuming the adolescent is not yet twenty years, and is even not mature enough to marry, I think it would give them too much sexual feelings because she would -- after all if I inject this -- I don't have any chance of pregnancy. So it would give them too much feelings to go for sex, yet they are still an inappropriate age to be having sexual intercourse." - VHT provider

"I don't feel comfortable at all [offering injectable contraceptives to adolescents]. Being a health worker and at the same time a mother, I would offer [injectables] because I will be thinking of the future of this girl as important. But again on the other side, I will be having feelings in my heart that am I not pushing this girl to make a mistake because she can now think I cannot conceive so I can do anything at any time." – Public provider

"Adolescents who are married, they are already living as husband and wife; it (the injectable) will be good for them. But for those ones who are not married, the bad part of it is that they will now not fear HIV and hepatitis B. Because what I know about youth, they fear pregnancy. They just fear to get pregnant. Now if there are these methods of injectables which are there for adolescent, if they use it, they will forget that I should use protection during sex because I may acquire HIV or Hepatitis B. You see, that is the bad part of it." – Pharmacy provider

More common however, were reservations related to parity, rooted in the misconception that the injectable causes infertility, which has origins in the delayed return to fertility common among DMPA users.

"The injection Depo is not recommended for the adolescent because it may interfere with their fertility since they have not produced in their life. So when it comes time for you to conceive, there may come a problem because the Depo takes a time long to leave the body system." – Private provider

"The young ones, we always advise them to use oral contraceptives because inject-a-plan [brand name of the socially marketed injectable] is meant for once you have at least three or four children. It can stop you from getting your normal menstruation period." – Private provider

"When they are married and the person has not yet delivered, it (the injectable) is not very advisable." – Pharmacy provider

Consistent with their reservations, more than one third of clinic-based providers felt that parental permission should be required (or is advisable) before offering family planning services to adolescents.

"Adolescents who are not married, I think parental permission for adolescents to use family planning is appropriate. The parent should be aware because as those people who use family planning methods say, methods have side effects. So if it starts before the parents, when she has no knowledge, the parents could have fears about what is happening." – VHT provider

Subcutaneous DMPA popular among providers

With respect to DMPA-SC specifically, more than three quarters of participants ($n = 33$) found the device easy to use, with the same number indicating they preferred it to intramuscular DMPA (DMPA-IM). Interviewees noted that the pre-packaged, all-in-one presentation offers advantages to providers, such as avoiding stock-outs of syringes, requiring less skill to administer, saving health workers' time, and minimizing the risk of a needle stick.

"It has its needle already attached. I don't have to withdraw the Depo or the medicine. So everything about it is easier or much better or more convenient."– NGO provider

"As I said, this issue of we don't have the syringe is not there because everything is connected and you can administer it by yourself. It does not really require much skill in injecting. Actually there is nothing I don't like about that."– NGO provider

Providers also identified benefits of DMPA-SC for women, including that the presentation readily lends itself to self-administration ($n = 21$), injections may be less painful due to the smaller needle ($n = 6$) and the perception that the lower dose DMPA-SC has fewer side effects ($n = 4$).

"I saw the needle was really very tiny, you don't experience much pain compared to the other injectable, and the (DMPA-IM) needle is a bit big." – NGO provider

"I think the product is very good because it is self-administered by the clients and side effects are not really serious like for other methods." – Public provider

"For me what I have liked about this [DMPA-SC], the first thing, it is private. You can use it privately. Secondly, the needle is very small for people who fear injections. Then you can do it even self-injection. Actually there is nothing, for me I feel there is nothing wrong with this."- Public provider

Most providers receptive to self-injection, perceive advantages for women

To gauge receptivity to self-injection, providers were asked whether they consider self-injection to be a good option for Ugandan women. By a margin of just under two to one, providers viewed self-injection favorably (*n* = 25), citing the benefits of greater convenience and time savings (*n* = 11), reduction in transport costs (*n* = 9), and better adherence to the reinjection schedule (*n* = 5). Two providers noted that offering self-injection may reduce provider workload. Even providers less receptive to self-injection readily identified advantages for women.

"Mostly I think the major part of the population in Uganda they are below poverty line so if someone can reduce the cost of transport, and get the injectable contraceptive which can be administered by themselves, it can really give them some [savings]." – Pharmacy provider

"In my location, I think it's going to be a good idea to help out women because most of them, during the season for digging (farming) they go really far away; we've had incidences that they miss out on their shots just because they were not close to the clinic. So if they have this, if they have Sayana Press with them, I think they can be able to carry it with them and inject themselves."- NGO provider

"Sometimes in the health centers you can go and you find that the health worker is not yet there, but if you are self-injecting yourself and you have got it enough with you at home, you will be using it without again need to look for health worker to help you inject you, all that."- Pharmacy provider

A number of providers (*n* = 11) spontaneously offered that self-injection is likely to enhance discretion for women who are hiding contraception use. When queried specifically about whether self-injection would be more discreet, nearly all the remaining providers (*n* = 27) thought self-injection would improve privacy.

"I think all the women should use [self-injection] because there are some men who don't advise their women to use family planning or to use any method.

So Sayana Press can help them. You can even go to your private room and just inject yourself."– Private provider

"Somebody who is concerned, maybe a neighbor, would say 'I saw your wife at the facility, is she sick?' You see? So it can bring problems."- Private provider

Even receptive providers raise concerns

For a minority of providers (*n* = 12) however, their initial reaction to the concept of self-injection was more skeptical. These providers, as well as a number of providers generally receptive to self-injection, cited a number of concerns, including appropriate hygiene (*n* = 13), storage (*n* = 11), and disposal (*n* = 6) practices.

"Normally those things have sterile procedures. If maybe the clients are not very clean the site may be infected."– NGO provider

"Storage at home. I could be having the kitchen where it is hot throughout the day. I think we have a temperature where we should keep this Sayana Press. When I have only one house, it's my bedroom, it's my storage, it's my kitchen. So it's like we are exposing this Sayana Press at very high temperature which can damage the product."– NGO provider

"What I see about this Sayana Press is convenient except the ways of disposing the waste. If it is not properly disposed, it can cause injuries at homes."– Public provider

In particular, some providers expressed a lack of confidence in women's ability to administer the injection properly. This included opinions that women would forget the injection steps or not do them correctly (*n* = 11), forget their reinjection date (*n* = 4), or choose an inappropriate injection site (*n* = 5).

"[Self-injection] is not so good because women are... they are not capable, intelligent enough to follow all the steps...It is better they go to the clinic or to the health workers to administer, not from home." – Private provider

"These women if you put your mind on learning the steps in self-injecting and if the health provider did not write for you your next date of injection, you may forget since you may be too busy doing house work... But if you are to remember it alone, you will forget due to so much house work that women usually do at their homes." – VHT provider

"And sometimes they may confuse the injection site. You see the drug has to be injected on the fatty tissue of the body, on the thigh and lower abdomen. So they can forget and end up injecting the wrong site and this may not be good for them."– VHT provider

Public sector clinic providers were disproportionately represented among the 12 individuals who were more skeptical about self-injection, with five of the eight public sector clinic providers expressing reservations. Conversely, public sector VHTs were disproportionally represented among those viewing self-injection favorably, with only one of eight VHTs expressing skepticism.

Mixed feelings about adolescent self-injection

Regarding self-injection for adolescents, a slight majority of interviewees ($n = 23$) opined that self-injection was a good or acceptable option for adolescents—although 7 of these had previously stated that they did not approve of giving the injectable to adolescents. In particular, providers cited the specific benefit of enhanced privacy and ability to conceal contraceptive use ($n = 21$), which some felt, was particularly important for adolescents who are attending boarding school.

"Because I think being in the health facility and also going to a family planning clinic, first of all [adolescents] fear being seen as I told you by the relatives, or the neighbors. But if they are now doing self-injection, they are more confident that nobody is seeing me."– Public provider

"I think Sayana Press would be very good for the adolescents since they can even go with it to school and administer without anybody noticing. Because adolescents go to the boarding school far away from home and the drug will cover them even if they come back home for holidays." – Public provider

Sixteen interviewees felt that adolescents should not be permitted to do self-injection. Beyond concerns about injectable use by adolescents, the most common reason for opposition was a belief that adolescents do not have the maturity to do the injection on their own. Others worried that self-injection, like use of contraceptives more generally, would lead to sexual promiscuity, and a few were concerned that self-injection would open the door to illegal injectable drug use.

"And for adolescents, they have to go to the health facility in order to get the injection because adolescents like taking things for granted. They may forget the procedure to follow when administering ..."– Private provider

"So someone like that (an adolescent), it is not appropriate for her because she might be given a method and she changes her mind to use another method. So the other method which she already had could expire unused. That is why I think that it (self-injection) is not very appropriate for adolescents."– VHT provider

"The adolescents will misuse the drug. Misusing, I mean like I had live sex (without a condom) and maybe I can get pregnant, so I will also give the injection again."– Pharmacy provider

"For the adolescents it would be beneficial but at the same time it would also cause a fear that once they get used to self-injection they may be introduced to some other drug like the drug use injection."– Private provider

Despite their general receptivity to self-injection (noted above), more than half of the VHTs (5 of 8) expressed reservations or concerns about self-injection by adolescents.

With regard to whether adolescents need parental permission to self-inject, providers were evenly divided with half indicating parental permission is needed and half indicating it is not. The rationales offered were similar to those for family planning use in general by adolescents.

"I would think the adolescent should get permission from her parents so that in case of any risks in future the parents would be aware. Because if she starts doing it on her own, if she starts injection on her own, without informing her parents, if the side effects like bleeding starts, who will help her?" – Public provider

"Some of the parents they are very tough. Yes, because if you tell your parents I'm injecting myself and obviously the parents will know that you have somebody somewhere. And some of them may even stop paying your school fees when, if you are still at school." – Pharmacy provider

Clinic providers best for training women

The vast majority of providers, regardless of the type of provider, identified clinic-based health workers as the most appropriate personnel to train women for self-injection, due to their medical expertise and contraceptive knowledge ($n = 33$).

"Health workers are the most appropriate to train because there is a bit of medical knowledge involved in the injection and involved in knowing about the drug.

Medical personnel may advise in an event that there's anything like swelling or maybe infection at the site which has not been administered well. A medical personnel can also give and can handle that." – Private provider

"Midwives who handle matters of family planning in the health center and in the area are appropriate and medical personnel with the knowledge on family planning."– VHT provider

That said, quite a few respondents recognized VHTs as capable of training women ($n = 15$), including nearly one third of those who first proposed clinic-based health workers ($n = 10$). VHTs are valued as trainers because of their close relationships with the community.

"Like you heard me say, first, those people (VHTs) are prior trained and have knowledge on how to administer Sayana Press. Secondly, the VHT is a person closer and known to the community as a person from whom we get these specific things, from whom we go obtain this particular assistance." – VHT provider

While all eight pharmacists identified health workers as the most appropriate trainers, five indicated, when queried, that pharmacy staff could also train women for self-injection. One disagreed however, noting that pharmacists don't have the time required to train women individually.

"The health workers in the pharmacy should also be trained so that any clients going there, they should also give that knowledge to them... As you are selling the products to the customers, the health workers must know more about the product because you cannot give a product to a client and the client will ask you very many questions and you have nothing to say. The client will not take that unless you have knowledge on that, then you can give and defend with the answers."– Pharmacy provider

"And the best people to train the women I would prefer those who work at the family planning section, maternity sites and antenatal care department because they are the ones who always interface with these women more often and they always carryout health education. Because like here at the pharmacy, no one can train these women since we provide a wide range of services and we do not have the time to talk to the clients for long." - Pharmacy provider

A few providers ($n = 3$) suggested that peer-to-peer training would be beneficial as it would provide role models to women.

"I would recommend that there should be regular outreaches on Sayana Press and demonstration. And maybe select one participant to come and demonstrate by herself to see how they administer Sayana Press so that women get more knowledge and get acquainted with the method."–NGO provider

By about two to one, providers felt that adolescents might prefer or benefit from separate training—away from adults—for reasons such as discomfort and shyness. They opined that, if trained with older women they might not ask questions or receive adequate training. A few providers noted that HIV and STI education should also be a focus of training for adolescents (but did not mention these topics as critical for adult women).

"The difference in the training needs maybe is there because there may be adolescents who are still very young like around 15 -16 years, and if you mix them with the older women, they may not ask any questions even if they have them, because of fear and not feeling free or comfortable."– VHT provider

"[The training of adolescents should be] a little bit special because these people should be training them not only on family planning methods but also train adolescents on preventing themselves from being exposed to HIV/AIDs and other STIs. So this means your knowledge again will have to go further onto this adolescent. Those one who will be providing the services to the adolescent, they should equip them with more knowledge than these one who train mothers."– Public provider

Post-training support and follow up important

About three quarters of providers ($n = 28$) mentioned that some form of proactive follow-up would be helpful to make sure clients remember the injection procedures and schedule. The most common form of follow up, identified by 19 interviewees, was home visits or community outreach to villages where women are self-injecting. Some specified that this form of follow-up would be most appropriate and feasible for the VHTs ($n = 11$). Others advocated that self-injecting clients be asked to return to the clinic periodically to demonstrate their mastery ($n = 6$). Some felt that phone calls to self-injecting clients would be appropriate support ($n = 6$)

"I think it would be easy if we follow them through the VHTs that are nearer to them because if the VHT near them, this VHT can go to a mother just like he is visiting the home, and will follow up these mothers from home that is one thing. The VHT can also ask

them how they are doing it and still remind them."– Public provider

"Women, especially those ones in the villages, when you inject them or you tell them to always come back to you after a certain period, they do come. So according to me, I recommend that all providers should tell whoever gets Sayana Press from them to always remember to come back to him/ her after a certain period -- maybe after 6 months -- so that you can still assess the person to see whether she is doing it rightfully. In that way, you would also be doing refresher training." – Pharmacy provider

The remaining participants ($n = 10$) were confident that, once trained, women would not need additional supervision or follow-up to do self-injection. They advised that follow up should be client-initiated, such that women return to the facility or pharmacy in case of problems.

"According to me, I feel if the women are cleared to start injecting from their homes, then they should tell them to always remember to come back to the health center in case they are forgetting the steps to follow in self-administering Sayana Press."– VHT provider

A number of providers recommended support in the form of a client instruction job aid and/or calendar be provided to remind women of the procedure and their next injection date ($n = 8$).

"Yeah that one [client support] will be a little bit hard but I think they need to be encouraged to at least have a place where they can record the next date for injection. So they should be provided with either a calendar or a book where they can write their next injection date so that they cannot forget."– Private provider

Nine providers were of the opinion that follow-up was particularly fundamental for adolescents because they need more encouragement and supervision to continue with the method.

"You know adolescent youth are not like adults. So for them they can change their mind anyhow so they need to be followed and talked with well. Advised."– Private provider

Discussion

This study suggests that informed choice is an ideal not yet realized when it comes to contraceptive services for adolescent clients in Uganda. Our findings regarding what methods providers consider appropriate or inappropriate for adolescents are largely consistent with what Chandra-Mouli and colleagues refer to as a 'condoms-only mindset' [28]. Be they motivated by concerns about STIs, promiscuity, or lingering suspicions about the safety of hormonal methods, the attitudes of our participants suggest that providers may impose restrictions on method choice for young, unmarried and/or nulliparous adolescent clients. While providers may feel they have the adolescent's best interests at heart in promoting condoms over other methods, adolescents may have older partners or engage in transactional sex, and may not be able to negotiate condom use in settings where gender norms promote inequality. Suspicion about the safety or appropriateness of high efficacy hormonal methods for adolescent women leaves them vulnerable to higher rates of contraceptive failure and method discontinuation associated with condoms and other short term methods [23, 29].

More specific to the main focus of this study, the parity and/or age restrictions on injectable use, which have no medical basis, present an obvious barrier to the offer of self-injection to this demographically-important population. Since fewer than half of providers see self-injection as a good option for adolescents, making self-injection available to adolescent clients will necessitate renewed efforts to overcome provider-imposed method restrictions and ease concerns about the ability of adolescents to self-inject safely. A number of promising interventions to reduce provider bias against adolescents have been proposed by the Beyond Bias Consortium, including: 1) clear directives and clarity from leadership regarding the importance of reproductive health services for adolescents; 2) provider education that involves communications training, values clarification, attitudinal conditioning or the pairing 'reluctant' providers with 'champions' in the provision of youth services, and using personalized anecdotes and exercises that encourage providers to see the world through an adolescent lens; and 3) a systems approach rather than one-off provider trainings to address the myriad conditions necessary for Youth-Friendly Services, such as expanded clinic hours, outreach to schools and communities, enhanced privacy, and reduced fees for adolescent clients [30].

With regard to self-injection for adult women, this study suggests that most providers view self-injection favorably, but with some reservations that will need to be addressed if the practice is to become widespread. In particular, provider concerns that women may be unable to self-inject competently should be addressed, with reference to the growing number of studies demonstrating its feasibility and acceptability, including for women in low resource settings and women with limited education [22, 31]. Identifying and featuring 'self-injection champions' is another strategy that may sway skeptical providers. Offering a client instruction guide and reinjection calendar may reassure health workers that women can self-inject independently. Concerns about safe storage and waste disposal may be assuaged by providing low cost impermeable containers to store the spent units until a convenient time to return the needles to a clinic, community health worker, or pharmacy.

With respect to other parameters for the design of a self-injection program, the vast majority of providers (of all types) identify clinic-based health workers as best placed to train women in self-injection. What providers may not recognize is that training women in self-injection can be time-consuming, particularly if training is conducted in a one-on-one fashion. The heavy workload of providers – particularly those in the public sector – may impinge on the availability of self-injection training. While less acceptable to providers in this study, permitting community-based health workers to train women may be a more realistic approach, and one that recent research suggests is feasible [8]. With regard to adolescents, a number of participants proposed that adolescents be trained separately from adult women, to reduce feelings of intimidation and discomfort. Making that proposal a reality likely entails offering self-injection training beyond the clinic, at outreach events or via programs that specifically target adolescent clients.

With respect to the private sector, though private clinic providers were not noticeably disinclined to endorse self-injection, it remains to be seen whether they will offer self-injection training, given their financial incentive to encourage repeat clientele in order to collect consultation fees. Training in commercial settings, such as pharmacies and drug shops, may be constrained by lack of a private setting for injections.

In terms of post-training support to self-injecting clients, most providers proposed proactive follow up to ensure that clients recall how and when to self-inject. This suggestion presents a number of challenges: First, many clients in Uganda are using methods discreetly, and much of the appeal of self-injection stems from the potential for enhanced confidentiality. In this setting, clients may not welcome a home visit or phone call from a family planning provider. Second, from a practical standpoint, the majority of women in Uganda do not have exclusive access to a cell phone, and providers are not resourced to provide home visits (or make calls to their clientele with phones). Tasking community health workers with follow up may be more practical and cost-effective, but will require strong coordination between clinic and field-based health workers. One option for client-initiated support currently being tested in Uganda is the offer of a toll-free hotline manned by trained self-injection counselors. If successful, this approach may satisfy the World Health Organization recommendation that self-injection be offered "in contexts where mechanisms to provide the woman with appropriate information

and training exist, referral linkages to a healthcare provider are strong, and where monitoring and follow-up can be ensured" [32].

Study limitations

As with all qualitative studies, our findings are not generalizable and may not apply to providers in other settings in Uganda and other countries. While attempts were made to solicit honest and forthcoming opinions, providers may have been subject to some degree of social desirability bias, offering opinions overly favorable to adolescent contraceptive use, injectable use, and/or self-injection.

Conclusion

Self-injection presents an opportunity to reduce the burden on the health system presented by heavy reliance on injectable contraception requiring quarterly clinic visits. For adolescents, the potential discretion and user control inherent in the practice of self-injection align with well-established priorities for improving adolescent access to contraceptive services. While our results reveal a level of cautious support for self-injection among providers in Uganda, their reservations about offering the service to adolescents suggest more needs to be done if self-injection is to be made available to women without regard to age, parity or marital status. In addition to including self-injection in healthcare training curricula, service delivery guidelines will need to be revised and existing providers will require continuous professional development to bring them up to speed with this self-care intervention. With about a dozen countries in sub-Saharan Africa currently poised to introduce self-injection as a delivery option, this study offers insights on provider perspectives that ministries of health may wish to consider, particularly if their goals include improving access to family planning for adolescents. Moving forward, policymakers and program implementers should design, implement, and evaluate self-injection interventions with the needs of adolescent clients uppermost in mind, recognizing that extra effort may be required to shift provider perspectives and assuage their concerns.

Abbreviations

AIDS: Acquired immune deficiency syndrome; DMPA: Depot medroxyprogesterone acetate; DMPA-IM: Intramuscular depot medroxyprogesterone acetate; DMPA-SC: Subcutaneous depot medroxyprogesterone acetate; HIV: Human immunodeficiency virus; IUD: Intrauterine device; NDA: National drug authority; NGO: Non-governmental Organization; STD: Sexually transmitted disease; STI: Sexually transmitted infection; VHT: Village health team

Acknowledgments

The coauthors would like to thank the research assistants in Gulu district who conducted the interviews and the health workers who shared their time and perspectives.

Funding

This work was funded by the Children's Investment Fund Foundation, London, United Kingdom [Request #333]. The funding sources did not play a role in study design; the collection, analysis, and interpretation of data; the writing of the report; or the decision to submit the article for publication.

Authors' contributions

JC oversaw the design and implementation of the study, finalized training materials and standard operating procedures (SOPs), co-facilitated the training of study staff, analyzed the findings, and drafted the manuscript. AN and JT contributed to the study staff training materials and the development of SOPs, co-facilitated the training of study staff, oversaw the in-country IRB submissions, oversaw all field work (data collection), and contributed to the manuscript. JL oversaw the IRB submissions, drafted SOPs for data collection, analyzed the findings, and contributed to the manuscript. CMC developed the protocol and designed the study staff training, and contributed to the manuscript. All authors read and approved the final manuscript.

Competing interests

The authors declare that they have no competing interests.

Author details

[1]PATH, PO Box 900922, Seattle, WA 98109, USA. [2]PATH, PO Box 7404, Kampala, Uganda. [3]St Catherine University, St. Paul Campus, 2004 Randolph Ave, St. Paul, MN 55105, USA.

References

1. Stout A, Wood S, Barigye G, Kaboré A, Siddo D, Ndione I. Expanding access to injectable contraception: results from pilot introduction of subcutaneous depot medroxyprogesterone acetate (DMPA-SC) in 4 African countries. Global Health: Science and Practice. 2018;6(1):55–72 https://doi.org/10.9745/GHSP-D-17-00250.
2. Jain, et al. Contraceptive efficacy and safety of DMPA-SC. Contraception. 2004;70:269–75.
3. Uganda Bureau of Statistics (UBOS) and ICF. 2017. Uganda Demographic and Health Survey 2016: Key indicators report. Kampala, Uganda: UBOS, and Rockville, Maryland, USA: UBOS and ICF.
4. PRB. 2017 World Population Data Sheet. Available at: http://www.prb.org/pdf17/2017_World_Population.pdf
5. Uganda Bureau of Statistics. The National Population and housing census 2014 – Main report. Uganda: Kampala; 2016.
6. PMA2020 / Uganda, Round 6: Family Planning Brief. https://www.pma2020.org/sites/default/files/PMA2020-Uganda-R6-FP-brief.pdf
7. Burke HM, et al. Observational study of the acceptability of Sayana ® press among intramuscular DMPA users in Uganda and Senegal. Contraception. 2014;89(5):361–7.
8. Burke HM, Chen M, Buluzi M, Fuchs R, Wevill S, Venkatasubramanian L, et al. Effect of self-administration versus provider-administered injection of subcutaneous depot medroxyprogesterone acetate on continuation rates in Malawi: a randomised controlled trial. Lancet Glob Health. 2018;6:e568–78. https://doi.org/10.1016/S2214-109X(18)30061-5.
9. Kohn JE, Simons HR, Della Badia L, Draper E, Morfesis J, Talmont E, et al. Increased 1-year continuation of DMPA among women randomized to self-administration: results from a randomized controlled trial at Planned Parenthood. Contraception. 2018;97(3):198–204. https://doi.org/10.1016/j.contraception.2017.11.009.
10. Cover J, Namagembe A, Tumusiime J, Nsangi D, Lim J, Dinah Nakiganda-Busiku. Continuation of injectable contraception when self-injected v. administered by a facility-based health worker: A non-randomized, prospective cohort study in Uganda. Contraception 2018. doi: https://doi.org/10.1016/j.contraception.2018.03.032.
11. Cover, J. et al. Continuation of self-injected v. provider-administered contraception in Senegal: a non-randomized, prospective cohort study. Under review at Contraception.
12. Amuyunzu-Nyamongo M, et al. Qualitative evidence on adolescents' views of sexual and reproductive health in sub-Saharan Africa: occasional report #16. New York: Guttmacher Institute; 2005. Available at: https://www.guttmacher.org/sites/default/files/pdfs/pubs/2005/03/01/or16.pdf
13. Biddlecom AE, et al. Adolescents' views of and preferences for sexual and reproductive health services in Burkina Faso, Ghana, Malawi and Uganda. Afr J Reprod Health. 2007;11(3):99–110.
14. World Health Organization. Making health services adolescent friendly: Developing national quality standards for adolescent friendly health services. 2012. Available at: http://www.who.int/maternal_child_adolescent/documents/adolescent_friendly_services/en/
15. United States Agency for International Development. High-impact practices in family planning (HIPs). Adolescent-friendly contraceptive services: mainstreaming adolescent-friendly elements into existing contraceptive services. Washington (DC): USAID; 2015. Available at: https://www.fphighimpactpractices.org/afcs
16. Hervish A, Clifton D. Status report: adolescents and young people in sub-Saharan Africa: opportunities and challenges. New York: United Nations Population Fund; 2012. Available at: http://www.prb.org/pdf12/status-report-youth-subsaharan-Africa.pdf
17. Kiapi-Iwa L, Hart GJ. The sexual and reproductive health of young people in Adjumani district, Uganda: qualitative study of the role of formal, informal and traditional health providers. AIDS Care. 2004;16(3):339–47.
18. Schwandt HM, et al. Contraceptive service provider imposed restrictions to contraceptive access in urban Nigeria. BMC Health Serv Res. 2017;17:278.
19. Ilene S, Speizer, et al. Do service providers in Tanzania unnecessarily restrict Clients' access to contraceptive methods? Int Fam Plan Perspect. 2000;26(1):13–20 & 42.
20. Nalwadda G, et al. Young peoples' interface with providers of contraceptive care: a simulated client study in two Ugandan districts. Contraception and Reproductive Medicine. 2016;1:15.
21. Nalwadda G, Mirembe F, Tumwesigye NM, Byamugisha J, Faxelid E. Constraints and prospects for contraceptive service provision to young people in Uganda: providers' perspectives. BMC Health Serv Res. 2011;11:220.
22. Cover J, et al. A prospective cohort study of the feasibility and acceptability of depot medroxyprogesterone acetate administered subcutaneously through self-injection. Contraception. 2016;95(3):306–11.
23. Prabhakaran S, Sweet A. Self-administration of subcutaneous depot medroxyprogesterone acetate for contraception: feasibility and acceptability. Contraception. 2012;85(5):453–7.
24. Cameron ST, Glasier A, Johnstone A. Pilot study of home self-administration of subcutaneous depo-medroxyprogesterone acetate for contraception. Contraception. 2012;85(5):458–64.
25. Stanwood NL, et al. Self-injection of monthly combined hormonal contraceptive. Contraception. 2006;73(1):53–5.
26. Williams RL, Hensel DJ, Fortenberry JD. Self-administration of subcutaneous depot medroxyprogesterone acetate by adolescent women. Contraception. 2013;88(3):401–7.
27. Cover, J. et al. Acceptability of contraceptive self-injection with DMPA-SC among adolescents in Gulu District, Uganda. International Perspectives in Sexual and Reproductive Health. Int Perspect Sex Reprod Health. 2017;43(4):153–62.
28. Chandra-Mouli, et al. A never-before opportunity to strengthen investment and action on adolescent contraception, and what we must do to make full use of it. Reprod Health. 2017;14:85.
29. Ann K. Blanc et al. Patterns and trends in Adolescents' contraceptive use and discontinuation in developing countries and comparisons with adult women. *International Perspectives in Sexual and Reproductive Health*, volume 35, Issue 2 June 2009.
30. Summer Starling, et al. Beyond Bias - literature review and expert interviews on provider Bias in the provision of youth contraceptive services: research summary and synthesis. April 2017. Camber Collective. Available at: https://www.thecompassforsbc.org/project-examples/beyond-bias-literature-review-and-expert-interviews-provider-bias-provision-youth.
31. Cover J, et al. Evaluating the feasibility and acceptability of self-injection of subcutaneous depot medroxyprogesterone acetate (DMPA) in Senegal: a prospective cohort study. Contraception. 2017;96:203–10. https://doi.org/10.1016/j.contraception.2017.06.010.
32. World Health Organization. Health worker roles in providing safe abortion care and post-abortion contraception, 2015. Available at: http://apps.who.int/iris/bitstream/10665/181041/1/9789241549264_eng.pdf#page=70.

3

Determinants of antenatal care attendance among women residing in highly disadvantaged communities in northern Jordan

Heba H. Hijazi[1*], Mohammad S. Alyahya[1], Amer M. Sindiani[2], Rola S. Saqan[3] and Abdulhakeem M. Okour[4]

Abstract

Background: One of the major reproductive health challenges among disadvantaged populations is to provide pregnant women with the necessary antenatal care (ANC). In this study, we suggest applying an integrated conceptual framework aimed at ascertaining the extent to which attendance at ANC clinics may be attributed to individual determinants or to the quality of the care received.

Methods: Using a cross-sectional design, data were collected from a sample of 831 women residing in nine sub-districts in three northern governorates of Jordan and designated according to national categorization as persistent poverty pockets. All of the sampled women were recruited from public maternal and child health centers and interviewed using a structured pre-tested survey. This tool covered certain predictors, ranging from the user's attributes, including predisposing, enabling, and need factors, to the essential components of the experience of care. These components assessed the quality of ANC in terms of five elements: woman–provider relations, technical management, information exchange, continuity of care, and appropriate constellation of services. Adequate ANC content was assessed in relation to the frequency of antenatal visits and the time of each visit.

Results: The results of multivariate logistic regression analyses show that the use of ANC facilities is affected by various factors related to the quality of service delivery. These include receiving information and education on ANC during clinic visits (OR = 9.1; 95% CI = 4.9–16.9), providing pregnant women with opportunities for dialogue and health talks (OR = 7.2; 95% CI = 4.1–12.8), having scheduled follow-up appointments (OR = 6.5; 95% CI = 3.5–12.0), and offering dignified and respectful care (OR = 5.7; 95% CI = 2.5–13.1). At the individual level, our findings have identified a woman's education level (OR = 1.2; 95% CI = 1.1–1.3), desire for the pregnancy (OR = 1.7; 95% CI = 1.1–2.7), and living in a district served by an ANC clinic (OR = 4.3; 95% CI = 2.3–8.1) as determinants affecting ANC utilization.

Conclusion: Taking women's experiences of ANC as a key metric for reporting the quality of the care is more likely to lead to increased utilization of ANC services by women in highly disadvantaged communities. Our findings suggest that the degree to which women feel that they are respected, informed, and engaged in their care has potential favorable implications for ANC.

Keywords: Utilization, Antenatal care, Disadvantaged communities, Poverty, Experience of care, Quality, Jordan

* Correspondence: hhhijazi0@just.edu.jo
[1]Department of Health Management and Policy, Faculty of Medicine, Jordan University of Science and Technology, P.O. Box 3030, Irbid 22110, Jordan
Full list of author information is available at the end of the article

Plain English summary

Millions of women in developing countries are more likely to experience life-threatening and pregnancy-related complications because of a lack of access to adequate and good-quality antenatal care (ANC). Indicators of adequate care, as recommended by the World Health Organization (WHO), include providing pregnant women with four antenatal visits, of which the initial contact should be scheduled during the first trimester of pregnancy. In Jordan, remarkable progress has been made to expand the coverage of ANC; however, disparities and inequity in access to quality ANC services among different socioeconomic groups are still evident and subject to debate. Thus, our study aims to explore barriers that prevent women who live in low-income settings from utilizing antenatal services adequately.

This study collected quantitative data from women aged 15–49 years residing in highly disadvantaged sub-districts in three northern governorates of Jordan. Data were gathered by means of a face-to-face interview using a health facility-based survey.

Among the 831 enrolled women, 36.6% had inadequate attendance at ANC services. Our findings indicate that utilization of ANC is embedded in the context of the healthcare delivery system, in which women's access to the necessary health education and engagement in one-to-one consultations were found to be significant predictors. Treating women with respect and dignity and providing them with scheduled follow-up appointments were also associated with ANC attendance.

As a result, to achieve significant changes in the delivery of ANC, it is extremely important for health authorities to pay more attention to the woman–provider interaction in increasing utilization of ANC and enhancing women's experience of pregnancy.

Background

ANC is a key strategy for reducing maternal morbidity and mortality directly by affording increased chances of the timely identification of high-risk pregnancies [1–3]. It also represents an entry point for the integrated use of skilled health personnel [4]. Empirical studies of preventive services have often found that regular monitoring of women during pregnancy is vital to reduce birth-related complications, provide supportive care, and promote safer motherhood [5, 6]. In contrast, low health service utilization throughout the prenatal period breaks the critical link in the continuum of care and contributes to poor birth outcomes [7].

In low- and middle-income countries (LMICs), ANC utilization has increased since the introduction of the 2002 WHO ANC model, known as 'focused' ANC (FANC) [8]. This model aims at delivering 'reduced but goal-orientated' clinic visits, at which essential interventions should be provided to pregnant women at specified intervals. With the FANC model, healthy women with no underlying pregnancy complications should be scheduled a minimum of four ANC visits, and more than four in the case of danger signs or pregnancy-related illnesses. For many of the essential interventions in FANC, it is crucial to initiate the care during the first trimester of pregnancy (up to 12 weeks of gestation), and schedule the second visit at 24 to 28 weeks of gestation and the third and fourth visits at 32 weeks and between 36 and 38 weeks of gestation, respectively [8, 9].

During the last decade, considerable research attention has been paid to determining the routine number of visits that are necessary to optimize the health of mothers and babies and enhance safety during pregnancy. Recently, however, a 2015 systematic review of randomized controlled trails has raised concerns that the reduced number of antenatal contacts is associated with an increased risk of perinatal mortality, particularly stillbirth [10]. Accordingly, in November 2016, the WHO began promoting a new model of ANC aimed at reducing perinatal deaths and improving women's experience of care by recommending a minimum of eight contacts [8].

While many may argue that increasing the frequency of antenatal visits would positively influence the health of mothers and newborns [8, 10], related literature has indicated that a reduced number of visits, but with targeted interventions at each visit, proved to be equally effective as monthly ANC visits [11]. In many resource-limited settings, increasing the number of ANC visits for women with uncomplicated pregnancies to more than four has not been found to be associated with improved birth outcomes [12, 13]. Considering that the optimum number of ANC visits in low-income settings depends not only on effectiveness but also on feasibility and other barriers to ANC access and supply [7], our study placed particular emphasis on investigating the delivery of 'reduced and goal-orientated' ANC.

In Jordan, only a few studies have examined factors that predict the utilization of ANC services. Importantly, previous research has generally focused on studying the association between the use of ANC facilities with a range of individual characteristics, such as a woman's age, occupation, parity, and level of education [14–17]. However, this may be imprecise and offers little insight into the context in which utilization occurs. Other attributes, including the accessibility, availability, and quality of ANC services, are also significant factors to consider. Hence, the main objectives of our study are to explore barriers that prevent women who live in highly disadvantaged communities from utilizing ANC services adequately, and to ascertain the extent to which their attendance may be attributed to the quality of the ANC service delivery or to the individual determinants of these women. Addressing such barriers is considered a matter of equality, social justice, and ethics, requiring policymakers to think differently about the poor and those at risk of social exclusion.

Jordan overview

The current national coverage rate for ANC is high in Jordan; almost all women (99%) receive ANC from medically trained personnel (doctors, nurses, or midwives) at least once during pregnancy [18]. While it is obvious that Jordan is on track to achieving its goal of expanding coverage of ANC services, most efforts to enhance the use of these services have focused on quantifiable issues, such as increasing the number of prenatal visits. Data on ANC are obtained mostly from household surveys, in which women who have had a live birth during the last five years preceding the survey are asked whether and from whom they received care. However, no information on the quality of ANC services is provided by the national surveys. Further, no specific data on ANC utilization are available for those who live in highly disadvantaged communities (i.e., poverty pockets).

To facilitate the geographic targeting of the poor, Jordan has developed a system for mapping poverty, using the Small Area Estimation Method to identify 'poverty pockets' across the country [19]. A poverty pocket represents a district or sub-district, which may be a village, a desert oasis, or a large, low-income locality within a metropolitan city or in the suburbs, where more than 25% of the population is below the poverty line [19]. Based on the Household Expenditure and Income Surveys (HEIS) data, most recently updated in 2010/2011, the absolute poverty line amounted to 814 Jordanian Dinars (JDs) annually or 67.8 JD per capita per month [19]. This measure continues to be used as the principal measure of poverty in Jordan, and the majority of the poor are still clustered around this line [19].

During the last decade, Jordan has made strenuous efforts in fighting poverty, within its limited resources and in the context of the global political and economic upheavals. However, figures released by the Ministry of Planning and International Cooperation (MoPIC), with the technical support of the United Nations Development Program (UNDP), show an increase in poverty rates from 13.3% in 2008 to 14.4% in 2010 [20]. The number of poverty pockets also increased from 22 pockets in 2006 to 32 and 36 poverty pockets in 2008, 2010, respectively [20].

Another worrisome finding reported by the United Nations Children's Fund (UNICEF) in 2016 is that a notable variation in the source of services across all social classes is apparent in Jordan. Women from lower wealth quintiles represent a larger share of women who access ANC services and deliver their babies at public facilities [21]. According to the National Strategy for the Health Sector in Jordan for the years 2015–2019, there are significant disparities with respect to the quality of health services between the health sector institutions and between different geographic regions [22]. This raises concerns about equitable access to quality ANC services among different socioeconomic groups within the country.

Conceptual framework

A woman's decision to seek ANC is not simply a matter of personal preference; the accessibility of services that either facilitate or impede utilization also has an important influence [23]. As outlined by the WHO, access to ANC services consists of several elements, including distance and/or time to a facility, the physical availability of services, cultural and social factors that may impede access, economic and other costs associated with use of services, and the quality of the services offered [24].

In a healthcare context, the use of services is a complex human behavioral phenomenon [25]. It reflects a point at which patients' needs meet the professional system [26]. During the last few decades, a number of models have been developed to identify factors affecting the utilization of healthcare services, the most widely used being the 1995 version of the Andersen's behavioral model [26]. According to this model, an individual's use of a service is considered to be a function of three components. These include predisposing factors, which represent the sociocultural characteristics of individuals that exist prior to their illness or condition; enabling factors in terms of the logistical aspects of obtaining care; and need factors that generate the necessity for healthcare services, such as the presence of diagnosed medical conditions and self-perception of health status.

Despite the importance of individual determinants affecting the utilization of care, it is well known that service attendance is strongly dependent on the quality of care experienced at healthcare facilities [26]. The philosophy behind providing pregnant women with FANC is to ensure access to goal-oriented and high-quality care for all women, not only those at risk, with targeted interventions at each visit [11]. Achieving improvements in the quality of ANC is multidimensional and requires increased attention to the process of care delivery, in which the experience of care should be evaluated based on globally determined and locally feasible criteria. In 2016, the WHO released a global framework for improving the quality of care throughout pregnancy, childbirth, and the postnatal period, quality being understood as the provision and experience of care from a health systems perspective [27].

Recent evidence has acknowledged that, if the quality of ANC is poor and women's experience is negative, women will not attend ANC services, regardless of the recommended number of contacts in the model [8, 28]. Accordingly, our study provides an additional consideration for identifying gaps in the experience of care that may lead to poor delivery of adequate care. Within the WHO framework, the experience of care consists of effective communication between healthcare providers with pregnant women; care that involves respect and the preservation of dignity; and access to social and emotional support that is sensitive to women's needs [27].

Inspired by the 2016 WHO framework and taking into account the study's main objectives, we suggest applying an integrated conceptual framework that incorporates both individual determinants for seeking care and the contextual characteristics of ANC service delivery. Specifically, our study aims to explore the effects of quality of care on the utilization of ANC and how the experience of care can lead to different access outcomes for women from lower-income backgrounds. As per Fig. 1, individual determinants are categorized as predisposing, enabling, and need factors; while variables related to the quality of ANC capture the essential components of the experience of care.

To assess the quality of ANC experienced, our study is directed by Bruce's framework for conceptualizing the quality of care in the provision of reproductive health services [29]. Within this framework, evaluating the quality of ANC requires the examination of five main elements, namely interpersonal relations between healthcare providers and clients; technical management; information exchange; continuity and follow-up; and an appropriate constellation of services [29].

Methods

Study design and sample

This study collected quantitative data from 14 sub-districts, identified by the MoPIC as poverty pockets, in northern Jordan. These sub-districts are spread over three northern governorates (the administrative division in the country), Irbid, Mafraq, and Jerash, and classified as rural and desert towns/villages. The modeling of the 14 sub-districts is compatible with the sampling frame of the HEIS 2011 and the social data pilot module survey launched by MoPIC and UNDP to measure vulnerability risk and social exclusion in the country. Over the last decade, nine of these sub-districts are classified as persistent poverty pockets, and five are classified as fluctuating ones [20]. To ensure that all poverty pockets shared the same characteristics, only persistent ones were included in our study. Furthermore, all of the sampled sub-districts are broadly similar in their level of socioeconomic wealth (i.e. sanitation, electricity, and water service) and age/gender structure.

Out of the nine selected sub-districts, five were served by public Maternal and Child Health (MCH) centers; however, the remaining four had no such service. Given that the target population of this study was users of reproductive health services at public MCH centers, and that these centers provide services to well-defined geographic

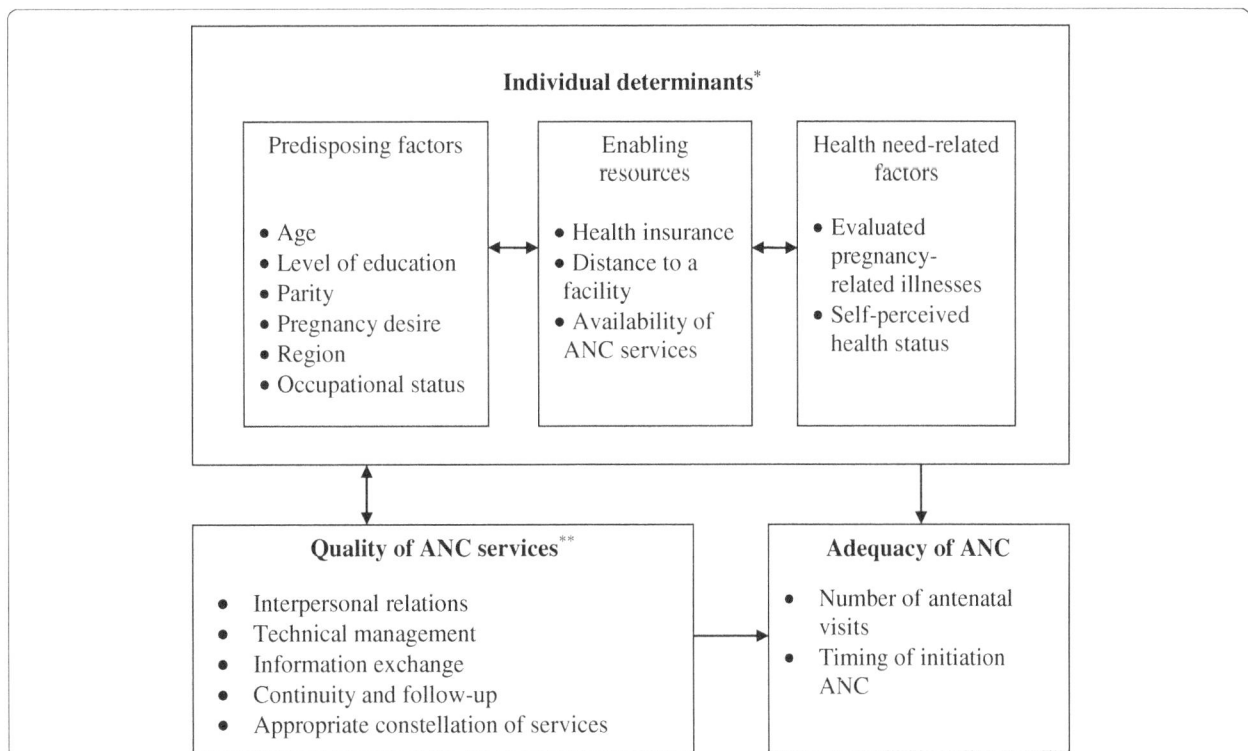

Fig. 1 Conceptual framework for analyzing determinants of ANC utilization among women residing in highly disadvantaged communities in northern Jordan
*Adapted from Andersen's behavioral model for health service use (Andersen, 1995)
**Adapted from Bruce's framework for assessing the quality of care (Bruce, 1990)

areas, the nearest center in each of the underserved sub-districts was targeted. Before starting the fieldwork, the names of MCH centers were obtained using a list provided by the Jordanian Ministry of Health (MoH). During this phase, new maps of all sub-districts were prepared, and the numbers of MCH centers were updated, listed, and documented.

The field work stage of data collection started in June 2015 and ended in July 2016. Using purposive sampling, efforts were made to ensure that all participating women met a number of inclusion criteria. In particular, a woman was eligible to participate only if she was a currently married woman, aged 15–49 years, had been living in one of the chosen highly disadvantaged sub-districts for at least the preceding four years, and had a household monthly income of 68 JDs or less per person and was receiving no other type of assistance. The primary users of services provided at the public MCH centers are married women of childbearing age from the middle and low socioeconomic classes, and thus most of the facilities' attendees were eligible for participation. Since the main focus of this study was to assess the quality of care as perceived by the women receiving the care, a number of exclusion criteria were applied. These included any currently married woman within the specified age group who had not had a live birth in the last two years preceding the survey ($n = 136$), was pregnant at the time of the survey ($n = 118$), did not have at least one ANC visit during the last pregnancy ($n = 21$), initiated ANC visits after the first trimester ($n = 190$), and obtained ANC from multiple/other facilities, or was a new registry ($n = 215$). Of the total 1511 women interviewed in the survey, with a 96% response rate, data from 831 participants were eligible for analysis.

The study instrument and variables
Data collection instrument
This study is based on original cross-section data collected by means of a face-to-face interview using a structured, pre-tested survey. The survey was adopted after reviewing the literature in the relevant research area. Prior to data collection, several steps were taken to assess the validity and reliability of the instrument. To examine content validity, a panel of eight experienced perinatal personnel was asked to review and refine each item in the instrument. This panel was composed of three obstetricians, three senior community midwives, and two researchers in the field of reproductive health. Further, the Pearson correlation coefficient was calculated to examine the test–retest reliability of the survey for a sub-sample of participants ($n = 28$). The questionnaire was administered again to the same sample three weeks later. The test–retest correlation coefficient for the instrument was 0.78 ($p < 0.001$), which is indicative of acceptable stability over time.

Outcome variable
In our analysis, the utilization of ANC services is classified into adequate versus inadequate as the outcome variable. To assess the overall adequacy of ANC, reviews of the medical records of respondents were conducted to obtain more accurate information about the basic ANC components received (i.e., frequency of antenatal visits and timing of each visit). Keeping in mind that this study was limited to the sample of women who initiated antenatal visits during the first trimester, ANC was defined as adequate if the woman with a normal pregnancy had at least four antenatal visits and more than four in case of complications; otherwise, it was defined as inadequate.

Explanatory variables
The study's explanatory variables consist of a number of covariates and predictors. Based on the previous conceptual framework and a review of the literature, several covariates were taken into consideration. These covariates embodied the background determinants of respondents: predisposing characteristics (i.e., age, education, parity, occupation, desire for the pregnancy, and region); enabling resources (i.e., health insurance, living in an area served by a MCH center, and the time taken to get to the nearest center); and need factors (i.e., evaluated pregnancy-related illnesses and self-perceived health status). Using a list of pregnancy-related complications, the participating women were asked to self-report the main illnesses that they had had during their last pregnancy. This list was identified by obstetricians and involved a number of medical conditions, including hypertension, diabetes, anemia, respiratory distress, abnormal vaginal discharge, pre-eclampsia, joint problems, and urinary tract infection.

Factors related to the perceived quality of ANC were included in the analysis as the main predictors of interest. These involved interpersonal relations (i.e., communication, understanding, and the presence of privacy); technical management (physical examination, availability of vaccines/supplements, and clinical tests); information exchange (clarity of providers' explanations, consultation time, and obtaining information and counseling on ANC); follow-up and continuity (i.e., scheduling of appointments and the sincerity of the provider); and an appropriate constellation of services (i.e., waiting time and opening hours).

Statistical analyses
Summary statistics were carried out to describe the study participants according to different characteristics. Differences in ANC attendance (i.e., adequate vs. inadequate use) were reported using chi-squared tests and two sample t-tests for categorical and continuous variables, respectively. Standardized residuals were examined for categorical variables to determine which cell

contributed to the statistically significant difference between the observed frequency and the expected one. Binary logistic regression models were performed to obtain adjusted odds ratios (ORs) for the outcome variable, using the SPSS 20.0 statistical package. Statistical significance was set at $p < 0.05$.

Results
Descriptive analysis
Analyses for characteristics of mothers using ANC services are presented in Table 1. The ages of the women at the birth of their last child ranged from 16 to 45 years,

Table 1 Baseline characteristics of the sample population ($N = 831$)

Variable	n (%)	Mean; SD
Age (years)		30.99; 7.47
≤ 23	185 (22.3)	
24–31	293 (35.3)	
32–39	229 (27.6)	
≥ 40	124 (14.9)	
Education (years)		10.41; 2.71
≤ 6	69 (8.3)	
7–9	240 (28.9)	
10–12	430 (51.7)	
> 12	92 (11.1)	
Parity		3.56; 2.06
1	154 (18.5)	
2–3	284 (34.2)	
4–5	254 (30.6)	
≥ 6	139 (16.7)	
Region		–
Irbid	213 (25.6)	
Jerash	170 (20.5)	
Mafraq	448 (53.9)	
Employment status		–
Unemployed	710 (85.4)	
Employed	121 (14.6)	
Health insurance		–
Uninsured	251 (30.2)	
Insured	580 (69.8)	
Total number of pregnancy-related illnesses		–
No health problems	380 (45.7)	
1–2 health problems	172 (20.7)	
≥ 3 health problems	279 (33.6)	
Self-perceived health status		–
Poor	208 (25.0)	
Average	403 (48.5)	
Excellent	220 (26.5)	

with a median age of 31 years. Forty-eight percent had received 10 or fewer years of schooling. The average total number of living children was 3.6, giving a range between 1 and 12 children. The majority of the respondents was housewives (85.4%) and had public sector insurance coverage (69.8%). The health status of 48.5% of participants was average during the last pregnancy, and 33.6% of the sample had had a high-risk pregnancy. Urinary tract infection, joint problems, and anemia were the three most common pregnancy-related illnesses among respondents, respectively. Concerning ANC attendance, 63.4% of women received the recommended care components, while 36.6% received inadequate ANC.

Differences in the usage of antenatal care services
Table 2 presents a comparative analysis of the differences between women who received the recommended basic ANC service components and those who did not, by individual determinants. Overall, there were statistically significant associations between all of the individual determinants and ANC attendance, except for employment and health status variables ($p = 0.644$ and $p = 0.837$, respectively). On bivariate analysis, the means of age and the number of living children variables were significantly lower among women who attended ANC adequately. Being more educated was also found to be positively associated with receiving adequate ANC services. Likewise, the proportions of women who had adequate use of ANC services were significantly higher among those who had wanted the pregnancy (67.6%), resided in Irbid governorate (72.8%), were insured (68.1%), lived in a neighborhood served by MCH services (71%), required less than 15 min to get to the nearest center (68.9%), and had a high-risk pregnancy (70.3%).

Differences in the overall ANC service adequacy were also observed by a number of factors related to the quality of care. As per Table 3, the highest percentages of adequate ANC attendance were among women who were often treated in a humane, respectful, supportive environment (82.7%) and those who were able to discuss their health problems/concerns with healthcare providers (81.0%). However, maintaining privacy during consultations was not significantly associated with the outcome variable ($p = 0.880$).

In relation to the technical management features, no significant differences were noticed between the two groups of interest, with the exception of the physical examination variable. Women who reported that a comprehensive physical exam was often performed at the center represented the highest rate of adequate ANC attendees (78.1%). Availability of vaccines/supplements at the facility and conducting clinical tests during the antenatal period were not found to be significantly associated with the utilization of ANC ($p = 0.404$ and $p = 0.879$, respectively).

Table 2 Comparison between adequate and inadequate utilization of ANC by individual determinants

Variables	Utilization of ANC		t-test/chi2	p-value
	Inadequate n = 304 n (%)	Adequate n – 527 n (%)		
Predisposing Characteristics				
Age in years[a] (Mean; SD)	(32.49; 7.04)	(30.12; 7.58)	4.45	<0.001
Years of education[a] (Mean; SD)	(9.69; 2.51)	(10.82; 2.73)	-5.91	<0.001
Parity[a] (Mean; SD)	(3.97;2.05)	(3.33; 2.04)	4.33	<0.001
Desire for the pregnancy				
Unwanted	128 (44.4)	160 (55.6)	11.74	0.001
Wanted	176 (32.4)	367 (67.6)		
Region				
Irbid	58 (27.2)	155 (72.8)	17.33	<0.001
Jerash	54 (31.8)	116 (68.2)		
Mafraq	192 (42.9)	256 (57.1)		
Employment status				
Unemployed	262 (36.9)	448 (63.1)	0.21	0.644
Employed	42 (34.7)	79 (65.3)		
Enabling Resources				
Health insurance				
Uninsured	119 (47.4)	132 (52.6)	18.17	<0.001
Insured	185 (31.9)	395 (68.1)		
Time taken to get to the nearest MCH center in minutes				
< 15 min	122 (31.1)	270 (68.9)	24.06	<0.001
15 -30	123 (36.6)	213 (63.4)		
>30	59 (57.3)	44 (42.7)		
Availability of ANC services				
Underserved	155 (48.7)	163 (51.3)	32.83	<0.001
Served	149 (29.0)	364 (71.0)		
Health Needs				
Total number of pregnancy-related illnesses				
No health problems	153 (40.3)	227 (59.7)	8.48	0.014
1-2 health problems	68 (39.5)	104 (60.5)		
≥ 3 health problems	83 (29.7)	196 (70.3)		
Self-perceived health status				
Poor	74 (35.6)	134 (64.4)	0.36	0.837
Average	146 (36.2)	257 (63.8)		
Excellent	84 (38.2)	136 (61.8)		

[a]t-test was run on the following variables: age, education, and parity
Bold text represents categories that are over-represented, indicating that they were more likely to utilize ANC services adequately

It is also interesting to note that there were statistically significant differences in the adequacy of ANC in terms of information exchange. In particular, the proportion of women who utilized ANC adequately was significantly higher among those who reported that the procedures and the diagnosis were often explained clearly by providers (73.2%), received enough information about ANC (86.9%), and had enough consultation time (78.7%).

By continuity and follow-up variables, the highest percentages of adequate ANC users were among women who often had follow-up appointments scheduled by health

Table 3 Comparison between adequate and inadequate utilization of ANC by factors related to the quality of service delivery

Variables	Utilization of ANC		chi2	p-value
	Inadequate n = 304 n (%)	Adequate n = 527 n (%)		
Interpersonal relations				
Dignified and respectful care was offered by healthcare providers				
Rarely	157 (62.5)	94 (37.5)	141.42	<0.001
Sometimes	77 (43.8)	99 (56.3)		
Often	70 (17.3)	334 (82.7)		
Providers were ready to discuss health problems/concerns with women				
Rarely	171 (58.6)	121 (41.4)	105.85	<0.001
Sometimes	70 (33.8)	137 (66.2)		
Often	63 (19.0)	269 (81.0)		
Privacy was maintained during consultations				
Rarely	94 (37.5)	157 (62.5)	0.26	0.880
Sometimes	36 (34.6)	68 (65.4)		
Often	174 (36.6)	302 (63.4)		
Technical management				
Comprehensive physical exams were performed				
Rarely	117 (50.4)	115 (49.6)	63.68	<0.001
Sometimes	105 (46.7)	120 (53.3)		
Often	82 (21.9)	292 (78.1)		
Vaccines/supplements were available at the facility				
Rarely	108 (39.6)	165 (60.4)	1.81	0.404
Sometimes	36 (33.0)	73 (67.0)		
Often	160 (35.6)	289 (64.4)		
Clinical tests were routinely conducted				
No	196 (36.8)	337 (63.2)	0.02	0.879
Yes	108 (36.2)	190 (63.8)		
Information exchange				
Information received on ANC was				
Little	175 (61.2)	111 (38.8)	171.19	<0.001
Fair	80 (46.8)	91(53.2)		
Enough	49 (13.1)	325 (86.9)		
Provider explanations were easily to understand				
Rarely	86 (65.6)	45 (34.4)	78.85	<0.001
Sometimes	68 (48.2)	73 (51.8)		
Often	150 (26.8)	409 (73.2)		
Consultation time was				
Short	136 (60.7)	88 (39.3)	101.62	<0.001
Average	78 (42.4)	106 (57.6)		
Enough	90 (21.3)	333 (78.7)		

Table 3 Comparison between adequate and inadequate utilization of ANC by factors related to the quality of service delivery
(Continued)

Variables	Utilization of ANC		chi2	p-value
	Inadequate n = 304 n (%)	Adequate n = 527 n (%)		
Continuity and follow-up				
Follow-up appointments were regularly scheduled by providers				
Rarely	180 (61.2)	114 (38.8)	157.43	<0.001
Sometimes	78 (40.2)	116 (59.8)		
Often	46 (13.4)	297 (86.6)		
A return visit was encouraged by healthcare providers				
Rarely	123 (55.4)	99 (44.6)	46.95	<0.001
Sometimes	23 (34.3)	44 (65.7)		
Often	158 (29.2)	384 (70.8)		
Appropriate constellation of services				
Time had to wait was				
Short	21 (33.9)	41 (66.1)	0.22	0.894
Average	124 (37.0)	211 (63.0)		
Long	159 (36.6)	275 (63.4)		
Hours of service were				
Inconvenient	76 (38.0)	124 (62.0)	0.23	0.633
Convenient	228 (36.1)	403 (63.9)		

Bold text represents categories that are over-represented, indicating that they were more likely to utilize ANC services adequately

workers (86.6%), and those who reported that they were encouraged by providers to make a return visit (70.8%). In contrast, no significant differences in the utilization of care were observed according to the appropriateness of the constellation of services, such as waiting time and service hours ($p = 0.894$ and $p = 0.633$, respectively).

Predictors of antenatal care attendance

Following the study's objectives, three models were employed to estimate the association between the explanatory variables (i.e., covariates and predictors) and the response variable (i.e., adequacy of ANC attendance). Table 4 summarizes the logistic regression estimation results for the three models. Each factor showing a statistically significant association with the response variable was interpreted controlling for the effects of other explanatory variables included in the model.

Initially, the first model was developed to investigate which of the individual's determinants are associated with receiving sufficient contents of ANC, and therefore only covariates were included in this model. As the figures in Table 4 indicate, the years of education showed a significant association with the use of ANC (95% CI = 1.09–1.23). For a one-year increase in women's education, the odds of utilizing ANC services increased by a factor of 1.15. Women's

desire to become pregnant was also found to have a positive association with the use of care, in which women who had a desire to get pregnant were 1.82 times more likely to attend ANC adequately compared to those who had an unwanted pregnancy (95% CI = 1.31–2.52). According to this model, mothers residing in the governorate of Mafraq were 52% less likely to have an adequate usage of ANC services than those living in Irbid (95% CI = 0.29–0.77). Our results also illustrated that, as the travel time to the nearest center increased, the odds of reporting an adequate use of ANC declined by a factor of 0.42 (95% CI = 0.26–0.69). Women who lived in a neighborhood served by MCH services were 2.73 times more likely to report adequate use of ANC (95% CI = 1.85–4.03). In respect of health needs variables, women who had experienced three or more previous pregnancy-related illnesses were 2.14 times more likely to attend ANC adequately compared to those had had a normal pregnancy (95% CI = 1.47–3.13).

To ascertain the extent to which the utilization of ANC services may be attributed to the quality of the ANC service delivery, only the predictors of interest were included in the second model. The results of this model demonstrated that women who often received dignified and respectful treatment from healthcare providers were 5.54 times more likely to utilize ANC adequately compared to

Table 4 Multivariate regression analysis predicting the utilization of ANC among women in highly disadvantaged communities in northern

Variables	Individual determinants (Model 1) Adjusted OR (95% CI)	Quality of service delivery (Model 2) Adjusted OR (95% CI)	Both (Model 3) Adjusted OR (95% CI)
Predisposing factors			
Age in years	0.98 (0.95-1.01)		0.98 (0.93-1.03)
Years of education	1.15** (1.09-1.23)		1.16* (1.06-1.27)
Parity	0.94 (0.84-1.05)		0.92 (0.77-1.09)
Desire for the pregnancy: (unwanted)			
Wanted	1.82** (1.31-2.52)		1.70* (1.06-2.72)
Region: (Irbid)			
Jerash	0.92 (0.57-1.51)		1.73 (0.86-3.51)
Mafraq	0.48* (0.29-0.77)		0.61 (0.30-1.23)
Employment status: (unemployed)			
Employed	0.80 (0.51-1.26)		1.45 (0.75-2.81)
Enabling recourses			
Health insurance: (uninsured)			
Insured	0.81(0.50-1.32)		0.72 (0.35-1.48)
Time taken to get to the nearest MCH center in minutes: (< 15 min)			
15-30	0.92 (0.66-1.29)		0.97 (0.60-1.56)
≥30	0.42* (0.26-0.69)		0.35* (0.17-0.70)
Availability of ANC services: (underserved)			
Served	2.73** (1.85-4.03)		4.34** (2.34-8.07)
Health needs			
Total number of pregnancy-related illnesses: (no health problems)			
1-2 health problems	1.01 (0.67-1.50)		0.80 (0.45-1.44)
≥ 3 health problems	2.14** (1.47-3.13)		1.66 (0.97-2.84)
Self-perceived health status: (poor)			
Average	1.03(0.70-1.51)		1.48 (0.85-2.59)
Excellent	0.94(0.61-1.44)		1.41 (0.76-2.60)
Patient-provider relations			
Dignified and respectful care was offered by healthcare providers: (rarely)			
Sometimes		2.09 (0.61-7.08)	1.80 (0.43-7.52)
Often		5.54** (2.60-11.81)	5.68** (2.45-13.13)

Table 4 Multivariate regression analysis predicting the utilization of ANC among women in highly disadvantaged communities in northern (Continued)

Variables	Individual determinants (Model 1)	Quality of service delivery (Model 2)	Both (Model 3)
	Adjusted OR (95% CI)	Adjusted OR (95% CI)	Adjusted OR (95% CI)
Providers were ready to discuss health problems/concerns with women: (rarely)			
Sometimes	2.37* (1.41-3.97)		2.28* (1.27-4.07)
Often	5.38** (3.28-8.82)		7.22** (4.06-12.82)
Privacy was maintained during consultation: (rarely)			
Sometimes		0.56 (0.12-2.63)	0.46 (0.09-2.52)
Often		0.70 (0.21-2.25)	0.38 (0.09-1.58)
Technical management			
Comprehensive physical exams were performed: (rarely)			
Sometimes		1.08 (0.61-1.93)	1.19 (0.61-2.33)
Often		1.45 (0.82-2.54)	1.58 (0.84-2.97)
Vaccines/supplements were available at the facility: (rarely)			
Sometimes		1.86 (0.41-8.43)	2.24 (0.43-11.82)
Often		1.87 (0.58-5.99)	3.63 (0.89-14.83)
Clinical tests were regularly conducted: (no)			
Yes		1.29 (0.84-1.97)	1.27 (0.77-2.08)
Information exchange			
Information received on ANC was: (little)			
Fair		1.11 (0.56-2.22)	1.16 (0.54-2.51)
Enough		7.34** (4.26-12.66)	9.12** (4.91-16.92)
Consultation time was:(short)			
Average		1.04 (0.29-3.69)	1.11 (0.26-4.81)
Enough		0.65 (0.29-1.46)	0.51 (0.21-1.27)
Provider explanations were easily to understand: (rarely)			
Sometimes		1.02 (0.53-1.96)	0.77 (0.37-1.62)
Often		1.97* (1.12-3.46)	2.38* (1.22-4.66)
Continuity and follow-up			
Follow-up appointments were regularly scheduled by providers: (rarely)			
Sometimes		3.03* (1.46-6.29)	3.65* (1.61-8.28)
Often		6.05** (3.51-10.43)	6.51** (3.52-12.01)

Table 4 Multivariate regression analysis predicting the utilization of ANC among women in highly disadvantaged communities in northern *(Continued)*

Variables	Individual determinants (Model 1)	Quality of service delivery (Model 2)	Both (Model 3)
	Adjusted OR (95% CI)	Adjusted OR (95% CI)	Adjusted OR (95% CI)
A return visit was encouraged by healthcare providers: (rarely)			
Sometimes		1.90 (0.89-4.07)	1.66 (0.72-3.83)
Often		2.42** (1.53-3.83)	1.82* (1.08-3.06)
Appropriate constellation of services			
Time had to wait was: (short)			
Average		0.86 (0.39-1.94)	0.63 (0.25-1.57)
Long		0.68 (0.31-1.50)	0.65 (0.27-1.57)
Hours of service were: (inconvenient)			
Convenient		0.94 (0.59-1.51)	0.96 (0.56-1.63)
Nagelkerke R²	0.205	0.574	0.660

*p < 0.05; **p < 0.001
The reference category is in parentheses

those who rarely had positive communication with providers (95% CI = 2.60–11.81). Additionally, the odds of reporting an adequate use of ANC services increased by factors of 2.37 (95% CI = 1.41–3.97) and 5.38 (95% CI = 3.28–8.82) for women who were sometimes and often able to discuss their health problem/concerns with healthcare providers, respectively.

According to the second model, women who received enough information and counselling on ANC were 7.34 times more likely to attend the targeted care as recommended compared to those who obtained little information (95% CI = 4.26–12.66). The odds of reporting adequate use of ANC also increased by a factor of 1.97 for women who perceived that the provider's explanations on pregnancy-related issues were clear compared to those who had poorer explanations (95% CI = 1.12–3.46).

Analysis of factors associated with the continuity of services revealed some significant results. The odds of reporting the adequate use of ANC were increased by factors of 3.03 (95% CI = 1.46–6.29) and 6.05 (95% CI = 3.51–10.43) for women who sometimes and often had regular follow-up appointments scheduled by healthcare providers, respectively. Women who were often encouraged to make a return visit were 2.42 times more likely to utilize ANC adequately compared to those who were rarely encouraged to come back (95% CI = 1.53–3.83). In contrast, variables related to technical management and the appropriateness of the constellation of services included in the second model did not show statistically significant associations with the outcome variable (Table 4).

All of the study's covariates and predictors were included in the third and final model, to identify if the quality of care was associated with the adequacy of ANC attendance, controlling for the influences of individual determinants. Based on this model, certain variables related to predisposing factors and enabling resources remained significant; however, health needs no longer had statistically significant associations with the response variable. As per Table 4, for a one-year increase in the woman's education, the odds of utilizing ANC services adequately increased by a factor of 1.16 (95% CI = 1.06–1.27). Likewise, women who had wanted the pregnancy were 1.7 times more likely to attend ANC adequately than those who had an unplanned pregnancy (95% CI = 1.06–2.72). Women who lived in a neighborhood served by MCH services were 4.34 times more likely to report adequate use of ANC (95% CI = 2.34–8.07). Our analysis also revealed that, as the travel time to the nearest center increased, the odds of reporting adequate utilization of ANC declined by a factor of 0.35 (95% CI = 0.17–0.70).

The results of the final model also illustrated that dimensions related to women–provider relations, information exchange, and follow-up and continuity were all significant predictors for the utilization of ANC services. Specifically, women who often received respectful and friendly treatment from healthcare providers were 5.68 times more likely to utilize ANC adequately compared to those who rarely had positive communication with providers (95% CI = 2.45–13.13). The odds of reporting adequate use of ANC services were also increased by factors of 2.28 (95% CI = 1.27–4.07) and 7.22 (95% CI = 4.06–12.82) for women who sometimes and often had opportunities for dialogue and health talks with staff, respectively.

Women's exposure to enough information, education, and advice on ANC during clinic visits had a significant positive association with ANC attendance (OR = 9.12; 95% CI = 4.91–16.92). Compared to mothers who reported limited understanding of providers' explanations on issues related to diagnosis and procedures, the odds of reporting adequate utilization of care increased by a factor of 2.38 for those who often received clear explanations (95% CI = 1.22–4.66).

Women who were often encouraged by health workers to continue antenatal visits at the same facility were 1.82 times more likely to utilize ANC adequately compared to those who were rarely encouraged to come back (95% CI = 1.08–3.06). Our analysis also indicates that the odds of reporting the adequate use of ANC were increased by factors of 3.65 (95% CI = 1.61–8.28) and 6.51 (95% CI = 3.52–12.01) for women who sometimes and often had regular follow-up appointments scheduled by healthcare providers, respectively. Similarly to the second model, technical management and the appropriateness of the constellation of services were not found to be significant predictors of ANC utilization (Table 4).

Discussion

This paper suggests applying an integrated conceptual framework to ascertain the extent to which the attendance at ANC clinics may be attributed to individual determinants among women from disadvantaged backgrounds or to the quality of service delivery. Empirical research on healthcare utilization has shown that users' characteristics account for an estimated 20 to 25% of the variance explained [30]. This is consistent with our findings, in which individual determinants (model 1) accounted for 21% of the systematic explained variance compared to 57.4% of the variance explained by the quality of ANC (model 2). Once the two models have been merged, the variance explained by the final model increased to 66.0%. This implies that the variations in the use of ANC facilities were mainly attributable to the quality of service as experienced by women at healthcare facilities.

One of the major concerns of current research is to explore the barriers that prevent women in highly disadvantaged communities from attending ANC adequately. According to the final model, adequacy of ANC coverage is affected by a number of health service and individual factors. In particular, our findings illustrate that the increase in the woman's level of education is a significant motivator for increasing the likelihood of her ANC attendance. This concurs with other studies demonstrating that the low level of a woman's education is associated with infrequent and no ANC, as well as delay in accessing medical help [1, 2, 9, 12, 31]. It makes sense that educated women are more likely to appreciate the benefits of ANC for their health and their children's well-being and to exercise autonomy and decision-making power. More years of schooling may also promote women's ability to approach health staff to ask questions and to discuss any possible health concerns.

The actual desire of women to become pregnant was also found to be an important factor in determining the adequacy of ANC. A study by Muhwava et al. [12] also supports this finding, revealing that wanted pregnancy was associated with increased odds of early initiation and adequate ANC attendance compared to unwanted pregnancy. Another study, done in Holeta in central Ethiopia [32], showed that women who reported an unplanned pregnancy were 67% less likely to attend ANC than those who reported they had planned the pregnancy. Researchers argue that unplanned pregnancy is highly likely to reflect a lack of access to education on family planning during antenatal visits [32, 33].

Not surprisingly, women's decision to use ANC services is affected by having the means available to utilize these services. Research findings from resource-poor sites (i.e., Malawi and Kenya) have indicated that a large distance to reach a health facility was associated with delayed initiation of ANC use and low frequency of care attendance [9]. One explanation for such behavior is women's desire to minimize the number of journeys to the facility and thereby their total expenditure on ANC. In the case of Jordan, in spite of policies promising free ANC, many women in disadvantaged communities tend to avoid clinic visits because they are unable to afford the associated travel costs. Considering that the actual ANC is being provided free of charge, this might explain the non-significant finding of the association between health insurance and ANC attendance in the study's models.

In the same context, our study revealed that living in a district served by an MCH clinic was a potential contributing factor to increasing the use of ANC among poor women in northern Jordan. These findings are in agreement with previous research conducted in underserved populations, where living closer to a health facility was found to be a motivator for ANC use, as absence from work and transportation costs might be minimized [34, 35].

At the health service level, our study highlights the importance of several factors in enhancing the frequency of ANC attendance, the most prominent of which is the information and education women received on ANC during one-to-one consultations. This assertion is supported by the literature, in which the provision of maternal health information by healthcare professionals has been reported to be an effective means of encouraging the use of ANC during pregnancy [9, 31]. Research has shown that improving women's access to the necessary health education is fundamental for increasing their knowledge of ANC benefits and helping them make informed decisions about their care [1, 36]. In a study by Asfawosen et al. [37], the mother's knowledge about pregnancy danger signs had the potential to impact positively on ANC utilization. A study by Erlindawati et al. [38] also illustrated that pregnant women who obtained enough information about ANC services had a lower percentage of inadequate utilization compared to those who received fair but limited information. In the literature, it has been reported that pregnant women with low quality of ANC and no counseling services were at risk of pregnancy complications owing to the lack of relevant information [39, 40]. According to a study by Ejigu et al. [40], receiving incomplete information about ANC was also among the reasons for mothers' dissatisfaction with the overall perceived quality of care offered in ANC clinics in northwest Ethiopia.

Women's attendance at ANC facilities was also found to be related to ease of understanding the provider's explanations on pregnancy-related issues. Researchers have asserted that the limited understanding women received during their visit to a health facility represents a 'missed opportunity' to inform women about the possible complications of pregnancy [41–43]. The delivery of clear advice and messages that explain how to prevent and manage problems (i.e., miscarriage, multiple births, and abnormal position of the baby) can result in better recognition of the importance of attending ANC in improving health outcomes for mothers and children.

It was not a surprise to find an association between the woman–provider relationship and the use of ANC services. This link is most apparent in studies showing that building a positive rapport with pregnant women can contribute to their achieving the recommended number of antenatal visits. In contrast, researchers have pointed out that having low-quality care because of providers' poor communication skills (which may include an abusive attitude on the part of staff) may negatively influence ANC attendance [32, 40, 44]. In the study by Birmeta et al. [32], one of the participating women stated that the reason for underutilization of ANC was that, "If you go to a health institution you will find a low quality of services and a lack of respect and mistreatment from some of the healthcare providers". Obviously, the lack of women's desire to return to the clinic could be largely based on their expectations about the care provided, which may depend on previous experience.

Similarly, this study demonstrated that providing pregnant women with opportunities for dialogue and health talks during visits had a central role in increasing their motivation to attend ANC adequately. Many have argued that allowing women to communicate their concerns to health staff may encourage them to start ANC earlier and to have at least four ANC visits [9]. It is also important to mention that women who have good relations with health staff may feel more supported to ask questions and talk about their reproductive concerns and problems [45].

Interestingly, our study illustrated that scheduling follow-up appointments is likely to have an impact on women's decision about future visits. It is widely known that healthcare providers exercise significant authority and their advice is generally trusted by women. In view of that, instructions about when to attend ANC communicated by health staff apparently influence ANC utilization. Similarly, a lack of encouragement to attend upcoming appointments can result in delays to accessing ANC [9]. In Jordan, a study conducted by Al-Qutob et al. [35] found that almost 80% of the women were satisfied with ANC when the return visit was scheduled by the midwife; moreover, their satisfaction level had improved when providers explained to them the advantages of the timed follow-up visit.

Policy considerations
Health education and information exchange
Our study provides additional evidence that it is critical for health authorities to put considerable efforts into enhancing the quality of ANC by providing pregnant women with proper counseling that includes supportive listening, advice giving, and relevant information. Engaging mothers as active participants in consultations would also help make changes in healthcare delivery from one based on provider-dominated dialogues to one that involves users in the decision-making process. This requires a transition in the role of health workers from one characterized by authority to one that depends on collaboration and partnership between patients and providers.

Antenatal information should also be given in a form that is easy to understand and accessible to the users of ANC services. Medical providers' explanations of reproductive health matters should be tailored to the different social contexts, including those with low levels of education and income. Healthcare workers at MCH centers need to ascertain that the pregnant women understand the information received during consultation well enough to make an informed decision.

Since the desire to have a pregnancy was found to be a significant factor in determining adequacy of ANC attendance, it may therefore be useful to focus on informing women about effective contraceptive methods that help prevent unintended pregnancy in these populations. Promoting family planning education and more widely disseminating knowledge on contraception need to be an integrated component of ANC coverage. This research also proposes that the MoH appoint a person in each of the MCH centers to work as a reproductive health counselor. This person would be able to present clear information about birth preparedness, complications readiness, danger signs, nutrition, breastfeeding, and maternal stress.

Our study suggests using radio reports and television spots as a means of raising public awareness regarding the benefits of antenatal visits for improving babies' and mothers' health. Such information could provide just enough knowledge to initiate action before the women's exposure to health education at clinics. Displaying educational posters in a prominent place at MCH centers is highly recommended.

Follow-up appointments and continuity of care
Given that women generally place trust in health staff's recommendations, repeated, structured follow-up appointments and encouragement for return visits are suggested as an effective approach to improve the continuation of ANC attendance. Issuing appointment cards showing the times of upcoming ANC visits would be one possible way to remind women about the date of attendance. The relevance of this schedule also needs to be explained by health workers.

Women's interpersonal relations with health staff
Recognition must be also given to the impact on women's willingness to attend ANC of respectful and friendly treatment offered by providers. This would call for special training courses targeted at improving the communication skills of health staff on how to deal with the centers' referents and how be more mindful, informative, and empathic. Treating women kindly and having sound interpersonal relations with them would be a key means of increasing the numbers of those turning to antenatal clinics to receive care.

It is also hugely important for healthcare providers to ensure an effective approach by giving women a chance to be heard and to encourage free discussion on their physical and psychological well-being. This study highly recommends health workers to spend more time with clients to obtain their medical histories, and to ask if they have previously experienced pregnancy-related complications. For this purpose, it is essential to increase the number of health staff working at ANC clinics.

Accessibility to antenatal care facilities
To achieve significant changes at the health service level, this research strongly suggests that the public sector develop health policies aimed at expanding the availability of MCH centers to cover underserved areas. Increasing the number of ANC clinics that are physically close to

those who live in disadvantaged conditions would help enhance their use. Likewise, the MoH can introduce mobile ANC in order to increase utilization of perinatal services and eliminate associated travel costs.

Conclusion

Whereas some researchers may consider the utilization of ANC services as a reflection of individual determinants, our study provides proof that this behavior is also embedded in the context of the healthcare delivery system. Specifically, our research has identified that attendance at ANC services was influenced by a number of factors, the most prominent of which are information exchange, follow-up and continuity of care, interpersonal relations with healthcare providers, and the availability of health facilities.

The results of this study have clarified that the interaction between women and providers is a key metric for the reported quality of ANC. The degree to which women feel that they are respected, informed, and engaged is considered an essential component of a successful strategy for improving mothers' experience with ANC and a way to motivate them to attend MCH clinics. In conclusion, our study reveals the strong association between how women perceive quality of care and their decision to attend reproductive health services. Strengthening the role of healthcare providers in counseling and health education would result in greater acceptance and sustained use of ANC.

Strengths and limitations

The potential limitations of this research were that the study may have been subject to recall bias, limited to women who were visiting the participating MCH centers at the time of the survey, and the tool did not include variables related to women's psychosocial and cultural factors. Future studies may also try to contact women who are not attending ANC at all and those who initiate ANC late (i.e., in the second or third trimester). Considering the importance of adaptation and implementation of the new ANC model within different health systems, clinical research investigating the contribution of the updated model to increasing the likelihood of positive pregnancy outcomes should be given priority. A need for research addressing the acceptability, feasibility, and cost-effectiveness of implementing the eight-contact model in low-resource settings is also obvious.

The strengths of this study include the use of a conceptual framework that takes contextual characteristics of ANC service delivery into account, the potential impact of such factors having been little explored in literature to date. Importantly, targeting contextual factors represents an opportunity to find areas that can be improved by policy formulation and implementation, unlike individual determinants, which are difficult to change. Analyzing women's perceptions of the care they have experienced by engaging stakeholders from disadvantaged communities would make the quality of care assessment more applicable to the expectations of users than that of health providers. By reviewing the medical records of respondents, the risk of recall bias is reduced, especially for measurement of the outcome variable.

Abbreviations

ANC: Antenatal Care; CI: Confidence Interval; DoS: Department of Statistics; FANC: Focused Antenatal care; HEIS: Household's Expenditure and Income Survey; JD: Jordanian Dinar; LMICs: Low and Middle Income Countries; MCH: Maternal and Child Health; MoPIC: Ministry of Planning and International Cooperation; OR: Odds Ratio; UNDP: United Nations Development Program; UNICEF: United Nations Children's Fund; WHO: World Health Organization

Acknowledgements

The authors would like to sincerely thank all women for their willingness to participate in this study. Special thanks are directed to Amneh Mohammad and Heba Abu-Awad for their efforts in data collection stage.

Funding

This research received no specific grant from any funding agency in the public, commercial or not-for-profit sectors. All the authors dedicated their additional working hours to develop this paper.

Authors' contributions

All authors contributed to study design, overall analysis and writing-up. All authors read and approved the final manuscript.

Competing interests

The authors declare they have no potential conflicts of interest with respect to the research, authorship, and/or publication of this article.

Author details

[1]Department of Health Management and Policy, Faculty of Medicine, Jordan University of Science and Technology, P.O. Box 3030, Irbid 22110, Jordan. [2]Department of Obstetrics and Gynecology, Faculty of Medicine, Jordan University of Science and Technology, P.O. Box: 3030, Irbid 22110, Jordan. [3]Department of Pediatrics and Neonatology, Faculty of Medicine, Jordan University of Science and Technology, P.O. Box: 3030, Irbid 22110, Jordan. [4]Department of Public Health and Community Medicine, Faculty of Medicine, Jordan University of Science and Technology, P.O. Box: 3030, Irbid 22110, Jordan.

References

1. Asamoah BO, Agardh A. Inequality trends in maternal health services for young Ghanaian women with childbirth history between 2003 and 2014. BMJ Open. 2017;7:e011663. https://doi.org/10.1136/bmjopen-2016-011663.

2.   Aminur R, Monjura KN, Tahmina B, Sayem A, Nurul A, Iqbal A. Trends, determinants and inequities of 4+ ANC utilisation in Bangladesh. J Health Popul Nutr. 2017;36:2. https://doi.org/10.1186/s41043-016-0078-5.

3.   Bitew T, Hanlon C, Kebede E, Medhin G, Fekadu A. Antenatal depressive symptoms and maternal health care utilisation: a population-based study of pregnant women in Ethiopia. BMC Pregnancy and Childbirth. 2016;16:301. https://doi.org/10.1186/s12884-016-1099-1.

4.   Liu X, Behrman JR, Stein AD, Adair LS, Bhargava SK, Borja JB, et al. Prenatal care and child growth and schooling in four low- and medium-income countries. PLoS One. 2017;12(2):e0171299. https://doi.org/10.1371/journal. pone.0171299.

5.   Kifle D, Azale T, Gelaw YA, Melsew YA. Maternal health care service seeking behaviors and associated factors among women in rural Haramaya District, eastern Ethiopia: a triangulated community-based cross-sectional study. Reprod Health. 2017;14:6. https://doi.org/10.1186/s12978-016-0270-5.

6.   United Nations Development Program. A social determinants approach to maternal health:discussion paper. 2011. http://www.undp.org/content/dam/undp/library/Democratic%20Governance/Discussion%20Paper%20MaternalHealth.pdf. Accessed 18 July 2017.

7.   Lincetto O, Mothebesoane-Anoh, Gomez P, Munjanja S. Chapter 2: Antenatal care. In: Lawn J, Kerber K, editors. Opportunities for Africa's newborns: practical data, policy and programmatic support for newborn care in Africa. Geneva: World Health Organization. 2006, 51–62. http://www.who.int/pmnch/media/publications/aonsectionIII_2.pdf. Accessed 22 June 2017.

8.   World Health Organization. WHO recommendations on antenatal care for a positive pregnancy experience. 2016.http://apps.who.int/iris/bitstream/10665/250796/1/9789241549912-eng.pdf. Accessed 20 February 2017.

9.   Pell C, Meñaca A, Were F, Afrah NA, Chatio S, et al. Factors affecting antenatal care attendance: results from qualitative studies in Ghana, Kenya and Malawi. PLoS One. 2013;8(1):e53747. https://doi.org/10.1371/journal.pone.0053747.

10. Dowswell T, Carroli G, Duley L, Gates S, Gülmezoglu AM, Khan-Neelofur D, Piaggio G. Alternative versus standard packages of antenatal care for low-risk pregnancy. Cochrane Database Syst Rev. 2015;7:CD000934. https://doi.org/10.1002/14651858.CD000934.pub3.

11. Miltenburg AS, van der Eem L, Nyanza EC, van Pelt S, Ndaki P, Basinda N, et al. Antenatal care and opportunities for quality improvement of service provision in resource limited settings: a mixed methods study. PLoS One 2017; 12(12): e0188279. https://doi.org/10.1371/ journal.pone.0188279.

12. Muhwava LS, Morojele N, London L. Psychosocial factors associated with early initiation and frequency of antenatal care (ANC) visits in a rural and urban setting in South Africa: a cross-sectional survey. BMC Pregnancy and Childbirth. 2016;16:18. https://doi.org/10.1186/s12884-016-0807-1.

13. Low P, Paterson J, Wouldes T, Carter S, Williams M, Percival T. Factors affecting antenatal care attendance by mothers of pacific infants living in New Zealand. N Z Med J. 2005;1216:1–10.

14. Abbas AA, Walker GJ. Determinants of the utilization of maternal and child health services in Jordan. Int J Epidemiol. 1986;15(3):404–7.

15. Obermeyer CM, Potter JE. Maternal health care utilization in Jordan: a study of patterns and determinants. Stud Fam Plan. 1991;22(3):177–87.

16. Shakhatreh FM, Abbas AA, Issa AA. Determinants of infant mortality and the use of maternity services in Jordan. Dirasat medical and biological sciences. 1996;23(2):59–69.

17. Alkhaldi SM. Predictors of antenatal care utilization in Jordan: findings from a national survey. Jordanian medical. Journal. 2016;50(2):69–79.

18. Department of Statistics [Jordan] and ICF International. Jordan population and family health survey 2012. 2013. https://dhsprogram.com/pubs/pdf/FR282/FR282.pdf. Accessed 15 July 2017.

19. United Nations Development Program. Jordan poverty reduction strategy: final report. 2013.http://www.jo.undp.org/content/dam/jordan/docs/Poverty/Jordanpovertyreductionstrategy.pdf. Accessed 15 July 2017.

20. United Nations Development Program, Department of Statistics, and Ministry of Planning and International Cooperation. Thinking differently about the poor "Findings from Poverty Pockets Survey in Jordan". 2012. http://www.undp.org/content/dam/jordan/docs/Poverty/Jordan_Poverty%20Pocket%20Report.pdf. Accessed 16 July 2017.

21. United Nations Children's Fund. Analyzing equity in health utilization and expenditure in Jordan with focus on maternal and child health services. 2016. https://www.unicef.org/jordan/ExecSummary_Analysing_equity_in_MCH_health_JordanMay2016.pdf. Accessed 16 July 2017.

22. The Higher Health Council. The national strategy for health sector in Jordan 2015–2019. 2016.http://www.hhc.gov.jo/uploadedimages/The%20National %20Strategy%20for%20Health%20Sector%20in%20Jordan%202015-2019.pdf. Accessed 19 July 2017.

23. Byrd TL, Law JG. Cross-border utilization of health care services by United States residents living near the Mexican border. Rev Panam Salud Publica. Pan Am J Public Health. 2009;26(2):95–100.

24. World Health Organization. Antenatal care in developing countries: promises, achievements and missed opportunities. 2003. http://apps.who.int/iris/bitstream/handle/10665/42784/9241590947.pdf?sequence=1. Accessed 19 July 2017.

25. Andersen RM. Revisiting the behavioral model and access to medical care: does it matter? J Health Soc Behav. 1995;36(1):1–10. https://doi.org/10.2307/2137284.

26. Babitsch B, Gohl D, Re-revisiting Andersen v LT. S behavioral model of health services use: a systematic review of studies from 1998–2011. GMS. Psychosoc Med. 2012; https://doi.org/10.3205/psm000089, URN: urn:nbn:de:0183-psm0000891.

27. World Health Organization. Standards for Improving Quality of Maternal and Newborn Care in Health Facilities. 2016. http://www.who.int/maternal_child_adolescent/documents/improving-maternal-newborn-care-quality/en/. Accessed 20 February 2018.

28. De Masi S, Bucagu M, Tunçalp Ö, Pablo Peña-Rosas J, Lawrie T, Oladapo OT, et al. Integrated person-centered health care for all women during pregnancy: implementing World Health Organization recommendations on antenatal care for a positive pregnancy experience. Global Health Sci Pract. 2017;5(2):197–201.

29. Bruce J. Fundamental elements of the quality of care: a simple framework. Stud Fam Plan. 1990;21(2):61–91.

30. Davidson PL, Andersen RM, Wyn R, Brown ERA. Framework for evaluating safety-net and other community-level factors on access for low-income populations. Inquiry. 2004;41:21–38.

31. Moore N, Blouin B, Razuri H, Casapia M, Gyorkos TW. Determinants of first trimester attendance at antenatal care clinics in the Amazon region of Peru: a case-control study. PLoS One. 2017;12(2):e0171136. https://doi.org/10.1371/journal.pone.0171136.

32. Birmeta K, Dibaba Y, Woldeyohannes D. Determinants of maternal health care utilization in Holeta town, Central Ethiopia. BMC Health Serv Res. 2013; 13:256.

33. Peer N, Morojele N, London L. Factors associated with contraceptive use in a rural area in western Cape Province. S Afr Med J. 2013;103:406–12.

34. Simkhada B, Teijlingen ER, Porter M, Simkhada P. Factors affecting the utilization of antenatal care in developing countries: systematic review of the literature. J Adv Nurs 2008; 61(3):244–260. doi: https://doi.org/10.1111/j.1365-2648.2007.04532.x PMID: 18197860.

35. Al-Qutob R, Mawajdeh S, Bin Raad F. The assessment of reproductive health services: a conceptual framework for prenatal care. Health Care Women Int. 1996;17(5):423–34.

36. Association of Reproductive Health Professionals. Breaking the contraceptive barrier: techniques for effective contraceptive consultations. Washington, DC: Association of Reproductive Health Professionals; 2008. http://www.arhp.org/Publications-and-Resources/Clinical-Proceedings/Breaking-the-Contraceptive-Barrier/System-Barriers. Accessed 2 August 2017.

37. Asfawosen A, Mussie A, Huruy A, Wondeweson T. Factors associated with maternal health care services in Enderta District, Tigray, northern Ethiopia: a cross sectional study. Am J Nurs Sc. 2014;3(6):117–25.

38. Erlindawati CJ, Isaranurug S. Factors related to the utilization of antenatal care services among pregnant women at health centers in Aceh Besar district, Nanggroe Aceh Darussalam province, Indonesia. J public health Dev. 2008;6(2):99–108.

39. Nwaeze IL, Enabor OO, Oluwasola TA, Aimakhu CO. Perception and satisfaction with quality of antenatal care services among pregnant women at the university college hospital, Ibadan. Nigeria Ann Ibd Pg Med. 2013; 11(1):22–8.

40. Ejigu T, Woldie M, Kifle Y. Quality of antenatal care services at public health facilities of Bahir-Dar special zone, Northwest Ethiopia. BMC Health Serv Res. 2013;13:443.

41. Nikie'ma B, Beninguisse G, Haggerty JL. Providing information on pregnancy complications during antenatal visits: unmet educational needs in sub-Saharan Africa. Health Policy Plan. 2009;24:367–76.

42. Anya S, Hydara A, Jaiteh L. Antenatal care in the Gambia: missed opportunity for information, education and communication. BMC Pregnancy and Childbirth. 2008;8:9.

43. Magoma M, Requejo J, Merialdi M, Campbell O, Cousens S, et al. How much time is available for antenatal care consultations? Assessment of the quality of care in rural Tanzania. BMC Pregnancy and Childbirth. 2011;11:64.

44. Ndwiga C, Warren CE, Ritter J, Sripad P, Abuya T. Exploring provider perspectives on respectful maternity care in Kenya: "work with what you have". Reprod Health. 2017;14:99. https://doi.org/10.1186/s12978-017-0364-8.

45. Sharan M, Valente TW. Spousal communication and family planning adoption: effects of a radio drama serial in Nepal. Int Fam Plan Perspect. 2002;28(1):16–25.

4

Reproductive health problems in rural South African young women: risk behaviour and risk factors

Hashini Nilushika Galappaththi-Arachchige[1,2]*（iD）, Siphosenkosi G. Zulu[3], Elisabeth Kleppa[1], Kristine Lillebo[1], Erik Qvigstad[2,4], Patricia Ndhlovu[5], Birgitte Jyding Vennervald[6], Svein Gunnar Gundersen[7,8], Eyrun Floerecke Kjetland[1,9] and Myra Taylor[9]

Abstract

Background: South African young women continue to be vulnerable, with high prevalence of teenage pregnancy, HIV, sexually transmitted infections (STIs) and female genital schistosomiasis (FGS). This study seeks to examine the underlying factors that may be associated with these four adverse reproductive health outcomes.

Methods: In a cross-sectional study of 1413 sexually active of young women, we explored these four adverse reproductive health outcomes by considering socio-demographic factors, socio-economic factors, sexual risk behaviour, substance abuse and knowledge about reproductive health by using a questionnaire. Consenting participants were asked about previous pregnancies and were tested for HIV, STIs and FGS. Multivariable regression analyses were used to explore the factors associated with these four reproductive health outcomes.

Results:

1. Early pregnancy: Among the young women, 44.4% had already been pregnant at least once. Associated factors were hormonal contraceptives, (adjusted odds ratio (AOR): 17.94, 95% confidence interval (CI): 12.73–25.29), and sexual debut < 16 years (AOR: 3.83, 95% CI: 2.68–5.47). Living with both parents (AOR 0.37, 95% CI: 0.25–0.57) and having a steady partner (AOR: 0.43, 95% CI: 0.24–0.76) were identified as protective factors against pregnancy.
2. HIV: HIV prevalence was 17.1%. The odds of having HIV were higher in intergenerational (AOR: 2.06, 95% CI: 1.05–4.06) and intragenerational relationships (AOR: 1.51 95% CI: 1.06–2.15), compared to age-homogenous relationships. Other associated factors were: condom use (AOR: 1.60, 95% CI: 1.16–2.20), number of times treated for an STI (AOR: 1.32, 95% CI: 1.02–1.71), and total number of partners (AOR: 1.14, 95% CI: 1.03–1.28).
3. STIs: Participants who had at least one STI (40.5%) were associated with total partner number (AOR 1.17, 95% CI: 1.06–1.30), and testing HIV positive (AOR: 1.88, 95% CI 1.41–2.50).
4. FGS: FGS prevalence (19.7%) was associated with previous anti-schistosomal treatment (AOR: 2.18, 95% CI: 1.57–3.05).

Conclusion: There is a high prevalence of pregnancy, HIV, STIs and FGS among sexually active young women in rural KwaZulu-Natal. Multidisciplinary approaches are urgently needed for educational and health literacy programs prior to sexual debut, and health care facilities, which should be made accessible for young women.

* Correspondence: hashiniga@gmail.com
[1]Norwegian Centre for Imported and Tropical Diseases, Department of Infectious Diseases Ulleval, Oslo University Hospital, Postboks 4956 Nydalen, 0424 Oslo, Norway
[2]Institute of Clinical Medicine, University of Oslo, Oslo, Norway
Full list of author information is available at the end of the article

Plain English summary

School-attending young women (16–20 years) from Kwa-Zulu-Natal, South Africa are highly affected by adverse reproductive health outcomes such as teenage pregnancy, HIV, sexually transmitted infections (STIs), and female genital schistosomiasis (FGS). Unlike the first three reproductive outcomes, FGS is caused by a fresh-water parasite that may cause discharge and sores in the genital tract in women. Affected women may present with lower abdominal pain or infertility. In this study we explore the teenage social and behavioural factors that are associated with these four adverse reproductive health outcomes. Early sexual debut, multiple partners, having an older partner, not living with both biological parents, and having previously received treatment for schistosomiasis were associated with adverse reproductive health outcomes. Implementing educational and health literacy programs, in addition to making health care facilities accessible may improve the health of young women.

Background

School-attending young women from KwaZulu-Natal (KZN), one of South Africa's poorest provinces, are markedly affected by reproductive health outcomes such as teenage pregnancy, HIV, sexually transmitted infections (STIs), and female genital schistosomiasis (FGS) [1–5].

In KZN, pregnancy among school-attending young women is very common, and about one third of young women have had a child by the age of 20 [1, 5]. This impacts on the mothers' schooling, and subsequent employment and earnings [6]. In turn, this also affects the child, who is born into poverty [6].

Worldwide, approximately 36.7 million are living with HIV and South Africa has the highest HIV prevalence in the world, with approximately 18% (7 million) of the global burden of HIV [7]. Young women aged 15–24 years are at particular risk of HIV and accounted for 20% of new HIV infections globally in 2015 and most of these are in Sub-Saharan Africa [8]. KZN has the highest HIV burden in South Africa with an estimated HIV prevalence of 44.4% reported in the antenatal survey of 2015 [9]. HIV prevalence in young women (15–24 years) is approximately four times that of men in the same age group, furthermore, in South Africa, young women acquire HIV at a much younger age than their male counterparts [10].

STIs, particularly *Chlamydia trachomatis*, *Neisseria gonorrhea*, *Trichomonas vaginalis* and syphilis, continue to be endemic in KZN, especially among sexually active young women [3, 11]. Many STI infections are asymptomatic [11]. Consequently, many do not seek care, and therefore remain untreated [12]. Untreated STIs may cause pelvic inflammatory disease (PID), increase the risk of ectopic pregnancies and cause infertility [13].

In *Schistosoma (S.) haematobium* endemic areas such as KZN, another neglected cause of reproductive morbidity in young women is female genital schistosomiasis [2, 14]. FGS is not caused by sexual intercourse, it is acquired through contact with contaminated fresh-water and can cause lesions in the reproductive tract [15]. Affected women may however suffer from symptoms similar to those of STIs (e.g. abnormal discharge) and can often be misdiagnosed [15, 16]. In addition, studies have shown that women with *S. haematobium* infection have 2–4 times increased odds of having HIV [17, 18].

Over the past decades, studies have shown that adverse reproductive health outcomes are largely due to a number of social and behavioural factors [19–24]. Moreover, relationship issues have also been found to contribute to risks for young women, such as the age difference between sexual partners (with an older male partner), multiple partners, and HIV positive partners [25]. In the absence of parental care and financial stability, young women may be more prone to involve themselves in transactional sex [26]. FGS is also multifactorial, with socio-economic factors playing a large role and lack of access to treatment (praziquantel) [2, 15, 27].

In this study we examine four common adverse reproductive health outcomes, (1) teenage pregnancy, (2) HIV, (3) STIs and (4) FGS, in sexually active young women in KZN. We explored these four outcomes by considering socio-demographic factors, socio-economic factors, sexual risk behaviour, substance abuse and knowledge about reproductive health. Furthermore, due to the similar clinical picture that FGS shares with STIs, we explored if there were any associations between the participants' knowledge about STIs and FGS. By understanding the underlying factors associated with these four adverse reproductive health outcomes, we may be able to help prevent these outcomes through intervention programs in collaboration with policy makers, health care workers, and educationists.

Methods
Study area and recruitment

The young women were part of a cohort of high-school students included in a cross-sectional study on female genital schistosomiasis in rural KZN, South Africa. The study investigated school-attending young women because schools provide a useful access point for mass treatment for schistosomiasis, as recommended by the World Health Organization. The study was undertaken in high schools from three districts in KZN. The recruitment took place from 2011 to 2013. Targeting high-schools with more than 300 pupils, situated in rural areas in Ilembe, uThungulu and Ugu districts, we randomly selected 70 schools in schistosomiasis-endemic areas (below 400 m altitude for the study) [28]. The included schools were visited during the least busy part of the school year, in order to have a minimal effect on their studies. Dates for possible investigations were provided by the teachers and subsequently discussed with the young women individually. All students from grade eight and above (16 years and older) were invited to participate in the recruitment phase of the study, however, only those who had been sexually active were included in the study. In order to determine who were sexually active, without disclosing this as the inclusion criterion, we used a questionnaire that also had many other questions. Furthermore, parents were informed about the study and participants who provided written informed consent were included. We excluded those who were pregnant, older than 20 years and those who did not consent to have a gynaecological examination. We further excluded those who had inconsistencies in the reported sexual debut age, age of menarche, and age of first pregnancy (e.g. if someone reported pregnancy before sexual debut or menarche). We calculated that with a sample size of minimum 1400 participants, we would have statistical power of 80% or more for detecting differences between groups of interest when at least 250 of the participants had a risk factor.

Questionnaire

A structured questionnaire, which was developed after reviewing the literature, was piloted among young school going women. The questionnaire was developed in English, translated into isiZulu (the local language) and translated back into English to ensure accuracy. It was used to interview all the consenting participants. Trained research assistants performed the interviews in their local language (isiZulu). The questionnaire contained questions designed to assess demographic, socio-economic and reproductive health factors. We asked questions on household characteristics, participants' relationship status, total number of lifetime partners, age of their oldest partner, sexual debut age and whether they had ever been pregnant. The questionnaire also enquired about contraceptive use (current hormonal and condom use), HIV and STIs related issues, such as: whether they had previously been tested for HIV, and whether they know what an STI is. We further asked about previous treatment history for both STIs and schistosomiasis. The age of alcohol debut and substance use was included as well.

Clinical examination and laboratory analyses

Prior to the gynaecological examination, the investigating clinician explained in detail about the procedure to each participant and answered any questions related to the examination. The examination started with a visual inspection of the vulva, vagina and cervix, followed by a photocolposcopic examination using an Olympus OCS 500 Colposcope with a mounted Olympus E420 (10 Mpx) single lens reflex (SLR) camera or a Leisegang colposcope with a mounted Canon EOS 650D (18 Mpx) SLR camera [29]. Lesions in the lower reproductive tract were described as: sandy patches, homogenous yellow sandy patches, rubbery papules, abnormal blood vessels, genital ulcers, leukoplakia, tumors and rubor [16]. A positive FGS diagnosis would be given if they had one of the characteristic FGS lesions, such as sandy patches, homogenous yellow sandy patches or rubbery papules [30].

Cervico-vaginal lavage samples (CVLs) were collected by spraying 10 mL saline on the cervix four times, followed by drawing this back into the syringe [16]. The CVL was analysed for *Neisseria gonorrhoea* and *Chlamydia trachomatis* using a strand displacement assay (ProbeTec CT/GC, Becton, Dickinson and Company (BD), Franklin Lakes, NJ, USA) [20]. The CVL was also analysed using an in-house PCR (Laboratory of Infection, Prevention and Control, University of KwaZulu-Natal (UKZN), Durban, South Africa) detecting *Trichomonas vaginalis* [20].

Thirty milliliters blood was collected in sterile acid-citrate-dextrose anti-coagulant Vacutainer tubes (BD) [19]. Using the South African Department of Health's protocol, HIV testing was done using the Bioline Rapid test HIV (New Jersey, United States) and confirmed using Sensa Tri-Line HIV Test Kit (Pantech, Durban, South Africa). Syphilis screening was performed at Laboratory of Infection, Prevention and Control, UKZN, Durban, South Africa, using rapid plasma reagin (RPR, Macro Vue test 110/112, BD), and positive tests were confirmed using *Treponema pallidum* hemagglutination assay (TPHA, Omega Diagnostics Group PLC, Alva, Scotland, UK) [23]. All serology was done on serum samples that had been stored at – 80 °C.

Statistical analysis

Teenage pregnancy was defined as having had at least one pregnancy (live birth, ectopic pregnancy, spontaneous abortion, or termination of pregnancy) before the age of 20. The STI-variable would be coded positive if the participant had tested positive for one or more STIs (*T. pallidum*, *T. vaginalis*, *N. gonorrhoea* or *C. trachomatis*). Further, we calculated the number of STIs for each of the participants, excluding participants who had any missing STI-results. To assess the risk entailed by having an older partner, we calculated the age difference between the young woman's current age and the age of the oldest partner. Then the age difference was further divided into age-homogenous (≤ 4 years age difference), intragenerational (5–9) and intergenerational relationships (≥10), as defined in the literature [31]. Level of education was categorised as secondary (grade 8–12) or tertiary education.

Statistical analyses were done using Statistical Package for Social Sciences (SPSS) version 24 (IBM, Chicago, IL, USA).

Due to the binary coding of the outcome variables, we used logistic regression (nonparametric) to evaluate the association between each of the four outcome variables and social and behavioural factors. We calculated odds ratio (OR) and the corresponding 95% confidence intervals (CI). Associations were considered statistically significant within a significance level of 0.05. This significance level was also used for inclusion of risk behaviour and social and behavioural factors in the multivariable logistic regression analyses. Due to a strong age-dependence, alcohol debut age was stratified for current age.

We created Venn diagrams using Venny version 2.1 (Juan Carlos Oliveros, http://bioinfogp.cnb.csic.es/tools/venny/) to evaluate the co-occurrence of adverse reproductive health outcomes [32]. We further assessed the social and behavioural factors associated with the two and three most common co-occurring reproductive health outcomes.

Results

General characteristics of the study population

In total, 1413 sexually active young women of median 18 years (range 16–20) were included in the study. Figure 1

shows the participant selection procedure. The characteristics of the participants' households are presented in Table 1.

The median age of menarche was 14 years (range 8–19) and the median age of first sexual debut was 16 years (range 10–20). At the time of the interview, 94.7% (1333/1407) of the young women reported having a steady partner and reported a median of two lifetime partners (range 1–22). The median age difference between the participants and their oldest partner was 3 years (range: less than 5 years and up to 40 years). The majority of the young women reported to have age-homogenous relationships (68.9% 966/1403), followed by intragenerational relationship (26.8% 376/1403) and intergenerational relationships (4.3% 61/1403). Only 2.1% (30/1408) reported receiving money or gifts for sexual favours and 7.5% (106/1409) reported having been sexually abused at some point in their lives. Less than half reported to have used a condom during their last sexual intercourse (40.0%, 494/1234). Hormonal contraceptives were used by 29.7% (418/1409) at the time of the study and of these, an injectable contraceptive was the most common contraceptive method (96.7%, 404/418).

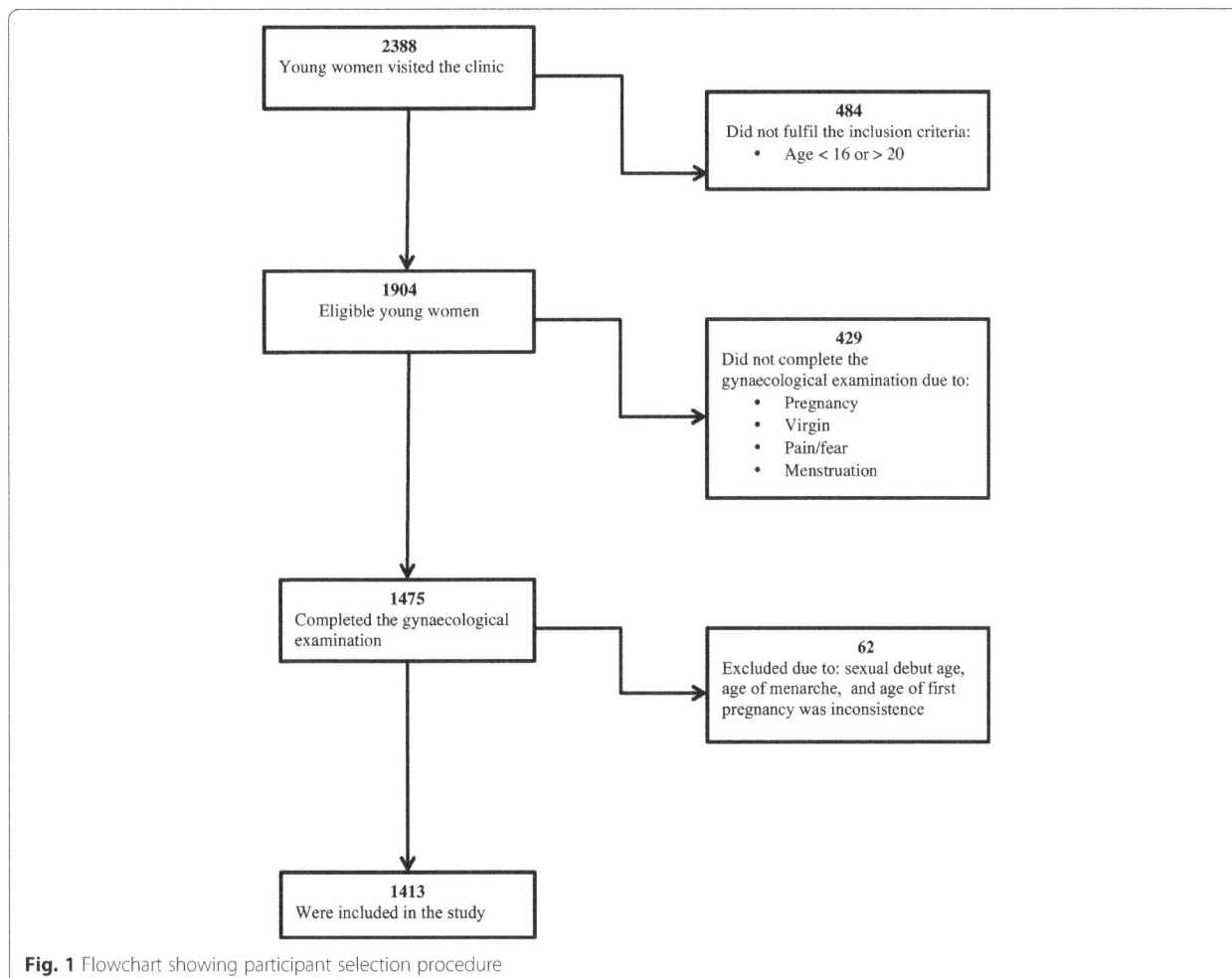

Fig. 1 Flowchart showing participant selection procedure

Table 1 Household structure, educational and socio-economic characteristics of the study participants

	Proportion of participants
Household structure	
Median number of people in the household (range)	6 (1–18)
Median number of adults (≥18 years) in the household (range)	4 (0–14)
Median number of children in the household (range)	2 (0–11)
Living with both of her biological parents	19.8% (279/1411)
Living with one of the biological parents or other adults	80.0% (1129/1411)
Did not have any adults in the household	0.2% (3/1411)
Participants 18 years or older were the only adult in the household	1.3% (19/1411)
Highest level of education in the household (excluding study participant)	
High School	88.0% (1236/1404)
Tertiary level of education	12.0% (168/1404)
Proportion of adults employed in the household	
No adults employed	43.1% (607/1408)
1–49% of adults employed	30.8% (424/1408)
≥ 50% of adults employed	26.1% (367/1408)

The median age for alcohol debut was 16 years (range 10–20). More than half, 59.0% (834/1413), reported to have tried alcohol. Illicit drugs were used by 3.8% (54/1411) of these young women, and 18.3% (258/1406) reported that their friends were using illicit drugs. The most common drug reported to be used by the participants was inhalation of benzine (4.3%, 61/1411), followed by smoking of cannabis (2.6%, 36/1410), inhalation of glue (1.1%, 15/1410) and taking ecstasy pills 0.6% (8/1410). Only one person reported use of injectable drugs.

Social and behaviour factors associated with teenage pregnancy

As many as 44.4% (627/1413) of the school-attending, sexually active young women reported having been pregnant at least once in their lifetime. One inclusion criterion for the study was admitting to being sexually active. Only 2.8% (39/1413) reported having been pregnant twice and one single participant reported having been pregnant three times. Miscarriage was reported by 1.3% (8/627), stillbirth by 1.6% (10/627) and 2.6% (16/627) reported that the child died during childhood. The median age of first pregnancy was 17 years (range 13–20). Social and behavioural factors associated with pregnancy are presented in Table 2. The odds of a participant having

Table 2 Logistic regression analysis of STIs, social and behavioural factors associated with pregnancy

Social and behavioural factors	Odds Ratio (95% CI)	Adjusted Odds Ratio (95% CI) [a]
Age in years	1.76 (1.60–1.95)[**]	2.10 (1.84–2.39)[**]
Living with both parents	0.57 (0.42–0.76)[**]	0.39 (0.26–0.59)[**]
Level of education in the household [b]	0.90 (0.66–1.23)	
Percentage of adults employed in the household	0.95 (0.86–1.04)	
Sexual debut before 16 years of age	1.56 (1.22–1.98)[**]	3.64 (2.56–5.17)[**]
Ever been sexually abused	1.17 (0.79–1.74)	
Ever been paid to have sex	1.65 (0.79–3.42)	
Number of lifetime sexual partners	0.97 (0.89–1.05)	
Have a steady partner now	0.56 (0.35–0.90)[*]	0.44 (0.25–0.78)[*]
Age difference to oldest sexual partner	1.01 (0.98–1.04)	
Age difference to older partner (years)		
Age-homogenous (0–4)	1	
Intragenerational (5–9)	1.09 (0.86–1.38)	
Intergenerational (≥ 10)	1.64 (0.98–2.77)	
Currently using hormonal contraceptive	16.18 (11.9–22.00)[**]	18.28 (12.99–25.74)[**]
Know what an STI is	1.23 (1.00–1.62)	
Tested positive for an STI at our clinic[c]	1.01 (0.82–1.26)	
Tested positive for HIV at our clinic	1.26 (0.95–1.66)	
Taking illicit drugs	1.00 (0.58–1.73)	
Alcohol debut age (stratified by current age)		
Current age 16	1.14 (0.67–1.94)	
Current age 17	0.95 (0.75–1.20)	
Current age 18	0.92 (0.77–1.11)	
Current age 19	0.90 (0.75–1.10)	
Current age 20	0.86 (0.70–1.06)	

CI confidence interval
[*]p < 0.05; [**]p < 0.001
[a]All variables in the table with p < 0.05 in univariate analysis were included in the multivariable analyses
[b]Categorised as secondary (grade 8–12) or tertiary
[c]Tested for C. trachomatis, T. vaginalis, N. gonorrhoea and T. pallidum

been pregnant were almost four-fold higher (p < 0.001) in those who reported sexual debut before 16 years of age. Current contraceptive use was more common among those who had been pregnant (p < 0.001). Those living with both parents had a reduced risk of being pregnant (p < 0.001) as did those who had a steady partner (p = 0.005).

Social and behaviour factors associated with HIV

We found that 17.1% (241/1351) of the young women tested positive for HIV infection and 74.1% (181/241) did not know that they were HIV positive. Social and behavioural factors associated with having HIV infection are presented in Table 3. HIV seropositivity was associated with reporting use of a condom during the last sexual intercourse ($p = 0.004$). However, among those who knew they were HIV positive, we did not see a significant association with condom use during last sexual intercourse ($p = 0.685$). The odds of HIV increased depending on their current age ($p = 0.006$), their number of total lifetime partners ($p = 0.008$), and the

number of times that they had been treated for an STI ($p = 0.038$). Furthermore, the odds of having HIV were higher in intragenerational and intergenerational relationships than in homogenous relationships ($p = 0.022$ and $p = 0.039$, respectively).

Social and behaviour factors associated with sexually transmitted infections

Chlamydia trachomatis was the most common STI with a prevalence of 24.8% (328/1325), followed by *Trichomonas vaginalis* at 17.9% (245/1371) and *Neisseria gonorrhoea* at 10.9% (145/1325). *Treponema pallidum* was the least common STI in this study group with a prevalence of 1.8% (24/1350). As many as 40.5% of the young women had one or more STIs. The numbers of concurrent STIs are presented in Tables 4, and 71.0% (991/1396) of the young women were aware of what an STI is. Few reported ever having received treatment for an STI (11.5%, 157/1360).

In a multivariable regression model, using positive test result for any of the four STIs (*C. trachomatis, T. vaginalis, N. gonorrhoea* and *T. pallidum*) as the outcome variable, we found that testing positive for HIV was significantly associated with testing positive for an STI (AOR: 1.88, 95% CI: 1.41–2.50, $p < 0.001$). Furthermore, we found that the total number of sexual partners was significantly associated with having an STI (1.17, 95% CI: 1.06–1.30, $p = 0.002$). None of the other social and behavioural factors were found to be associated with having an STI and therefore these data are not reported.

Social and behavioural factors associated with female genital schistosomiasis

We identified sandy patches in 19.7% (279/1413) of the young women and 18.7% (264/1410) reported having received anti-schistosomal treatment at some point in their life, whereas 35.2% (496/1410) could not recall whether they had received such treatment. In the multivariable analysis, controlling for the employment rate in the household, the only factor that remained associated with having FGS was previous anti-schistosomal treatment (AOR: 2.18, 95% CI: 1.57–3.05, $p < 0.001$). None of the other social and behavioural factors were found to

Table 3 Logistic regression analysis of STIs, social and behavioural factors associated with HIV

Social and behavioural factors	Odds Ratio (95% CI)	Adjusted Odds Ratio (95% CI)[a]
Age in years	1.31 (1.16–1.47)[**]	1.21 (1.06–1.40)[*]
Living with both parents	0.55 (0.36–0.86)[*]	0.65 (0.40–1.10)
Level of education in the household [b]	0.71 (0.45–1.11)	
Percentage of adults employed in the household	0.96 (0.85–1.09)	
Sexual debut before 16 years of age	0.97 (0.87–1.07)	
Number of lifetime sexual partners	1.27 (1.13–1.42)[**]	1.17 (1.04–1.31)[*]
Have a steady partner	1.13 (0.58–2.18)	
Age difference to older partner (years)		
Age-homogenous (≤ 4)	1	1
Intragenerational (5–9)	1.58 (1.16–2.15)[*]	1.51 (1.06–2.15)[*]
Intergenerational (≥ 10)	2.46 (1.37–4.40)[*]	2.06 (1.05–4.06)[*]
Ever been sexually abused	1.55 (0.96–2.49)	
Ever been paid to have sex	2.12 (0.96–4.70)	
Condom used during last sexual intercourse	1.50 (1.11–2.04)[*]	1.60 (1.16–2.20)[*]
Using hormonal contraceptive	0.84 (0.62–1.15)	
Know what an STI is	1.24 (0.89–1.71)	
Number of times treated for an STI	1.60 (1.27–2.01)[**]	1.32 (1.02–1.71)[*]
Taking illicit drugs	1.99 (1.07–3.69)[*]	1.43 (0.65–3.11)
Alcohol debut age		
16	2.32 (0.92–5.80)	
17	1.27 (0.93–1.70)	
18	1.07 (0.81–1.40)	
19	1.23 (0.97–1.56)	
20	1.08 (0.86–1.35)	

CI confidence interval
[*] $p < 0.05$; [**] $p < 0.001$
[a] All variables in the table with $p < 0.05$ in univariate analysis were included in the multivariable analyses
[b] Categorised as secondary (grade 8–12) or tertiary

Table 4 Number of concurrent sexually transmitted infections

Number of STIs[a]	Participants (%)[b]
No STIs	719/1259 (57.1)
Single STI	401/1259 (31.9)
Two concurrent STIs	115/1259 (9.1)
Three concurrent STIs	23/1259 (1.8)
Four concurrent STIs	1/1259 (0.1)

[a] Tested for *C. trachomatis, T. vaginalis, N. gonorrhoea* and *T. pallidum*
[b] Participants with any missing lab results were excluded

be associated with having FGS and therefore these data are not reported.

Co-occurrence of reproductive adverse outcomes

As shown in Fig. 2, we found that 76.6% (1082/1413) had experienced an adverse reproductive health outcome (the sum of all cells in Fig. 2). Of these, 55.5% (600/1082) experienced a single outcome (the sum of all non-overlapping cells in Fig. 2), 33.3% (360/1082) experienced two outcomes (the sum of all the two-overlapping cells in Fig. 2), 9.7% (105/1082) experienced three outcomes (the sum of all the three-overlapping cells in Fig. 2) and 1.6% (17/1082) experienced four outcomes (the cell where all four outcomes overlap in Fig. 2, indicated by the darkest shade of grey). We were not able to do any further statistical sub-analyses in the latter group due to the small sample size.

The three most commonly co-occurring outcomes were pregnancy, STIs and HIV (the cell indicated by the medium shade of grey in Fig. 2, $n = 49$). Adjusting for age, hormonal contraceptive use and number of STI treatments in a multivariable regression analysis, we found that significant factors for experiencing these three reproductive health outcomes concurrently, were "thinks she has an STI now" (AOR 3.27, 95% CI: 1.20–8.92, $p = 0.21$) and total number of lifetime partners (AOR 1.35, 95% CI: 1.04–1.76, $p = 0.026$).

Of the participants who experienced only two adverse outcomes at the same time, we identified having been pregnant and having an STI to be the most commonly co-occurring outcomes (the cell indicated by the lightest shade of grey in Fig. 2, $n = 146$). In a multivariable

regression analysis, we found that current use of hormonal contraceptive and age were significantly associated with having undergone teenage pregnancy and having a current STI (AOR: 3.74, 95% CI: 2.61–5.35, $p < 0.001$ and AOR: 1.20, 95% CI: 1.03–1.40, $p = 0.021$, respectively).

Discussion

In this study, we explored four common adverse reproductive health outcomes, defined as (1) teenage pregnancy, (2) HIV, (3) sexually transmitted infections (STIs) and (4) female genital schistosomiasis (FGS), in sexually active young women in Kwazulu-Natal (KZN). To our knowledge, these outcomes have not been reported together before.

We found that living with biological parents was a strong protective factor against pregnancy, and may signify that parental supervision, monitoring and care are important factors that can reduce teenage risk behaviour [33, 34]. Use of hormonal contraceptives is an essential protective factor against unwanted pregnancies, however we found that those who were currently using hormonal contraceptives had higher odds of having been pregnant. This suggests that following the first pregnancy, the health care workers may have advised the use of hormonal contraceptives, and their parents may have further encouraged this [33–35]. This may also explain why our data showed low numbers of participants who reported being pregnant a second and third time. Unfortunately, overall contraceptive use among our participants remained low, which may indicate that teenagers do not seek or receive this service from the local clinics. It can be

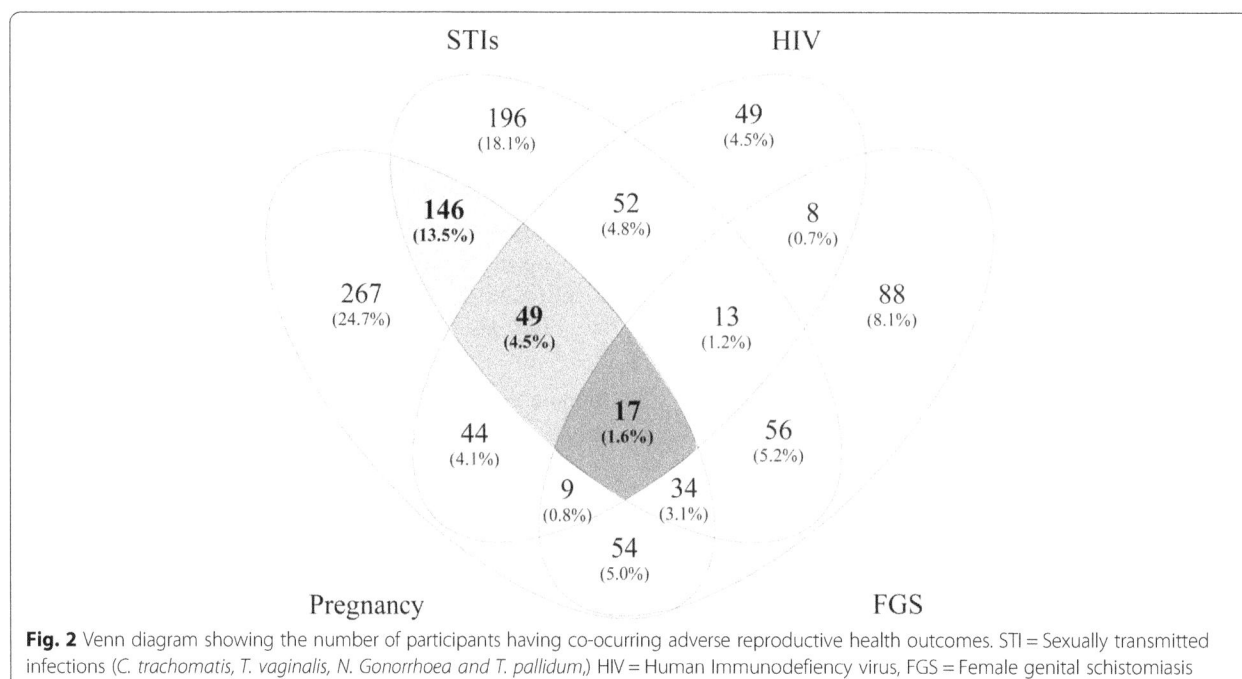

Fig. 2 Venn diagram showing the number of participants having co-ocurring adverse reproductive health outcomes. STI = Sexually transmitted infections (*C. trachomatis, T. vaginalis, N. Gonorrhoea and T. pallidum,*) HIV = Human Immunodefiency virus, FGS = Female genital schistomiasis

difficult to admit sexual activity to health care workers in the first years following sexual debut and this may result in missed opportunities for preventive care [36]. Among those who used contraceptives, an injectable contraceptive was the most common birth control method. Even though contraceptives are available free of charge in public health care settings, these women were living in rural areas and may neither have had a clinic nearby nor the funds to reach the nearest clinic [6]. Furthermore, young women who reported having a steady partner were less likely to have been pregnant. This could be because they had a stable relationship and were making shared decisions and exercising safer and healthier sexual practices [37].

Our study shows that most of the young women reported living with their biological mother, or with other adults although they were not their biological parents. Sadly, only less than one quarter reported living in a household with both biological parents. This may be a consequence of the HIV epidemic that has negatively affected the household structure in HIV endemic areas, where single or widowed females are the heads of the households [20]. It has also been reported that increasing numbers of children end up living with relatives rather than their biological parents or parents may have left their children with relatives in order to find work in the cities [20]. In our study, the presence of parents in the household reduced the odds of having HIV infection. However, when adjusted for other factors, this did not remain a protective factor for HIV. Similar to other studies, we found that having multiple partners and having an older partner increased the odds of testing positive for HIV [25, 38, 39]. A study from KZN found that a woman's perceived risk of HIV infection from her partner was the most powerful predictor of condom use [40]. This may be reflected in our study as we see a significant association between condom use during last sexual intercourse and testing positive for HIV. However, we did not find an association between condom use and knowing whether they were HIV positive.

Confirming recent epidemiological studies from KZN, we found that the STI prevalence among young women remained high [3, 11]. In 2014, Naidoo et al. found that in KZN, women younger than 25 years, non-cohabitating and unmarried were at higher risk of getting an STI [3]. In agreement with previous studies, we found that young women who had multiple partners were more likely to be diagnosed with one or more STIs [25, 39, 41]. Very few in our study, reported ever receiving treatment for an STI. Most women with an STI infection do not experience any symptoms and consequently most infections would remain untreated [42]. Furthermore, there is increasing evidence that the "youth unfriendliness" of the primary health care facilities in South Africa may be a contributing factor to why young women do not seek help [43].

Genital lesions (sandy patches) caused by *S. haematobium* were found in almost one fifth of the young women. We found that the risk of having FGS was higher in those who had taken tablets to treat schistosomiasis previously. This may suggest that treatment did not work or that the lesions had already become chronic at the time when treatment was taken [44]. The findings suggest that the anti-schistosomal interventions have been insufficient and that reinfection has been common. Unfortunately, in South Africa, despite having high *S. haematobium* prevalence, there is no current national schistosomiasis control programme.

More than a third of the study participants had experienced multiple adverse reproductive health outcomes. Of particular public health importance, is the co-occurrence of pregnancy and STIs or HIV, which affected 21.2% of our study population. This combination may represent a particularly harmful synergy, putting both the young women and their children at increased risk for perinatal and postnatal morbidity and mortality [45]. The South African antenatal HIV prevalence survey from 2015 found that in KZN, there was an increase in HIV prevalence among pregnant women (age 15–49 years) from 37.4% in 2011 to 44.4% in 2015 [9], which corresponds well with our findings (Fig. 2). Unfortunately, the survey did not include data on STIs.

More than half of the young women had tasted alcohol but as few as 4% admitted that they had used illicit drugs. Previous studies have found substance use among young people, especially alcohol and illicit drugs to influence what they do sexually, and it is thought to place them at increased risk of practicing unsafe sex [46]. However, in our study, the number reporting alcohol and substance abuse was too small to explore these as risk factors.

Distressingly, in this study we found that young women who had sexual debut before the age of 16 years had almost four-fold higher odds of having been pregnant than those who debuted later. These adverse reproductive health outcomes can be prevented by early initiation of educational programs on puberty, sex and sexual risk behaviours prior to sexual debut (e.g. promote contraceptive use) [47]. Furthermore, our results clearly show that there is a lack of interaction between the young women and health clinics (e.g. low number of people used contraception, few had ever been tested for HIV). Making youth-friendly health services easily accessible to young people is an important factor to improve the health of young women by enabling free access to testing, treatment and contraception [43, 47, 48].

These results are not representative of the wider population, as these were school-attending, sexually active, young women. Furthermore, this is a cross sectional study which limits conclusions about the causality of the associations. Participants were tested for HIV, some STIs and

FGS. However, the social and risk behaviour were self-reported and could not be confirmed independently [49]. Human papillomavirus and herpes simplex were only tested in a sub-sample and were therefore not included in this analysis even though they are important STIs. The difficulty of diagnosing FGS is a well-recognized problem, as sandy patches can be found anywhere in the genital tract as well as in the sub-mucosa [16]. Consequently, we may have under-estimated the FGS prevalence.

Conclusion

These results confirm that there is a high prevalence of pregnancy, HIV, STIs and FGS among sexually active, school-attending young women living in rural KwaZulu-Natal, South Africa. Factors such as early sexual debut, multiple partners and older partners remained a significant risk factor for adverse reproductive health outcomes in young women. There is also an alarming co-occurrence of pregnancy and STIs or HIV. Furthermore, national school mass drug treatment programmes should be implemented to offer regular treatment to schools in schistosomiasis-endemic areas. Educational programs should be implemented to inform about safer sexual practices prior to sexual debut. Youth friendly health care facilities should be made more easily accessible for young women to obtain effective diagnosis, treatment and care.

Abbreviations

FGS: Female genital schistosomiasis; HIV: Human immunodeficiency virus; KZN: KwaZulu-Natal; PCR: Polymerase chain reaction; STI: Sexually transmitted infections

Acknowledgements

The authors would like to thank Roy Manyaira for data management and the team at the BRIGHT research clinic (http://brightresearch.org/) for their hard work. We would also like to thank all the South African young women who participated in this study.

Funding

The research leading to these results has been funded by the European Research Council under the European Union's Seventh Framework Programme (PIRSES-GA-2010-269245), University of Copenhagen with the support from the Bill and Melinda Gates Foundation (Grant # OPPGH5344),the Norwegian Research Council (Grant # 213702), the South-Eastern Regional Health Authority of Norway (Grants # 2014065 and 2016055), and Oslo University Hospital, Norway.

Authors' contributions

EFK, MT, SGG, BJV and PDN designed and conceived the study. HNGA, EK, KL, SGZ and EFK conducted the study and collected data. HNGA and MT analysed the data. HNGA, SGZ, EK, KL, MT, EQ, PDN, BJV, SGG and EFK wrote the paper. All authors read and approved the final manuscript.

Ethics approval and consent to participate

All participants were above 16 years of age and signed individual, written informed consent, according to South African legislation. Parents were informed about the study. The participants were made aware of their right to withdraw at any time during the study. The study was approved by the Biomedical Research Ethics Committee (BREC), University of KwaZulu-Natal

(Ref BF029/07), KwaZulu-Natal Department of Health (Reference HRKM010-08) and the Regional Committee for Medical and Health Research Ethics (REC), South Eastern Norway (Ref 469-07066a1.2007.535). The Departments of Health and Education in Ugu, Ilembe and Uthungulu districts, KwaZulu-Natal, gave permission for this study. The ethical committees, BREC (annual renewal) and REC, were aware that minors (aged 16 and 17) were participating in the study and specifically approved independent minor consent without parental consent. Each participant was assigned a unique identification number to ensure privacy and to keep the study data confidential. The same identification numbers were used for lab results and colposcopic images. We followed the South African syndromic protocol to diagnose and treat clinical signs and findings at the point of care. The current study area is categorized as moderately endemic for schistosomiasis according to the World Health Organization (prevalence of 10–50%), and all consenting participants received a single oral dose of 40 mg praziquantel per kg [33]. HIV testing was undertaken according to the South African Department of Health protocol and pre-and post testing counselling was offered to all participants. Anti-retroviral treatment is provided at no cost in South African health facilities and participants if HIV positive were referred for treatment to the local facilities.

Competing interests

The authors declare that they have no competing interests.

Author details

[1]Norwegian Centre for Imported and Tropical Diseases, Department of Infectious Diseases Ullevaal, Oslo University Hospital, Postboks 4956 Nydalen, 0424 Oslo, Norway. [2]Institute of Clinical Medicine, University of Oslo, Oslo, Norway. [3]Department of Infection Prevention and Control, Nelson R Mandela School of Medicine, College of Health Sciences, University of KwaZulu-Natal, Durban, South Africa. [4]Department of Gynaecology, Women and Children's Division, Ullevaal University Hospital, Oslo, Norway. [5]Imperial College London, Hammersmith Campus, London, UK. [6]Section for Parasitology and Aquatic Pathobiology, Faculty of Health and Medical Sciences, University of Copenhagen, Copenhagen, Denmark. [7]Research Unit, Sorlandet Hospital, Kristiansand, Norway. [8]Department of Global Development and Planning, University of Agder, Kristiansand, Norway. [9]Discipline of Public Health Medicine, Nelson R Mandela School of Medicine, College of Health Sciences, University of KwaZulu-Natal, Durban, South Africa.

References

1. Rosenberg M, Pettifor A, Miller WC, Thirumurthy H, Emch M, Afolabi SA, Kahn K, Collinson M, Tollman S. Relationship between school dropout and teen pregnancy among rural south African young women. Int J Epidemiol. 2015;44(3):928–36.
2. Galappaththi-Arachchige HN, Amlie Hegertun IE, Holmen S, Qvigstad E, Kleppa E, Sebitloane M, Ndhlovu PD, Vennervald BJ, Gundersen SG, Taylor M, et al. Association of Urogenital Symptoms with History of Water Contact in Young Women in Areas Endemic for S. haematobium. A cross-sectional study in Rural South Africa. Int J Environ Res Public Health. 2016;13(11)
3. Naidoo S, Wand H, Abbai NS, Ramjee G. High prevalence and incidence of sexually transmitted infections among women living in KwaZulu-Natal, South Africa. AIDS Res Ther. 2014;11:31.
4. Waxman AM, Humphries H, Frohlich J, Dlamini S, Ntombela F. Young women's life experiences and perceptions of sexual and reproductive health in rural KwaZulu-Natal South Africa. Cult Health Sex. 2016;18(10):1122–36.
5. South Africa Demographic and Health Survey 2016 [http://www.statssa.gov.za/publications/Report 03-00-09/Report 03-00-092016.pdf]. Accessed 1 June 2017.
6. Neal SE, Chandra-Mouli V, Chou D. Adolescent first births in East Africa: disaggregating characteristics, trends and determinants. Reprod Health. 2015;12:13.
7. The Gap Report 2014 [http://www.unaids.org/sites/default/files/media_asset/UNAIDS_Gap_report_en.pdf]. Accessed 1 June 2017.
8. Global AIDS update 2016 [http://www.unaids.org/sites/default/files/media_asset/global-AIDS-update-2016_en.pdf]. Accessed 1 June 2017.

9. 2015 National Antenatal Sentinel HIV & Syphilis Survey Report [http://www. health.gov.za/index.php/shortcodes/2015-03-29-10-42-47/2015-04-30-08-18-10/2015-04-30-08-21-56?download=2584:2015-national-antenatal-hiv-prevalence-survey-final-23oct17]. Accessed 1 June 2017.

10. Shisana O, Rehle T, Simbayi LC, Zuma K, Jooste S, Zungu N, Labadarios D, Davids A, Ramlagan S, Onoya D, et al. South African National HIV prevalence, incidence and behaviour survey, 2012: HSRC Press; 2014.

11. Moodley D, Moodley P, Sebitloane M, Soowamber D, McNaughton-Reyes HL, Groves AK, Maman S. High prevalence and incidence of asymptomatic sexually transmitted infections during pregnancy and postdelivery in KwaZulu Natal, South Africa. Sex Transm Dis. 2015;42(1):43–7.

12. Wilkinson D, Abdool Karim SS, Harrison A, Lurie M, Colvin M, Connolly C, Sturm AW. Unrecognized sexually transmitted infections in rural South African women: a hidden epidemic. Bull World Health Organ. 1999;77(1):22–8.

13. Moodley P, Sturm AW. Sexually transmitted infections, adverse pregnancy outcome and neonatal infection. Semin Neonatol. 2000;5(3):255–69.

14. Kabuyaya M, Chimbari MJ, Manyangadze T, Mukaratirwa S. Efficacy of praziquantel on Schistosoma haematobium and re-infection rates among school-going children in the Ndumo area of uMkhanyakude district, KwaZulu-Natal, South Africa. Infect Dis Poverty. 2017;6(1):83.

15. Kjetland EF, Leutscher PD, Ndhlovu PD. A review of female genital schistosomiasis. Trends Parasitol. 2012;28(2):58–65.

16. Kjetland EF, Ndhlovu PD, Mduluza T, Gomo E, Gwanzura L, Mason PR, Kurewa EN, Midzi N, Friis H, Gundersen SG. Simple clinical manifestations of genital Schistosoma haematobium infection in rural Zimbabwean women. Am J Trop Med Hyg. 2005;72(3):311–9.

17. Downs JA, van Dam GJ, Changalucha JM, Corstjens PL, Peck RN, de Dood CJ, Bang H, Andreasen A, Kalluvya SE, van Lieshout L, et al. Association of Schistosomiasis and HIV infection in Tanzania. Am J Trop Med Hyg. 2012; 87(5):868–73.

18. Kjetland EF, Ndhlovu PD, Gomo E, Mduluza T, Midzi N, Gwanzura L, Mason PR, Sandvik L, Friis H, Gundersen SG. Association between genital schistosomiasis and HIV in rural Zimbabwean women. AIDS. 2006;20(4):593–600.

19. Pascoe SJ, Langhaug LF, Mavhu W, Hargreaves J, Jaffar S, Hayes R, Cowan FM. Poverty, food insufficiency and HIV infection and sexual behaviour among young rural Zimbabwean women. PLoS One. 2015;10(1):e0115290.

20. Heuveline P. Impact of the HIV epidemic on population and household structure: the dynamics and evidence to date. AIDS. 2004;18(Suppl 2):S45–53.

21. Mittal K, Goel MK. Knowledge regarding reproductive health among urban adolescent girls of Haryana. Indian J Community Med. 2010;35(4):529–30.

22. Pazol K, Whiteman MK, Folger SG, Kourtis AP, Marchbanks PA, Jamieson DJ. Sporadic contraceptive use and nonuse: age specific prevalence and associated factors. Am J Obstet Gynecol. 2015;212(3):324. e321–328

23. Morojele NK, Kachieng'a MA, Mokoko E, Nkoko MA, Parry CD, Nkowane AM, Moshia KM, Saxena S. Alcohol use and sexual behaviour among risky drinkers and bar and shebeen patrons in Gauteng province, South Africa. Soc Sci Med. 2006;62(1):217–27.

24. Hemovich V, Crano WD. Family structure and adolescent drug use: an exploration of single-parent families. Subst Use Misuse. 2009;44(14):2099–113.

25. Gregson S, Nyamukapa CA, Garnett GP, Mason PR, Zhuwau T, Carael M, Chandiwana SK, Anderson RM. Sexual mixing patterns and sex-differentials in teenage exposure to HIV infection in rural Zimbabwe. Lancet. 2002; 359(9321):1896–903.

26. Zembe YZ, Townsend L, Thorson A, Ekstrom AM. "Money talks, bullshit walks" interrogating notions of consumption and survival sex among young women engaging in transactional sex in post-apartheid South Africa: a qualitative enquiry. Glob Health. 2013;9:28.

27. Evan Secor W. Water-based interventions for schistosomiasis control. Pathog Glob Health. 2014;108(5):246–54.

28. Appleton CC, Gouws E. The distribution of common intestinal nematodes along an altitudinal transect in KwaZulu Natal, South Africa. Ann Trop Med Parasitol. 1996;90(2):181–8.

29. Holmen SD, Kjetland EF, Taylor M, Kleppa E, Lillebo K, Gundersen SG, Onsrud M, Albregtsen F. Colourimetric image analysis as a diagnostic tool in female genital schistosomiasis. Med Eng Phys. 2015;37(3):309–14.

30. Kjetland EF, Norseth HM, Taylor M, Lillebo K, Kleppa E, Holmen SD, Andebirhan A, Yohannes TH, Gundersen SG, Vennervald BJ, et al.

31. Leclerc-Madlala S. Age-disparate and intergenerational sex in southern Africa: the dynamics of hypervulnerability. AIDS. 2008;22(Suppl 4):S17–25.

32. Oliveros JC: Venny. An interactive tool for comparing lists with Venn's diagrams. In. 2007–2015.

33. Kincaid C, Jones DJ, Sterrett E, McKee L. A review of parenting and adolescent sexual behavior: the moderating role of gender. Clin Psychol Rev. 2012;32(3):177–88.

34. DeVore ER, Ginsburg KR. The protective effects of good parenting on adolescents. Curr Opin Pediatr. 2005;17(4):460–5.

35. Deptula DP, Henry DB, Schoeny ME. How can parents make a difference? Longitudinal associations with adolescent sexual behavior. J Fam Psychol. 2010;24(6):731–9.

36. Cuffee JJ, Hallfors DD, Waller MW. Racial and gender differences in adolescent sexual attitudes and longitudinal associations with coital debut. J Adolesc Health. 2007;41(1):19–26.

37. Maharaj P, Munthree C. Coerced first sexual intercourse and selected reproductive health outcomes among young women in KwaZulu-Natal, South Africa. J Biosoc Sci. 2007;39(2):231–44.

38. Crosby RA, DiClemente RJ, Wingood GM, Cobb BK, Harrington K, Davies SL, Hook EW 3rd, Oh MK. HIV/STD-protective benefits of living with mothers in perceived supportive families: a study of high-risk African American female teens. Prev Med. 2001;33(3):175–8.

39. Ramjee G, Wand H. Geographical clustering of high risk sexual behaviors in "hot-spots" for HIV and sexually transmitted infections in Kwazulu-Natal, South Africa. AIDS Behav. 2014;18(2):317–22.

40. Maharaj P, Cleland J. Risk perception and condom use among married or cohabiting couples in KwaZulu-Natal, South Africa. Int Fam Plan Perspect. 2005;31(1):24–9.

41. Heeren GA, Mandeya A, Jemmott JB, Chiruka RT, Marange CS, Batidzirai JM, Gwaze AR, Tyler JC, Hsu J. Multiple partners and condom use among students at a south African University. J Evid Based Soc Work. 2014;11(5): 437–44.

42. Peters RP, Dubbink JH, van der Eem L, Verweij SP, Bos ML, Ouburg S, Lewis DA, Struthers H, McIntyre JA, Morre SA. Cross-sectional study of genital, rectal, and pharyngeal chlamydia and gonorrhea in women in rural South Africa. Sex Transm Dis. 2014;41(9):564–9.

43. Geary RS, Gomez-Olive FX, Kahn K, Tollman S, Norris SA. Barriers to and facilitators of the provision of a youth-friendly health services programme in rural South Africa. BMC Health Serv Res. 2014;14:259.

44. Kjetland EF, Kurewa EN, Ndhlovu PD, Midzi N, Gwanzura L, Mason PR, Gomo E, Sandvik L, Mduluza T, Friis H, et al. Female genital schistosomiasis--a differential diagnosis to sexually transmitted disease: genital itch and vaginal discharge as indicators of genital Schistosoma haematobium morbidity in a cross-sectional study in endemic rural Zimbabwe. Tropical Med Int Health. 2008;13(12):1509–17.

45. Adachi K, Klausner JD, Xu J, Ank B, Bristow CC, Morgado MG, Watts DH, Weir F, Persing D, Mofenson LM, et al. Chlamydia trachomatis and Neisseria gonorrhoeae in HIV-infected pregnant women and adverse infant outcomes. Pediatr Infect Dis J. 2016;35(8):894–900.

46. Cavazos-Rehg PA, Krauss MJ, Spitznagel EL, Schootman M, Cottler LB, Bierut LJ. Substance use and the risk for sexual intercourse with and without a history of teenage pregnancy among adolescent females. J Stud Alcohol Drugs. 2011;72(2):194–8.

47. Bearinger LH, Sieving RE, Ferguson J, Sharma V. Global perspectives on the sexual and reproductive health of adolescents: patterns, prevention, and potential. Lancet. 2007;369(9568):1220–31.

48. Mayaud P, Mabey D. Approaches to the control of sexually transmitted infections in developing countries: old problems and modern challenges. Sex Transm Infect. 2004;80(3):174–82.

49. Boynton PM, Greenhalgh T. Selecting, designing, and developing your questionnaire. BMJ. 2004;328(7451):1312–5.

Classification of the lesions observed in female genital schistosomiasis. Int J Gynaecol Obstet. 2014;127(3):227–8.

5

Barriers and facilitators to humanizing birth care in Tanzania: findings from semi-structured interviews with midwives and obstetricians

Lilian T. Mselle[1*], Thecla W. Kohi[2] and Justine Dol[3]

Abstract

Background: In Tanzania, the provision of humanized care is increasingly being emphasized in midwifery practice, yet studies regarding perceptions and practices of skilled health personnel towards the humanization of birth care are scare. Previous reviews have identified that abuse and disrespect is not limited to individuals but reflects systematic failures and deeply embedded provider attitudes and beliefs. Therefore, the current study aims to explore the perceptions and practices of skilled health personnel on humanizing birth care in Tanzania by identifying current barriers and facilitators.

Methods: Semi-structured interviews were held with skilled health personnel including midwives ($n = 6$) and obstetricians ($n = 2$) working in the two district hospitals of Tanzania. Data were analyzed using thematic coding.

Results: Skilled health personnel identified systematic barriers to providing humanizing birth care. Systematic barriers included lack of space and limited facilities. Institutional norms and practices prohibited family involvement during the birth process, including beliefs that limited choice of birth position as well as disrespected beliefs, traditions, and culture. Participants also acknowledged four facilitators that improve the likelihood of humanized care during childbirth in Tanzania: ongoing education of skilled health personnel on respectful maternal care, institutional norms designed for continuous clinic support during childbirth, belief in the benefit of having family become active participants, and respecting maternal wishes when appropriate.

Conclusion: To move forward with humanizing the birth process in Tanzania, it will be essential that systematic barriers are addressed as well as changing the mindset of personnel towards respectful maternal care. It will be essential for the government and private hospitals to revalue their labour wards to increase the space and staff allocated to each mother to enhance family-integrated care. Additionally, in-service training as well as incorporation of respectful maternal care during pre-service training is key to changing the culture in the labour ward.

Keywords: Material services, Birth care, Humanizing birth, Qualitative, Tanzania, Skilled health personnel

* Correspondence: nakutz@yahoo.com
[1]Department of Clinical Nursing, Muhimbili University of Health and Allied Sciences, Dar es Salaam, Tanzania
Full list of author information is available at the end of the article

Plain English summary

In Tanzania, many women report not experiencing respectful care from skilled health personnel when they give birth at a hospital. Previous findings suggest that there are many factors that influence whether a skilled health personnel can provide quality birth care to women including physical space and staff limitations as well as deeply embedded provider fear, attitudes and beliefs. Therefore, we decided to explore the beliefs and behaviours of nurse midwives and obstetricians in Tanzania with the goal of identifying current difficulties as well as existing enablers that allow them to provide quality care. For this study, we interviewed six nurse midwives and two obstetricians working in the two District hospitals of Tanzania. Data were analyzed using thematic coding. Only two obstetricians were interviewed because of limited number of skilled health personnel in the area. We found that participants identified barriers including physical space issues, engrained traditions within the hospitals that limited family involvement, not providing a woman the choice for the position during birth, and disregard for belief, traditions and culture of mothers. Participants also acknowledged four enablers that allow them to provide respectful maternal care during childbirth included receiving training on the need to provide respectful maternal care, hospital policies to provide continuous support and quality care, personal belief in the value of having family involved, and respecting maternal wishes during childbirth when appropriate. It will be essential for the government and private hospitals revalue their labour wards to increase the space and staff. In-hospital training and pre-service education is key to changing the culture in the labour ward.

Background

It is well known that disrespect and abuse in maternity care is a global problem [1] with a growing emphasis on humanizing birth care to change this and improve the care women receive during childbirth [2]. According to the World Health Organization (WHO), respectful maternal care (RMC) is defined as "care organized for and provided to all women in a manner that maintains their dignity, privacy and confidentiality, ensures freedom from harm and mistreatment, and enables informed choice and continuous support during labour and childbirth" (p.3, [3]). Humanizing birth occurs when woman who are giving birth are put in the centre, with full control of the experience, working with the skilled health provider as equals to ensure evidence-based care [2]. In order for women to have a humanizing birth experience, RMC is a necessary but not sufficient requirement, yet understanding RMC can lead to a greater understanding of barriers and facilitators to fully experience humanizing birth care. Humanizing care during childbirth privileges respect towards women's sense of dignity and autonomy

without compromising their active involvement in the process of birth [2, 4].

The recognition of the need for RMC and humanizing birth care has been growing in recent years. In 2015, the WHO issued a statement on the prevention and elimination of disrespect and abuse during facility-based childbirth that called for greater action, dialogue, research and advocacy on this important public health and human rights issue [5]. Following that in 2016, The Lancet published a called to action on improving quality maternity care for every woman, everywhere [6]. Most recently, the WHO provided recommendations on intrapartum care for a positive childbirth experience where RMC was indorsed as a way to reduce maternal morbidity and mortality, improve women's experience of childbirth, and reduce health inequalities [3]. However, in order for RMC to be implemented and to fully humanize birth care, it takes more than awareness – changes need to occur in the healthcare system as well as within individual maternal healthcare providers.

Recent systematic reviews have explored disrespect and abuse during labour and delivery from the perspective of healthcare providers and women [7–9]. These reviews highlight that abuse and disrespect is not limited to individual behaviours by midwives, but reflects systematic failures and deeply embedded provider attitudes and beliefs [7–9]. In a study with Kenyan midwives, they acknowledged that there were health system challenges, including infrastructure gaps and limited staff, that hindered their ability to implement a rights-based approach to maternity care despite a desire by providers' to do so [10]. In a study exploring both women and midwives perspectives of disrespect during delivery care in Ethiopia, Burrowes and colleagues [11] found that while disrespect and abuse was present, the midwives reported that the abuse was unintended and reflected challenges of the healthcare system or occurred due to medical necessity.

In Tanzania, several studies highlight the importance of quality of care during childbirth [12, 13]; however, the prevalence of disrespect and abuse in a variety of healthcare and community settings is a widespread problem [12, 14–17]. For example, two qualitative studies in urban Tanzania have revealed that all participants reported experiencing or hearing about others experiences of both respectful and disrespectful or abusive care during facility based childbirth [16, 18]. However, there has been limited discussion with the midwives on their perceptions of providing RMC during childbirth in Tanzania. Women's experience of disrespect and abuse by midwives contribute to poor access of skilled birth care in the health facility [19], denying women rights to quality maternal care [20] and contributes to maternal mortality and mortality [21].

Using participatory methods to understand and promote a culture of respectful maternal care may be key to sustainable changes [22]. Therefore, it is essential to explore the perceptions and experiences of midwives and maternal skilled health providers to understand the existing gaps and to contextualization of humanized birth care that is culturally sensitive and appropriate. The objective of this qualitative study was to describe the perceptions and practices of nurse midwivesand obstetricians (hereafter referred jointly as skilled health personnel) on humanizing birth care and barriers and facilitators to respectful maternal care in Tanzania.

Methods
Study Design & Setting
This study is part of a larger project exploring community and skilled health personnel perceptions and practices on humanizing birth care in Tanzania. The study was conducted in the two District hospitals in the Mwanza and Mara regions in the Lake Zone, Tanzania. Districts hospitals in Tanzania are the first referral level in the health system referral pyramid where necessary drugs, equipment, and skilled staff are supposed to be available to provide comprehensive EmOC. Further up in the health pyramid, there are regional hospitals, followed by zonal referral hospitals, and at the highest level are the national hospitals. The Lake Zone was chosen as it is one of the regions of Tanzania with the highest maternal mortality rates, with Mara having a maternal mortality ratio of 362 per 1000 births and 305 per 1000 births in Mwanza according to the 2012 census [23].

Participants and data collection
The aim of this study was to explore the perceptions and experiences of humanizing birth care in Tanzania. Therefore, eight skilled health personnel including six midwives and two obstetricians were conveniently selected from two hospitals in the Lake Zone. Only eight skilled health personnel were interviewed, however qualitative sample size has no rule it depends on what the researcher wants to know, the purpose of the research study, and what can be done with available time and resources. It is further recommended that the minimum samples for qualitative research should be based on expected reasonable coverage of the phenomenon given the purpose of the study and interest [24]. The inclusion criteria were midwives or obstetricians working in the labour ward for a minimum of two years providing birth care and agreed to participate in the study. A midwife in charge of the labour ward (not part of the interviewed midwives) identified midwives and obstetrician who met the inclusion criteria. Throughout this paper, the term "skilled health personnel", as defined by the 2018 WHO [25], is used to include both nurse midwives and obstetricians because of the desire not to

separate out the nurse midwives and obstetricians specific findings.

The purpose of the study and principles of confidentiality were explained to participants, and thereafter, a convenient time for an interview was arranged. Semi structured interviews [26] with midwives and obstetricians who were on duty during the data collection period were conducted. A semi-structured interview guide was used focusing on skilled health personnels'perceptions and experiences of humanizing birth care (see Table 1). The guide with open-ended questions and probes used was flexible to allow the interviewer to explore issues of relevance as they emerged [27]. Interviews were conducted in aprivate, quiet room within the hospital premise at the end of the participants shift. In each interview, the participant was a major speaker and the researcher served as a guide and facilitator. The level of openness of the interviewees varied but seemed to be generally good. All interviewees agreed to the use of an audio-recorder and interviews lasted between 30–45 min. Notation of nonverbal expressions of the informants during the interview was taken during and immediately after the interview.

Data analysis
Semi-structured interviews were transcribed verbatim into Kiswahili, and then translated into English by hired research assistants fluent in both languages. It was essential to translate transcripts into English to ensure access of data to non-Kiswahili speaking members of the research team. Data were analyzed using thematic coding using the English transcripts with initial codes collected and reviewed, duplicates removed, and similar codes grouped together [28, 29]. Codes and corresponding quotes were reviewed and re-labeled if necessary [30]. The semi-structured interviews yielded significantly rich data whereby no additional themes seemed to emerge, suggesting sufficient data to develop themes [30].

Table 1 Interview guide for Midwives and Obstetricians

SN	Interview question and probes
1	Could you please explain what kind of support do you provide to mothers during labour and delivery? (Which position did women usually assume during delivery?, who decides for delivery position?, Do women have opportunity to choose position that they would like to assume during delivery?
2	How do women's relatives involved during labour and delivery? (Could a woman choose to be with her husband during labour?, What barriers?)
3	How do you maintain women's privacy during labour and delivery?
4	How do you incorporate women's cultural, spiritual and tradition believes in caring during labour and delivery?
5	What happens to the baby after delivery?

Ethical consideration

This study was approved by the National Institute of Medical Research in Tanzania (Ref. no. NIMR/HQ/R.8a/Vol.IX/2143). All participants gave informed written consent to be interviewed. Participants were informed that their interviews would be recorded and agreed for their anonymous quotes to be used.

Results

Barriers

Four barriers were reported by participants regarding provision of humanized and respectful maternal care. This included two systematic barriers that are beyond the ability of skilled health personnel to address on their own. These are physical space and facilities limitations, and institutional norms and practices that limit family involvement. However, it also included two individualized barriers as initiated by the skilled health personnel, including beliefs that choice of birth position should be limited as well as disrespect for belief, traditions and culture of the mother.

Space and facility limitations

Participants reported that physical space and hospital facilities limited the ability to provide high respectful and compassionate care. The limitation of mother's movement during labour due to limited space was reported by one of the participants:

"It is impossible [for mothers to walk around in the labour room] given limited space in our labour room. The room has a little space for a bed and small table". (Skilled health personnel 1)

Physical space and facility size also limited the ability to provide privacy to mothers, which is a primary tenant to respectful maternal care.

"[For privacy] delivery rooms have partitions. There are some partitions but the other end of the room, especially those aluminum and glass partition, do not ensure privacy of a delivering mother. Privacy does not mean only being unseen by other people when giving birth but any mother who enters the labor room expects to be alone with the midwife". (Skilled health personne l7)

Participants also acknowledged that the lack of space would need to be addressed if improvements were to be made to providing more humane birth care.

"(...) our health facilities are very small. Rooms are not separated; you can easily cross from one woman to another. I think if we would like to have such things we need to make some improvements". (Skilled health personne l3)

"We really do not allow them [family members] to stay with mothers during delivery because we have so many women, so you cannot allow every woman who comes in the labour room to stay with their relative, there is no place for them to stay". (Skilled health personnel 5)

Participants were also concerned with the limited staff that impacted the quality of maternal care provided, saying that the number of mothers who presented at the hospital for delivery exceeded the staff available during the shift to provide sufficient maternal care. The limited staff and space also limited the ability for mothers to stay long after delivery, with most mothers being discharged within 12 to 24 h after delivery.

Institution norms and practices

Institutional norms and practices were reported as barriers that limited acceptance and encouragement of family involvement, which is a key pillar in humanizing the birth process. Participants reported that the process of humanized birth care is not fully embedded in the hospital culture. For instance, it is not common practice for family members to be involved during the birth process:

"(...) few private hospitals in Tanzania allow this". (Skilled health personnel 1)

Because of this, the norm is for family members who bring the woman to the hospital for delivery to be sent home and encouraged only to visit and bring items for the mother during limited visiting hours.

"We do not allow them [family members] to come in, once they brought in a woman we deal with her by ourselves". (Skilled health personnel 1)

"Because of our rooms is difficult to find a relative in the room all the time, we have nurses there who can provide details to relatives when they require them, but because of our rooms relatives do not stay to the end. Until the woman is delivered the relatives are outside and are not allowed to enter in the room. They will get all the details they want from nurses. Until after when the baby is born and the condition of the mother is stabilized, there is no chance for any relative to enter the room". (Skilled health personnel 3)

Participants also reported that they were fearful of the repercussions of having family members involved in the birth process, for themselves, their patients, and for their profession. They expressed that husbands and family members might not understand what they are doing and perceive it as abusive or harsh:

"(...) he [husband] might see the way we are handling his wife as inappropriate and react accordingly". (Skilled health personnel 4)

It may also lead to breach of confidentiality of their clients' information:

"(...) besides, when the relatives are too involved at this critical time, they may divulge sensitive medical information to the mother and share the medical records publicly by passing it to other people (...)". (Skilled health personnel 8)

In terms of the fear related to their profession, one skilled health personnel explained that despite the recognition that family members should be involved, they still feared a negative outcome.

"Panic can emerge as the result of the spouse beholding the critical health condition of the woman in labour, where the mother is experiencing excessive bleed or the midwife is pressing the woman's abdomen to push the baby out. These situations may be perceived by the spouse as coercive or abusive. This perception may cause the spouse to consider legal action against the hospital. So, yeah, much as everyone has rights, we strive to avoid such problems by encouraging minimal spouse involvement." (Skilled health personnel 8)

Beliefs that choice of birth position should be limited

It was learnt from the participants that they preferred women to deliver in the lithotomy position as it makes it easier for the skilled health personnel to assist with delivery and helps the baby deliver smoothly.

"Lithotomy position for pregnant woman is better because it will be easy to see as the baby protrudes through the woman's vulva. (...) it is also good for the midwife to check the cervix of the mother who is about to give birth compared to when the mother is in the lateral position. In my view, the lithotomy position is better because less time will be spent for child delivery". (Skilled health personnel 5)

Another participant also shared that lithotomy is a professionally sanctioned position:

"[The lithotomic position] is the professionally sanctioned standard position (...) it is the most

accommodating in that it gives the mother considerable pushing power and allows the mother to grab her legs when [pushing], which is the safest way". (Skilled health personnel 8)

"(...) what I was taught is that that is [lithotomy] a good position and it helps a mother to give birth well and exactly depending to how a baby lies. You can help her well and you can receive the baby in good condition and it makes the mother to be more comfortable. (...) I have also read that lithotomy position is best and delivery can be conducted easily".(Skilled health personnel 3)

Skilled health personnel expressed that because of this preference, they often told the woman to get into this position during delivery, rather than allowing her to decide the position she would prefer to use when giving birth:

"You are [midwife] the one who tells the woman which position she should lie for easy delivery because other women it is their first delivery so they do not know". (Skilled health personnel 4)

"We [midwives] have experience with that position, the one which she lies on her back". (Skilled health personnel 3)

"Many women give birth lying on their backs. Many say that they feel more comfortable when they deliver they get strength. (...) we normally don't ask but we instruct them how to lie". (Skilled health personnel 6)

"[Some mothers prefer] to sit, others prefer a delivering posture the same as they are in the toilet. But others prefer to lie in sideways. I think that, on the side of the woman, the best posture is that which she feels comfortable. As a service provider, I prefer the lithotomy position, especially when we want to maintain the mother's cleanliness. This allows me to control a mother when assisting her during delivery. So it is a two-sided perspective". (Skilled health personnel 7)

Disrespect for traditions and culture

Participants reported disrespect or disregard for the traditions and culture of the women who come to give birth. They acknowledged that they do not recognize the tradition norms but instead encourage the westernized, evidence-based medicine that is provided in hospital. Participants explained their hesitation with the use of herbs used by women to facilitate labour:

"Our perspective is that herbs are not scientifically tested. Although the herbs help in accelerating contraction, they have side effects. (...) we don't know exactly its composition. Actually, the issues of tradition and customs is not given due weight. I personally do not take it as a serious issue. I work as I was trained. (...) we may be performing our duties as Europeans. I take the medical training that I received is of European norms and principles. So, we take that understanding expecting mothers who has come to the hospital for treatment or childbirth has left her traditions and customs at home. She has agreed with European norms. She may perform her traditions and customs when she goes back home. I have not asked any mother about her observance regarding childbirth according to her tribe". (Skilled health personnel 7)

Participants also explained how their previous experience with women using traditional medicine had done more harm than good for the mother and baby, and thus they devalued their importance. One skilled health personnel shared the story about the dangers of using traditional medicine:

"Most women use herbs to facilitate uterine contractions. (...) we need contractions but with normal required intensity and frequency. (...) most of the expecting mothers use herbs before coming to the hospital and they end up with fetal distress, because she may have good contractions but with an unopened cervix. In this situation, contractions do not go with labor progress (...)". (Skilled health personnel 7)

Facilitators
Despite the barriers described for humanizing birth care, participants also acknowledged several facilitators that are currently in place that could improve the provision of respectful maternal care during childbirth. This included systematic facilitators such as the ongoing education of skilled health personnel on the need to provide respectful maternal care and institutional norms designed for continuous clinic support during childbirth. Additionally, personal factors among the skilled health personnel that encourage respectful maternal care include the belief in benefit of having family to become active participants as well as respecting maternal wishes during childbirth when appropriate and safe.

Ongoing education of skilled health personnel on respectful maternal care
Despite the barriers and institutionalized barriers, skilled health personnel described receiving education on key behaviours that reflected respectful maternal care.

Skilled health personnel reported receiving training on different delivery positions as well as the need to respect the rights of the mother during the delivery:

"(...) even in class we were told the mom [can] choose [the position] how to push". (Skilled health personnel 1)

"As we were taught, we have to allow the woman to assume the position which she is comfortable to give birth, although most of time we advices them to lie with their back. But if she wants to squat, you have to allow her". (Skilled health personnel 3)

"(...) we were educated about importance of maintaining privacy, ensuring the woman in labour is constantly supported physically and emotionally by providing psychological support and managing pain (...)". (Skilled health personnel 1)

Institutional norms designed for continuous clinic support during childbirth
Participants provided insight into current practices within the hospital that involve providing continuous support for mothers during childbirth. While not always provided as evidenced through above barriers, participants noted that throughout the birth process, the skilled health personnel attempted their best to provide continuous care:

"(...) women are helped from the first stage until the fourth stage of labour and we stay with her until she is discharged and she becomes free with her relatives". (Skilled health personnel 1)

"During a typical delivery, the doctors, while they were not always present during every uncomplicated delivery, they were close by and active in complicated deliveries or during operations". (Skilled health personnel 4)

The participants explained the delivery process for mothers who come for birth. They commonly assess the woman during admission determining what stage of labour she is in:

"(...) when a woman arrives at the reception, we always receive her quickly and do quick assessment, we prioritize women because they arrive many at once. (...), you have to check what kind of women you have because some are in true labour pain and close to deliver or sometimes we like to ask those who have urge to push". (Skilled health personnel 1)

If she is in the first stage of labour, she is placed in the observation room and re-assessed every four hours or until she notifies a skilled health personnel a change in her labour status. If she is in second stage of labour, they bring her immediately to the labour room where she is continuously monitored until delivery:

"When the mother arrives with labour pain, I receive her and start physical examinations. I check her to ensure her blood pressure is not high which can cause problems during delivery. After doing that then I do abdominal examinations and PV examination to asses if the cervix is open or not and if yes by how much; so that to determine the progress of labour or she will be taken to labour room directly, because others arrive already in second stage (...). After completing examinations I then check her health status; if she has tested or not. I test her if she hasn't been tested to know if she has acquired infection or not (...)". (Skilled health personnel 4)

The privacy is attempted to be maintained during delivery:

"(...) here at our facility we use curtains to maintain privacy. If a woman wants to give birth, we must make sure all curtains are set. In our labour ward, there are partitions so we close the curtains very well". (Skilled health personnel 2)

Once the baby is delivered, they assess the baby and transfer the mother and her baby to the postnatal ward for recovery.

"[After the baby is born] we look up at the child's scoring, appearance (...) we also look at how the baby is crying and then we wrap up the baby. Thereafter we weight the child on a scale. After these procedures, we instantaneously carry the baby to a parched area and immediately put her to breastfeeding".(Skilled health personnel 7)

Thus, current practices in the labour ward attempt to offer continuous support to mothers and their babies, despite the barriers faced by skilled health personnel. Providing a dehumanized birth experience was not expressed as a desire by any skilled health personnel.

Belief in benefit of having family to become active participants

Despite space limitations in the labour wards, participants acknowledged the benefit to the woman to have family members be active participants during the delivery process. Skilled health personnel gave the following justifications when explaining the benefits to having family members involved:

"(...) if the partner is present from the beginning of labour up to delivery, then he will understand what the mother has been through and hence be able to help her while at home". (Skilled health personnel 4)

"(...) a partner being present during labor is to help the expectant mother emotionally and to encourage the mother to push. (...) there are few midwives and most of the time they are outnumbered by the expectant mothers. There may be up to seven expectant mothers on beds with only one midwife making it difficult for her to work on time and with efficiency". (Skilled health personnel 3)

"(...) normally they come with their mothers. I think her mother should be there. Because she understood, she is able to guide her (...)". (Skilled health personnel 6)

Respecting maternal wishes when appropriate

As skilled health personnel were taught behaviours related to respectful care, they reported that they would respect maternal wishes when it was appropriate. Participants explained that they might not understand some of the decisions that women made. However, if the decision did not limit their ability to provide quality and safe care to the mother and the baby, they would allow the mothers' wishes to be followed. A skilled health personnel explained that despite suggesting the lithotomy position, if a mother wants to give birth in another position, she obliges:

"(...) if she tells us her best position then we have to support her in that position for her to give birth comfortably". (Skilled health personnel 3)

Likewise, another participant explained how they dealt with traditional beliefs and practices:

"In my perspective, we are not that thoughtful of the traditional practices but we are always accommodative of the mother and family wishes, if there are any. Whether it's the longing to pack up the placenta back home or this and that, one should simply let the mother fulfil her wish". (Skilled health personnel 7)

Discussion and implications for midwifery and health policies

Overall, skilled health personnel identified several barriers that limited their ability to provide humanized birth care including systematic issues, including physical space and institutional norms and practices as well as personal barriers, including beliefs that choice of birth position should be limited and disrespect for tradition. Nevertheless, several facilitators were identified that are currently in place that can move the process of humanizing birth forward, including ongoing education of midwives on respectful maternal care, institutional norms designed for continuous clinic support during childbirth, belief in the benefit of having family become active participants, and respecting maternal wishes when appropriate.

The current findings are consistent with the recent systematic review by Bradley et al. [8] that highlighted that abuse and disrespect is not limited to individual skilled health personnel but reflects systematic failures and deeply embedded provider attitudes and beliefs [7, 8]. In Bradley et al.'s conceptual framework based on their meta-analysis of women's perceptions of intrapartum care in Sub-Saharan Africa, macro-level factors (colonial legacy, structural inequality, and health system policy & drivers) and meso-level factors (medicalization of birth, midwifery history and training, hierarchical and institution-centred, work environment and resources, poverty and inequality, gender inequality/status of women) influence and shape the inter-personal dynamics happening at a day-to-day micro-level for skilled health personnel [8]. For instance, in our study, we found that skilled health personnel desired women to accept Western norms around birthing position, echoing the colonial legacy and the ongoing medicalization of birth in these countries, reflecting macro- and meso-level factors. Challenges remain in shifting the attitudes and behaviours of all skilled health personnel to embrace evidence-based practices to enhance the humanizing birth experience, even if it varies from Western-based medicine.

To move forward with humanizing the birth process, there is a need to address the barriers and enhance the facilitators as identified by the skilled health personnel. First, it will be essential that individual level issues are addressed. Individual level barriers included currently held beliefs that choice of birth position should be limited and ongoing disrespect for tradition. Yet skilled health personnel also identified corresponding facilitators, including holding the belief in the benefit of having family become active participants and respecting maternal wishes when appropriate. It is clear from our findings that there is a desire to offer respectful maternal care and a humanizing child birth experience, yet it has not fully emerged in practice. There exists some discord around what skilled health personnel think and desire to happen, versus what is actually happening in the unit. For example, some participants reported that privacy was consistently provided to mothers, yet others reported that due to institutional barriers, this was not always provided. This is not unique to our study, as Warren

et al. [31] found that both respect and disrespect were considered common among midwives in Mali.

It is essential to change the mindset of skilled health personnel towards humanizing birth care, particularly around the delivery position and respecting tradition if it does not impact safety and quality of care. One of the facilitator mentioned was that skilled health personnel are taught about different delivery positions and that women should be allowed to choose which position they would like to assume during delivery, yet the culture on the labour wards does not encourage this in practice. The issues of skilled health personnel exercising power and control, particularly through controlling the position a women assumes and limiting movement, to assert their professional identity, and to take charge of both women and the birth process has been acknowledged elsewhere [8]. This behaviour is thought to be related to the need for skilled health personnel to maintain a particular social status compared to the women (the skill health personnel's role and social distance and 'othering') [8]. In a systematic mapping by Filby et al. [7] of midwife-identified barriers in providing quality care, they identified professional, social, and economic barriers, which resulted in burn out and moral distress for midwives when not addressed. Therefore, it will be important to target their concern related to maintaining their professional identity as skilled health personnel as well as ensure they are offered the professional and social support needed to provide humanizing birth care to mothers.

However, the physical space within the current labour wards significantly limits skill health personnel's ability to provide a humanizing birth experience. If there is limited space and a need to enhance women's privacy, it is impossible to allow family members to join the mother during the delivery process despite the acknowledgement by participants that this would be beneficial. Additionally, the limited staff also hinders the ability to provide quality care, despite the desire to provide continuous support and quality care. The issue of space limitations related to humanizing birth care due to poor infrastructure or the health care system is not unique to Tanzania [4, 10, 11, 32] and remains a larger issue that needs to be addressed moving forward. In order to provide a humanizing birth experience in Tanzania and beyond, consideration of changes to the physical space is warranted related to systematic issues.

Education to individual skilled health personnel alone is not sufficient without education occurring also at the administration and policy level, where the power to influence change at the systematic level can occur. Without this, even skilled health personnel who want to provide a humanizing birth experience to mothers are limited by space and institutional norms that hinder these opportunities [4]. As seen in the *Heshima* project in Kenya, when providing education to both providers and managers related to respectful maternal care, there was an increase in knowledge and practices among providers for understanding client rights and client-centered care [10]. However, the authors noted that challenges remained due to peer influence, whereby the existing work culture limited the ability of healthcare providers to change behaviour, even if they so desired [10]. To encourage humanizing birth care, more than just individual factors related to skilled health personnel need to be addressed but includes systematic issues that need to be considered moving forward. Interventions targeting both skilled health personnel and administrations have shown some success in reducing disrespect and abuse in Tanzania [15, 33], yet further research is needed to fully understand how women's values, belief and providing respect and autonomy during the birth process can be achieved. The WHO identifies that in order for RMC to occur, there needs to be systematic resources in place, including trained and skilled health personnel, adequate physical infrastructure, and accountability within the ward [3].

Limitations

While this study was conducted with rigor and provides important insights into the humanizing birth care barriers and facilitators in Tanzania, there are some limitations that should be acknowledged. First, the study was conducted at two district hospitals in two regions of Tanzania where participants were employed. Participants may be unlikely to report any disrespectful care that either they or their colleagues engaged in due to fear of repercussion. However, all attempts were made to ensure confidentiality and participants were informed that their responses would not be shared with their employers. While there is always the risk of social acceptability bias, that is that the health care providers would try to minimize their lack of respectful care when speaking to other health care providers, this may have been minimized by the fact that the nurse-midwives who conducted the interviews did not work in the hospitals where the research was conducted and that they had extensive experience in conducting health research and trying to probe for the interviewee's real perspectives. Furthermore, despite this risk, participants identified several barriers that limited respectful maternal care, suggesting that participants were honest in their responses. Nevertheless, data from interviews should be interpreted with some caution as conducting interview at the health facility there is a risk of 'courtesy bias', or participants providing what they believe are acceptable responses rather than their own opinions.

Another limitation is that this study included only two obstetricians because of a low number of skilled health personnel in this category available in the district hospitals in this area of study. Nevertheless, it was important

to capture the perspective of both obstetrician and nurse midwives as both categories of skilled health personnel provide ongoing care to mothers within these hospitals. As both nurse midwives and obstetricians are involved in providing birthing care at these District hospitals, our sample reflects the skilled health personnel involved in providing humanizing birth care and their interpretation of facilitators and barriers.

A final limitation is that analysis of interviews was completed in English from translated transcripts, which may have impacted the analysis. However, transcripts were verified by research team members fluent in Kiswahili to ensure adequate translations and all codes and themes were discussed amongst the researchers who were able to review the original transcripts. Additionally, after every interview, researchers had opportunity to listen to the audio recorded interviews, reflecting on the interview sessions and information gathered in the reflection sessions, which were used during analysis to complement interpretation of themes.

Conclusion

The findings of our study provide valuable insight into the current perceptions and practices by skilled health personnelon humanizing birth care in Tanzania. Several barriers were identified in providing respectful maternal care including systematic and personal barriers, yet several facilitators existed that could be encouraged and enhanced to address the barriers. To humanize the birth process in Tanzania, it will be essential for the government and private hospitals to revalue their labour wards to increase the space and staff allocated to each mother to enhance family-integrated care. Additionally, in-service training as well as incorporation of respectful maternal care during skilled health personnel training is key to changing the culture in the labour ward.

Acknowledgements

The authors would like to thank and acknowledge the contribution of the midwives and obstetricians who gave their time to be interviewed for this study. Further, Dr. Amalberga Kasangala and Saturini Manangwa for collecting data in Mara region.

Funding

Funding for this research was provided by UNFPA through the Ministry of Health Community Development, Gender, Elderly and Children (MOHCDGEC), Dar es Salaam, Tanzania. The funders did not have any role in the study design, data collection, analysis, interpretation of data or in writing the manuscript.

Authors' contributions

LTM and TWK were involved in the planning of the original study, collecting the data, doing the analysis. JD led the analysis and LTM and TWK provided verification of analysis. JD and LTM drafting the manuscript that was critically reviewed by TWK. All authors contributed and approved the final manuscript.

Competing interests
The authors declare that they have no competing interests.

Author details
[1]Department of Clinical Nursing, Muhimbili University of Health and Allied Sciences, Dar es Salaam, Tanzania. [2]Department of Nursing Management, Muhimbili University of Health and Allied Sciences, Dar es Salaam, Tanzania. [3]Faculty of Health, Dalhousie University, Halifax, Canada.

References
1. The White Ribbon Alliance for Safe Motherhood. Respectful maternity care: The universal rights of childbearing women. The White Ribbon Alliance for Safe Motherhood. 2011;1–6. http://whiteribbonalliance.org/wp-content/uploads/2013/10/Final_RMC_Charter.pdf. Accessed 13 July 2017.
2. Wagner M. Fish can't see water: the need to humanize birth. Int J Gynecol Obstet. 2001;75:25–37.
3. World Health Organization. Intrapartum care for a positive childbirth experience. Geneva: World Health Organization; 2018. http://apps.who.int/iris/bitstream/handle/10665/260178/9789241550215-eng.pdf;jsessionid=6543E90288D4B72DEF9FC547FA29F2C4?sequence=1.
4. Behruzi R, Hatem M, Fraser W, Goulet L, li M, Misago C, et al. Facilitators and barriers in the humanization of childbirth practice in Japan. BMC Pregnancy Childbirth. 2010;10:25.
5. WHO. The prevention and elimination of disrespect and abuse during facility-based childbirth. 2015.
6. Koblinsky M, Moyer CA, Calvert C, Campbell J, Campbell OMR, Feigl AB, et al. Quality maternity care for every woman, everywhere: a call to action. Lancet. 2016;388:2307–20.
7. Filby A, Mcconville F, Portela A. What prevents quality midwifery care? A systematic mapping of barriers in low and middle income countries from the provider perspective. PLoS One. 2016;11:1–20.
8. Bradley S, McCourt C, Rayment J, Parmar D. Disrespectful intrapartum care during facility-based delivery in sub-Saharan Africa: a qualitative systematic review and thematic synthesis of women's perceptions and experiences. Soc Sci Med. 2016;169:157–70.
9. Mannava P, Durrant K, Fisher J, Chersich M, Luchters S. Attitudes and behaviours of maternal health care providers in interactions with clients: a systematic review. Glob Health. 2015;11
10. Ndwiga C, Warren CE, Ritter J, Sripad P, Abuya T. Exploring provider perspectives on respectful maternity care in Kenya: "Work with what you have". Reprod Health. 2017;14:99.
11. Burrowes S, Holcombe SJ, Jara D, Carter D, Smith K. Midwives' and patients' perspectives on disrespect and abuse during labor and delivery care in Ethiopia: a qualitative study. BMC Pregnancy Childbirth. 2017;17:263.
12. Mselle LT, Moland KM, Mvungi A, Evjen-Olsen B, Kohi TW. Why give birth in health facility? Users' and providers' accounts of poor quality of birth care in Tanzania. BMC Health Serv Res. 2013;13:174.
13. Shimpuku Y, Patil CL, Norr KF, Hill PD. Women's perceptions of childbirth experience at a Hospital in Rural Tanzania. Heal Care Women Int. 2013;34:461–81.
14. Kruk ME, Kujawski S, Mbaruku G, Ramsey K, Moyo W, Freedman LP. Disrespectful and abusive treatment during facility delivery in Tanzania: a facility and community survey. Health Policy Plan. 2018;33:e26–33.
15. Ratcliffe HL, Sando D, Lyatuu GW, Emil F, Mwanyika-Sando M, Chalamilla G, et al. Mitigating disrespect and abuse during childbirth in Tanzania: an exploratory study of the effects of two facility-based interventions in a large public hospital. Reprod Health. 2016;13:79.
16. McMahon S, George AS, Chebet JJ, Mosha IH, Mpembeni RN, Winch PJ. Experiences of and responses to disrespectful maternity care and abuse during childbirth: a qualitative study with women and men in Morogoro region, Tanzania. BMC Pregnancy Childbirth. 2014;14:268.
17. Sando D, Ratcliffe H, McDonald K, Spiegelman D, Lyatuu G, Mwanyika-Sando M, et al. The prevalence of disrespect and abuse during facility-based childbirth in urban Tanzania. BMC Pregnancy Childbirth. 2016;16:236. https://doi.org/10.1186/s12884-016-1019-4.
18. Shimoda K, Horiuchi S, Leshabari S, Shimpuku Y. Midwives' respect and disrespect of women during facility-based childbirth in urban Tanzania: a qualitative study. Reprod Health. 2018;15:1–13.
19. Otis KE, Brett JA. Barriers to hospital births: why do many Bolivian women give birth at home? Rev Panam Salud Pública. 2008;24:46–53. https://doi.org/10.1590/S1020-49892008000700006.
20. Physicians for Human Rights. Deadly Delays: Maternal mortality in Peru: A Rights-Based Approach to Safe Motherhood. 2007. https://s3.amazonaws.com/PHR_Reports/maternal-mortality-in-peru2007.pdf
21. United Nations Population Fund. The state of the world's midwifery: a universal pathway. Geneva: A women's right to health; 2014.
22. Ratcliffe HL, Sando D, Mwanyika-Sando M, Chalamilla G, Langer A, McDonald KP. Applying a participatory approach to the promotion of a culture of respect during childbirth. Reprod Health. 2016;13:80.
23. National Bureau of Statistics (NBS) and Office of Chief Government Statistician (OCGS). The United Republic of Tanzania. Dar es Salaam: Mortality and Health Report 2015; 2015.
24. Patton M. Qualitative Research & Evaluation Methods. Thousand Oaks: SAGE Publications; 2002.
25. World Health Organization. Definition of skilled health personnel providing care during childbirth. Geneva: The 2018 joint statement by WHO, UNFPA, UNICEF, ICM, ICN, FIGO and IPA; 2018.
26. Kvale S. Interviews: an introduction to qualitative research interviewing. Thousand Oaks: SAGE Publications; 1996.
27. Minichiello V, Aroni R, Timewell E, Alexander L. In-depth interviewing. 2nd edition. Longman: Pearson Education Australia; 1995.
28. Braun V, Clarke V. Using thematic analysis in psychology. Qual Res Psychol. 2006;3:77–101.
29. Attride-Stirling J. Thematic networks: an analytic tool for qualitative research. Qual Res. 2001;1:385–405.
30. Polit D, Beck C. Nursing research. 9th ed. Philadelphia: Lippincott Williams & Wilkins; 2012.
31. Warren N, Beebe M, Chase RP, Doumbia S, Winch PJ. Nègènègèn: sweet talk, disrespect, and abuse among rural auxiliary midwives in Mali. Midwifery. 2015;31:1073–80.
32. Shakibazadeh E , Namadian M, Bohren MA, Vogel JP, Rashidian A, Nogueira Pileggi V, Madeira S, Leathersich S, Tuncalp Ö, Oladapo OT, Souza JP, Guulmezoglu AM. Respectful care during childbirth in health facilities globally: a qualitative evidence synthesis. BJOG 2018;125: 932–42.
33. Kujawski SA, Freedman LP, Ramsey K, Mbaruku G, Mbuyita S, Moyo W, et al. Community and health system intervention to reduce disrespect and abuse during childbirth in Tanga region, Tanzania: a comparative before-and-after study. PLoS Med. 2017;14:1–16.

6

Attitudes toward sexual and reproductive health among adolescents and young people in urban and rural DR Congo

Fidèle Mbadu Muanda[1], Ndongo Parfait Gahungu[2], Francine Wood[3] and Jane T. Bertrand[4*]

Abstract

Background: In the Democratic Republic of Congo (DRC), onset of sexual intercourse is initiated during adolescence, however only two in ten sexually active unmarried women are using modern contraception. Improving adolescents' and young peoples' knowledge and practices related to sexual and reproductive health (SRH) is necessary to improve health outcomes. However, little is known about the SRH attitudes and needs among young people in the DRC. The study aims to contribute to the available evidence by examining adolescents' and young people's insights on their cultural norms, practices and attitudes towards SRH services.

Methods: Fourteen focus group discussions were conducted with a total of 224 adolescents and young people aged 15–24 years in urban and rural areas of the DRC. The topics discussed and age groups of participants differed somewhat in the urban and rural areas. Data were analyzed to identify themes in the participants' discussion of their attitudes towards SRH.

Results: Regardless of age differences, common themes emerged. Both in rural and urban areas premarital sex was largely sanctioned by peers but not adults; adolescents feared pregnancy and had limited knowledge of contraceptive methods. Many were misinformed that certain common pharmaceutical products (e.g., decaris) prevent pregnancy. Key barriers to accessing contraception from health facilities and pharmacies included shame and stigma; urban participants also cited cost and judgmental attitudes of health providers.

Conclusion: Addressing the SRH needs of adolescents and young people can have life-long protective benefits. Increasingly decision-makers and gatekeepers in the DRC are accepting the concept of providing SRH services and information to young people. This study shows the pressing need for information and services for young people in both urban and rural areas. The continued expansion SRH programming to all health zones and the developed of the National Strategic Plan for Health and Wellbeing of Adolescents and Youth 2016–2020 are steps toward that goal.

Keywords: Contraception - sexual and reproductive health, Adolescents - young people - Democratic Republic of Congo (DRC), Qualitative research, Focus group discussion

* Correspondence: bertrand@tulane.edu
[4]Department of Global Health Management and Policy, Tulane University School Public Health and Tropical Medicine, 1440 Canal Street, New Orleans, LA 70112, USA
Full list of author information is available at the end of the article

Plain English summary

Evidence suggests adolescents in developing countries face a range of challenges when they choose to access sexual and reproductive health services. We conducted a study in selected health zones in urban and rural areas in the Democratic Republic of Congo to explore cultural norms, attitudes, and practices of adolescents and young people regarding sexual and reproductive health (SRH) services. We held focus group discussions in selected health zones with young people aged 15–19 years in the urban areas and 18–24 years in rural areas. We found that young people in urban and rural areas have very similar attitudes towards SRH services, practices and cultural norms. Young people were accepting of premarital sex, feared pregnancy, had limited knowledge of contraceptive methods, erroneously used common pharmaceutical products to prevent pregnancy, experienced barriers when purchasing contraception from health facilities and pharmacies; and felt shame and stigma. Urban adolescents (only) experienced cost-related barriers; and only urban young women more frequently cited judgmental attitudes of providers. In the rural areas, adolescents felt that using contraception was the responsibility of the woman. In order to improve the use of services, these norms, practices and attitudes of the young people need to be taken into account and addressed in the design and delivery of programs to young people and adolescents.

Background

The Democratic Republic of Congo (DRC), with a population of 79.9 million, has the third highest total fertility rate (TFR) in the world; 6.5 children, varying from 5.4 (urban) to 7.3 (rural) [1]. By 2050, it will be the 8th most populous country in the world [2]. It is among the poorest countries of the world ranking 178 out of 188 countries for the Human Development Index [3].

Similar to other high fertility countries, the population of the country is young; 52% are under 15 years [1]. Early sexual experience and early childbearing contribute to maintaining high levels of fertility. According to the 2013–14 Demographic and Health Survey (DHS), 27% of women aged 15–19 have begun childbearing: 21% are mothers and 6% are currently pregnant [1]. Half of women initiate sexual intercourse by age 16.8; men on average at 17.6 years [1]. Modern contraceptive use is low: only two in ten sexually active unmarried women are using modern contraception, with the male condom being the most popular method [1]. Prior research indicates that adolescent women experience greater unmet need of contraception than their adult counterparts [4, 5].

Globally, the DRC ranks 8th in the top ten countries with the greatest number of women aged 20–24 who gave birth by age 18 [6]. Even within the region, the adolescent fertility rate (124 per 100 women aged 15–19 years) for the DRC is high in comparison to that of sub-Saharan Africa (109 per 1000) [7]. Consistent with these findings, modern contraceptive use among women 15–24 in the DRC (15.5%) is among the lowest in sub-Saharan Africa [1, 5].

Adolescent pregnancy and childbearing both threaten the health of the young woman and limit her future opportunities for education and employment. Research from multiple countries shows that adolescent pregnancy can be detrimental to the health of the mother and newborn because of the higher risk of maternal complications including postpartum hemorrhaging, eclampsia, preterm delivery and systemic infections [4, 8, 9]. Newborns have a higher chance of suffering low birth weight and early neonatal death. In addition, pregnancies during adolescence can have negative social and economic effects on families and communities [10, 11]. Despite the high proportion of adolescents and youth between ages 15–24 years, little research has been conducted on sexual and reproductive health (SRH) among this group in the DRC [12, 13]. Rather, much of the evidence on young people's contraception use and preferences for reproductive health services have been conducted in other countries [14–17].

Multiple factors contribute to high fertility norms in the DRC, including high adolescent fertility. Romaniuk points to social, cultural and economic factors: low levels of education among the population, especially girls; the low status of women, who become legally subordinate to their husbands at the time of marriage; few alternative economic opportunities; strong cultural norms that encourage large families; expectations from the husband's family for numerous children in return for the dowry paid for the woman, among others [18]. The DRC is a predominantly Christian country, with a large percentage belonging to the Catholic Church [1]. Although the dictates of the Catholic Church against "artificial contraception" are sometimes cited, the Catholic Church is not a major barrier to contraceptive service use [19].

In the past 5 years the number of programmatic initiatives to address adolescent and young people's sexual and reproductive health has steadily increased in the DRC, largely in urban areas (e.g., Kinshasa, the capital city) [20]. Whereas the DHS surveys provide valuable quantitative data on pregnancy rates, age at first sex, percentage using modern contraception, and related indicators, the emerging programmatic efforts will benefit from the rich, insightful findings that characterize qualitative research. To date, there is a dearth of qualitative research in the published literature on attitudes and behaviors among adolescents and young people in the DRC. The current article is intended as a means of building this literature.

The objective of this analysis is to present, compare and contrast the attitudes and perceptions of adolescents and young people in an urban and a rural context of the DRC on issues related to marriage, pre-marital sex, pregnancy prevention and contraceptive use.

Methodology

The data for this analysis came from two different studies - one conducted in the capital city of Kinshasa (urban), the other in three rural health zones participating in the ASSP (*Accès au Soins de Santé Primaire*) Project. A single individual (first author on this paper) served as study director for both, thus bringing consistency in the methodological approach to data collection and analysis. The objective of the primary study was to collect qualitative data from both urban and rural sites on barriers to contraceptive use among adult women and men in these communities, the results of which have been published elsewhere [12, 13]. We took advantage of having the research teams in the field (especially in the remote rural areas) to also explore SRH attitudes among young women and men in these same communities.

Although the age groups and topics discussed were not identical, the authors considered it valuable to compare and contrast the views of adolescents and youth from these very different settings on SRH issues.

Study setting and population

In Kinshasa, we purposely selected two health zones that were centrally located, densely populated and had better than average access to contraceptive services (to reduce the influence that lack of access could play on the non-use of contraceptive methods): Kalamu II and Bumbu.

In each of three rural provinces – Maniema, Kasai, North Ubangi – we selected one "strong" and one "weak" health zone, based on a widely used measure of output in family planning programs, couple-years protection (CYP) [21]:

1. Maniema: Alunguli (strong) and Kampene (weak)
2. Kasai: Mutoto (strong) and Mweka (weak)
3. North Ubangi: Bili (strong) and Bosobolo (weak)

We were interested in comparing the attitudes of young people from urban and rural areas, given the differential fertility of the two. For example, the adolescent birth rate in Kinshasa as of 2013–14 was 67 per 1000 women 15–

19 years old, compared to Kasai (148 per 1000), Maniema (161 per 1000), and Nord Ubangi (166 per 1000) [1].

Recruitment

In Kinshasa, the data collection team worked with nurses to invite a convenience sample of adolescents to participate in individual and confidential interviews to determine their eligibility. Invitations to participate in the focus group discussions (FGD) were extended to adolescents who fulfilled the eligibility criteria: to be 15–19 years old, unmarried, and sexually active (have had sexual intercourse within the last 3 months). In the rural area the research team with the assistance of community leaders recruited youth from the community who met the following eligibility criteria: 18–24 years old, unmarried, with no children.

FGD guide

The framework of Sexual and Reproductive Health Lifestages provides a theoretical basic for the topics covered; the phases included pre-sexual, sexual & pre-reproductive, and sexual & reproductive [22]. Each question from the guide would allow for participants to directly answer the question or make related comments not necessarily on the guide (e.g., provider attitudes toward adolescents who seek contraceptive services).

Because the research team anticipated that adolescents and young people living in urban areas would have greater exposure to issues related to contraception than those living in remote rural areas, the urban FGD guide focused on: knowledge of contraceptive methods, teenage pregnancy; obstacles and barriers to contraceptive use; attitudes to teenage pregnancy and the use of contraceptive methods; and the social acceptability of contraceptive use. The rural FGD guide included a series of topics that would provide greater context to sexual behavior and need for contraception, such as the desire for a family, preferred family size, attitudes toward pre-marital sex, and adolescent's motivation to engage in premarital sex; the guide also touched on knowledge of modern methods, and perceptions of provider attitudes towards adolescents' use of contraceptives.

Data collection

The data collection team for each FGD consisted of a moderator and a note-taker who were experienced in FGD. Prior to the data collection, they participated in a refresher training on FGD methodology, the study protocol, questions to cover, translation of specific questions into the local language, and pre-testing of the guides.

The urban FGD were conducted in February 2015, the rural FGD in August 2015. In Kinshasa, we conducted eight FGD among males and females aged 15–19 years old with 10 participants per group. In the rural area four FGD were organized in each of 6 health zones, with 12 participants each. The focus group method allowed all, regardless of their ability to read or write, to participate. In both the urban and rural areas, the groups were composed of members of similar age, sex, and marital status. The homogeneity of each group created an atmosphere where participants were comfortable and readily shared their perspectives.

Data analysis

The sessions were conducted in the local language and audiotaped. The transcribers listened to the tapes in the local language and then transcribed them into French. Subsequently the research team coded the participants' responses by theme and sub-theme, to facilitate thematic content analysis. Once the data were coded, the team developed a matrix that captured the key ideas by theme, location, and gender. In addition, they identified verbatim quotes that succinctly captured common responses for use in the article. In this paper, we present key findings for urban and rural groups separately, indicating the gender of the respondents. Unpublished reports of these findings are available in French [21, 23].

Ethical approval

The study received IRB approval from Tulane University [urban (14-669918); rural (717117)] and the University of Kinshasa School of Public Health [urban (ESP/CE/057/2014); rural (ESP/CE/0901/2015)].

Prior to data collection, the moderator clarified study objectives and ensured confidentiality for participants. Each participant in the urban and rural health zones signed a consent form, prior to participation in the FGD.

Results

Characteristics of study participants

In total, we recruited 224 participants: 112 females and 112 males. In Kinshasa, there were a total of 80 participants aged 15–19 years: 40 males aged and 40 females. All participants were unmarried and majority (90%) had some secondary school education. Their median age was 18 years and majority reported not having children (94%).

In the rural area, 144 participants aged 18–24 years were recruited: 72 females and 72 males. We did not collect data on the socio demographic characteristics of the rural participants. However, the data from the 2013–2014 DHS show that 43% of young people aged

15–24 years from rural areas of these provinces have some secondary or higher education and 63% are employed [1]. The DHS also shows that Kinshasa has the highest percentage of young people with secondary or higher education (89.9%) and North Ubangi has the lowest (43.4%) [1]. The DRC as a country is predominantly Christian, including Catholics, Protestants, Evangelicals, and Kimbanguists [1].

Urban population

Both males and females aged 15–19 from Kinshasa were very open and forthcoming with their attitudes on multiple issues related to pregnancy and contraceptive use.

Attitudes towards pregnancy

Pregnancy was a recurrent theme in the FGD with the urban population. Overall, adolescent girls and boys were afraid of pregnancy occurring at an early age.

I would like to be older before getting pregnant, because then I can take better care of my child. (Female, Kalamu II)

I would rather that I am older before I give birth, because I must first study. If I get pregnant today, I will dishonor my parents. (Female, Bumbu)

I think it's not good get pregnant when we are very young because we will have complications at the birth. (Female, Bumbu)

I have a child now, when I gave birth I lost all my friends, I have no time to go out and I take care of my child by myself. (Female, Kalamu II)

If you are young and you have a child but you live with your parents, it is a burden for them because they still have to take care of your child and yourself too. (Female, Bumbu)

I prefer to have a child later because if I have a child now, I will lose the chance to marry a good husband, the man I can love. (Female, Kalamu II)

On the other hand, some adolescent girls who preferred to have an early pregnancy explained that:

I would like to give birth very early because when the age advances, there are complications to bring [a baby] into the world. (Female, Bumbu)

The advantage of giving birth early is that even if I die very early, at least I will have left a child on the earth. (Female, Kalamu II)

I think that giving birth very early has an advantage. My big sister gave birth very early and now her child is 10 years old and they can grow up together. (Female, Kalamu II)

It is not good to delay the first pregnancy, because of menopause. In time it reached our mothers at the age of 45, but nowadays menopause could as early as 30 and 35, which is why girls prefer to give birth very early. (Female, Bumbu)

For the adolescent boys, their fear of pregnancy stemmed from the financial implications, the reaction of their parents, the acquisition of a "bad" reputation in the neighborhood, and dishonor and shame pregnancy would bring to their family especially their parents. Some shared that pregnancy could interrupt their education and that of the girl.

We're afraid of impregnating someone's daughter because we are young and do not have opportunities. This may be a burden for our parents. (Male, Kalamu II)

I'm really scared to make a girl pregnant. The news is going to spread everywhere and it will be a disgrace to my parents and myself. (Male, Bumbu)

In some families, as soon as you impregnate someone's daughter pregnant, you have to compensate her and sometimes we can even go to jail. (Male, Kalamu II)

In the case where a girl became pregnant, some of the adolescent boys shared that they would marry her.

If I impregnate a girl, I must marry her because she's the woman I love. (Male, Bumbu)

If a girl is pregnant with my child, I will only take the child. However, if she is well educated, then I will marry her. (Male, Kalamu II)

If a woman had a prior pregnancy, majority of the adolescent boys would not marry her for a variety of reasons.

I am afraid to marry a woman who has already given birth. I am afraid that the father of the child will want to have a relationship with the woman. (Male, Kalamu II)

I cannot marry a woman who has already given birth because children are unnecessary burdens, I will marry a woman who has not yet given birth. (Male, Bumbu)

I will marry a woman who has children only with me and not a woman who already has a child. (Male, Kalamu II)

It is not certain that my wife's child will be grateful after I have raised him/her. (Male, Bumbu)

My parents always told me not to marry a woman who already has a child. (Male, Bumbu)

Barriers to modern contraceptive use

In the urban population, both adolescent males and females experienced barriers that prevent them from accessing and using modern contraception. Both groups mentioned lack of information or misinformation of contraceptives, as well as community disapproval. Adolescent girls cited the judgmental attitudes of health providers; adolescent boys mentioned fear of side effects and stigma surrounding contraception use.

Lack of information and misinformation about contraceptive methods Although both males and females had some knowledge about contraceptive methods, the FGD suggest that lack of knowledge and misconceptions about contraception are barriers to use. Adolescent girls seemed to have more knowledge of the different types of contraceptives than males; most could name at least one method, including condoms, pills, the Depo injection or the implant, in that order. However, they also cited pharmaceutical products, such as antimalarial (Quinine and Tetracycline) and deworming medications (Decaris, Vermox, Tanzol), which they believed to prevent pregnancy but do not. They also erroneously named traditional methods (calendar/rhythm and withdrawal) as modern.

I know girls who use condoms to avoid getting pregnant and also to avoid certain diseases. There are also girls who take medication like decaris adult or child. (Female, Kalamu II)

Virtually all the adolescent boys were familiar with the condom but were far less familiar with other modern methods. Some had knowledge about natural methods (withdrawal and the calendar method). Similar to adolescent girls, adolescent males incorrectly cited pharmaceutical products- Decaris, Tetracycline and Vermox- as modern methods. Additionally some males indicated other ways to avoid pregnancy: having the girl drink a lot of water or sit over a basin after sexual intercourse to get rid of the semen in her vagina.

When I have sex without a condom, I drink a lot of water and the girl drinks a lot of water. We do not use drugs because medications can give complications and water does not. (Male, Bumbu)

I know a drug, Decaris, which a woman takes after sex. Once she urinates, there will be nothing left. (Male, Bumbu)

Some males further explained that adolescents lacked information on where to access contraceptive methods.

Some women do not use modern methods of contraception due to ignorance, because they have no idea where to go to get them. (Male, Kalamu II)

Attitudes towards contraceptives Both adolescent boys and girls had similar attitudes toward contraception. Overall, most girls felt that using a contraceptive method to prevent pregnancy was smart.

I use contraceptive methods and my friends think I'm smart because many of them have children. (Female, Bumbu)

They will think we are smart, because the person who is not intelligent is the one who does not protect herself and can get pregnant. (Female, Bumbu)

Most adolescent girls also felt that unmarried adolescent girls have the right to use contraceptives because they have sex and thus need to prevent early and unwanted pregnancy.

All girls have the right to use contraceptive methods to protect themselves against diseases. (Female, Kalamu II)

We, girls, have the right to protect ourselves from getting pregnant. (Female, Bumbu)

A girl who is not yet married must use contraceptive methods to protect herself from early pregnancy because she also has sex like married people. (Female, Kalamu II)

All adolescents in the urban FGD knew someone who had used a contraceptive method, citing the condom, pill, Depo injection and implant.

I know a young woman in the neighborhood who uses the condom to avoid getting pregnant. (Female, Bumbu)

To avoid getting pregnant, I know a girl who uses depo provera. (Female, Kalamu II)

My big sister uses the depo provera injection. (Female, Kalamu II)

By contrast, a minority of adolescent girls felt that only married women should use contraceptives.

I think a girl who is not yet married cannot use a contraceptive method. (Female, Kalamu II)

Regarding adolescent boys, the majority felt that contraceptive use was important to protect against early pregnancy and STI/HIV.

Condoms are important and it's good to use them because they protect against diseases and early pregnancies. (Male, Bumbu)

For me, I think the condom really protects against pregnancies, because prostitutes always use the condom and do not get pregnant. (Male, Kalamu II)

The condom protects against pregnancy because after sex, sperm remains in the plastic and does not go into the woman's body, and the woman cannot get pregnant. (Male, Bumbu)

Most of these adolescent boys indicated that their preferred method was the condom. But paradoxically, most expressed a negative attitude towards using condoms.

People say that the condom reduces sexual pleasure. With some girls, as soon as you show her a condom, she reacts by saying that you suspect she has a disease. (Male, Kalamu II)

For me the condom does not protect completely because it sometimes tears during sex especially if it is not of good quality. (Male, Kalamu II)

Me, when I have sex with a girl with a condom, I do not feel pleasure that's why I do not use condom. (Male, Bumbu)

Some boys shared that their use of condoms was dependent on the nature of the sexual encounter.

I use the condom only when I'm with another girl I do not know or a prostitute, but I do not use it when I'm with my girlfriend. (Male, Kalamu II)

I can meet a girl along the way and I am attracted. If I must have sex at this time, I am not going to use the condom because I did not plan to meet that girl that day (Male, Bumbu)

Fear of side effects emerged as another reason for an adolescent's nonuse of modern contraceptives.

We are often told that the lubricant from the condom causes disease. Moreover even when you open the condom you smell a bad odor, it proves that the lubricant on the condom has microbes. (Male, Kalamu II)

Community disapproval and stigma Several adolescent girls shared that females experience shame and embarrassment when they attempt to purchase contraceptives from health centers or the pharmacy, due to community disapproval of adolescents' participating in sexual activities.

I think girls are ashamed go and get condoms in a health center. (Female, Bumbu)

Girls are sometimes ashamed of going to the pharmacy to buy the condom or the pill in front of everyone,

people will think they have sex and that's why they want to protect themselves. (Female, Kalamu II)

One adolescent girl shared that at times she feels shame from even bringing up the topic of contraceptives to family members:

We cannot talk to family members, they may think that I'm having sex, on the contrary I feel comfortable speaking with the big sisters [other girls or women] in the neighborhood (Female, Kalamu II)

Similarly, adolescent boys experienced embarrassment and shame from buying condoms and going to the health centers.

When we go to buy condoms in a pharmacy and meet an adult who came to buy medicine, we are ashamed to go inside and buy the condoms. (Male, Kalamu II)

Perceptions of attitudes and knowledge of health providers The anticipated reception from health providers was another reason for the nonuse of modern contraception and services at the health center. Many adolescent girls shared that personnel at pharmacies treated them poorly, at times were indiscrete and were reluctant to sell them modern contraceptives.

I know of girls who have purchased contraceptives in pharmacies, but sometimes when you want to buy condoms, the pharmacist asks us to tell the person who sent us, they prefer to sell to adults. (Female, Bumbu)

For certain contraceptives, the pharmacist does not sell them, he says that in case of problems it is he that will be arrested. (Female, Kalamu II)

Instead, adolescent girls preferred to visit health centers because they felt that the doctors and nurses were more knowledgeable and had a higher level of training on reproductive health services in comparison to pharmacists.

I prefer the health center because I can meet with a nurse, but at the pharmacy that's not the case, because pharmacists let other people sell in their place and these people do not know the drug. (Female, Bumbu)

At the health center, the doctors will examine you and then he will prescribe you medication while in the pharmacy you go directly to purchase drugs without the doctor's prescription. (Female, Kalamu II)

I prefer the health center, because it gives information on how to protect against pregnancies and disease. (Female, Bumbu)

Even though adolescent girls preferred health centers, they cited the unwillingness of many health personnel, including doctors and nurses, to provide modern contraception to adolescents.

For us minors, it is difficult for nurses or doctors to give us contraceptive methods. (Female, Bumbu)

Cost of modern contraception A number of adolescent girls and boys cited cost of modern contraceptives and the inability to afford the services at the health center as barriers to their use. The prices of methods and services vary depending on the location of the service. Several adolescent females shared that:

Some girls lack money to go to the health center. (Female, Kalamu II)

Other contraceptive methods are expensive and the price varies from US $10 to US $20, which is not within our reach. (Female, Kalamu II)

Adolescent males shared the same sentiment; one participant suggested that condoms be given out for free.

I think that women do not use these methods because they do not have the means to obtain them, they have no money. (Male, Bumbu)

For me, the condom must be free. Sometimes, I even don't have 100 Fc ($0.10 U.S.). At the moment when I want to have sex with my girlfriends, I do it without a condom. (Male, Kalamu II)

Rural population

While adolescents from the urban areas were aged 15–19 years, the respondents from the rural areas were aged 15–24 years. Regardless of the age difference, common themes were identified in the urban and rural FGDs. Both discussed barriers to the use of contraceptive methods, perceptions of provider attitudes towards adolescents' use of contraceptives and

the social acceptability of the use contraception among adolescents. In addition, young people in the rural FGD expressed their views on their preferred family size and marriage, their motivation to engage in premarital sex and the social norms around premarital sex.

Desire for a marriage and pregnancy

The majority of the young women in the rural areas preferred to get married between the ages of 18 and 20 years.

I must marry when I am about 20 years old because it is the age of maturity, and I can give birth without problems. At this age, I will be an adult and I will be able to manage my home well. (Female, Alungi)

I will get married after high school so that my future husband respects me. Also then I can go to university, find work and earn a living. (Female, Bili)

I want to get married at 19 because I want to give birth early. (Female, Bosobolo)

The young men participating in the FGD shared that they preferred to get married between the ages of 20 and 25.

I prefer to get married at 20 years old because first, I need to go to school and find a job before I get married in order to feed my family; I have to have money. (Male, Bosobolo)

We want to get married at married at 24 because we think we will be mature at this age. (Male, Mweka)

A minority of young men and women wanted to get married early so they could have children early.

I'm going to get married quickly because I am afraid of dying early and impregnating someone's daughter. I want to be a young dad like my parents who were married at a young age. (Male, Alunguli)

The majority of the young women wanted to have more than 6 children. Many who desired large families believed that with more children, they are more likely to have multiple sources of financial support in their old age; others felt it would help combat the fear of losing a child at a young age.

I also want to have many children because among them, one can become a mason and build a house for us [parents], another can plow/cultivate a field, another can even go study and go abroad where he can properly support his family and our future will be assured. (Female, Mutoto)

Males gave similar responses:

I must give birth to more children, 8 or 9, because not all of them will live, there will also be those who die. (Male, Bosobolo)

I will have many children because one of the children may have lots of money and will help me in my old age. (Male, Alunguli)

A minority of young women and men wanted fewer than six children because of financial and economic reasons:

I will only have three children because I will be capable of providing for them, raising them because if you have many children, you need a lot of money too. (Female, Bili)

"I think I will have 4 children because here in Mweka it is not easy to find work, you must have few children to allow you to educate them and to feed them well" (Female, Mweka)

I will not have many children because life is expensive, it is necessary that we do not follow our parents, me I would like to take good care of my children. (Male, Mweka)

I will not have more than five children. If they are many, it will be difficult to finance their education, to feed them, to lodge and to clothe them. If I am not able to bear the costs, then they could find themselves in the street. (Male, Alunguli)

Attitudes towards premarital sex

The majority of young men and women had a favorable opinion towards their peers who engaged in sexual activity before marriage for multiple reasons:

For me having sex with boys before marriage is a proof that one is beautiful because the men come to you. (Female, Kampene)

We live together, if you do not have sex like the others, we will laugh at you and say that in marriage you will not be a good wife, that's why we encourage sex before marriage. (Female, Mweka)

Girls have sex because they seek to practice before marriage, they do so out of curiosity and so that they are loved by the boy. (Female, Mutoto)

People think that if we do not have sex before marriage, we will not have children in the marriage and will have difficulty conceiving (Female, Mweka)

Young women in the community may engage in sex for financial benefits and lack of parental supervision.

Our parents are retired and they cannot do anything for us. The boy provides money, I know it comes at a cost, because he is not a family member (brother/father). When he asks to have sex, I will agree. (Female, Alunguli)

Some girls have sex because they imitate their colleagues who do it. When they see their girlfriends wear clothes that they bought with the money they got from boys, they will mimic them. (Female, Bili)

Because parents don't monitor their children and the bad company that girls keep, they [girls] have sex before marriage (Female, Mutoto)

Young men were also favorable to premarital sex - out of curiosity, peer pressure, a test of virility, a chance to gain experience, and their reward for giving a girl gifts.

Me, I'm doing it [having sex] because I'm curious to know about the body of the girl and also to know if I am sexually active. (Male, Alunguli)

In our community, we are not waiting for marriage before having sex. When we see that our friends do it, we also begin to imitate that. (Male, Mweka)

A boy must have sex to test his manhood. His body must be in motion to be in good health. And girls respect us when we have sex. (Male, Bili)

We have sex because if we are not experienced, the woman can leave us because of sexual dissatisfaction. She will look for another man to satisfy her and so we must learn now so we don't get a divorce one day. (Male, Kampene)

We sometimes have sex before marriage because we are told that if we do not have sex before we are 18, we will be impotent and people will mock us on our wedding day. (Male, Mutoto)

I have sex because girls ask for money and if they don't have sex, then we waste/lose our money. (Male, Bosobolo)

By contrast, a few young men and women had an unfavorable opinion of premarital sex. Their explanations focused on the health consequences, religious reasons and stigma surrounding premarital sex.

If your friends learn that you have sex with boys, they will consider you a prostitute and you will feel shame. (Female, Bosobolo)

My friends tell me not to have sex before marriage because there are many diseases in the world. (Male, Bili)

I sometimes advise friends to finish their studies before having sex because they can jeopardize their future if the girl becomes pregnant, and then religion forbids sex. (Male, Bili)

Whereas the majority of young people accepted premarital sex, they felt that adults in the community disapproved of sex.

When the mothers of the village see us with boys, often they are not happy. They advise us to finish our studies and be careful about unwanted pregnancies. (Female, Bosobolo)

Adults are unhappy when they see us with boys and tell us that sex causes STIs and HIV. (Female, Mutoto)

The young men indicated that adult disapproval of premarital sex stemmed from socio-cultural factors and risks associated with sex.

Parents do not want their children to have sex before marriage, especially if their child is a girl. The custom here is that if the girl is a virgin when she gets married, the girl's parents are given a gift, a goat. It is an honor for the parents and for the church where the girl prays. (Male, Mutoto)

Our parents often tell us this: we [the parents] do not understand why young people today want to have sex before marriage when in our time we did not do it. (Male, Bili)

Adults are not happy [if their children have sex] because parents have suffered a lot to raise their children. They expect to be helped by their children in their old age. With sex before marriage, young people are at risk of contracting diseases and compromising their future. (Male, Bosobolo)

A few of the males cited cases where the adults in the community might condone sex before marriage:

An adult in my village told me to have sex with the girls so that they would respect me. The old man said, if you do, you will be a strong and powerful man and the girls will respect you especially if it is satisfying. (Male, Alunguli)

For some irresponsible parents, when their daughter is friends with a boy who has money, they say nothing and they sometimes encourage them. (Male, Mweka)

Barriers to modern contraceptive use

Young people in the rural population experienced barriers to contraceptive use similar to those found in Kinshasa: lack of knowledge and misinformation of contraceptive methods, negative attitudes towards contraceptives, and judgmental attitudes among health providers.

Lack of knowledge and misinformation The young women and men in the rural FGD were knowledgeable about some forms of contraception. Young women tended to know at least one method, including condoms, the calendar method, Depo injection, implants, the pill, abstinence, and withdrawal. Young women did not express a preference for any one method over another: their choice would depend on the situation. Young people incorrectly cited some pharmaceutical products, such as Decaris, Paracetamol, Tanzol Ampicillin as contraceptives. A few sought advice from parents, doctors, nurses and friends.

> Me, when I need to avoid pregnancy, I go to my sister's house in the neighborhood who tells me this: just take 2 or 3 paracetamol tablets before intercourse and you will not get pregnant. (Female, Bosobolo)

> Often I go to my mother who teaches me how to calculate my dates [calendar method]. (Female, Kampene)

The methods most commonly mentioned by the young men were condoms, rhythm, withdrawal and abstinence.

> I am positive that my friends have sex. I just advise them to wear a condom to prevent pregnancy or disease. (Male, Mweka)

> The most appropriate method for us boys is the condom. This method is good especially for girls who have an irregular cycle because we do not know their cycle. (Male, Bili)

> To avoid pregnancy, we must also follow the dates of the girls because during the month, the woman has a bad [fertile] period. (Male, Bosobolo)

> There is a method of throwing semen on the ground instead of directly in the female organ [vagina]. (Male, Mutoto)

For information or advice, young men would consult health providers at health centers, their parents or teachers.

> When we need information, we will go in the health facilities to speak with the health staff. At school, we must consult the teachers. They are experts, they tell us how to protect ourselves against diseases. (Male, Kampene)

> I ask my family members because they have had children before and they have a lot of information on how to avoid sex. (Male, Bili)

> When I need information on how to avoid a pregnancy, I go to a health facility with doctors or nurses. They advise us to use the condom during sex to avoid pregnancy. (Male, Bili)

Attitudes towards contraceptive methods Male attitudes were a major barrier to use. Most young men agreed that it was important to use contraceptives but felt it was the girl's responsibility to prevent pregnancy.

> It's the girl who is responsible for the contraception. She knows her monthly cycle and she must say when she cannot have sex with a man because she is in her fertile period. (Male, Mweka)

> It is the girl who is responsible because she can refuse the gifts given to her by the boy, also she knows her menstral cycle. (Male, Kampene)

A few males who thought it was also their own responsibility:

> The boy is responsible because he asked the girl to have sex. He must take every precaution to avoid pregnancy. (Male, Bosobolo)

Perceptions of provider attitudes towards youths' contraceptive use Majority of the young women felt that the health providers had a negative attitude towards their use of contraception, which discouraged them from using services:

> At the hospital, I was getting the Depo Provera injection. The doctor asked me if I had given birth before: I told him no and he forbade me to continue taking it. He said it is forbidden to girls who have not yet given birth, because it makes them sterile. He told me to keep track of my dates (calendar method). (Female, Bosobolo)

> The nurses do not receive us well because when we ask questions, they see us as bad girls who seek prostitution, thus I cannot ask the nurses or the doctors. (Female, Mweka)

Conversely, young males had mixed experiences with providers:

> The providers receive us well at the health center, they like people who come asking for advice on preventing pregnancy. (Male, Mweka)

One day I went to the health center to ask for information about sex, a nurse who scolded me. And so, I will not be returning over there for fear of being scolded again. (Male, Alunguli)

Discussion

The bustling city of Kinshasa with over 11 million people and the relatively isolated rural areas of the DRC seem worlds apart, yet the SRH problems facing young people are surprisingly similar. Despite differences in age of the participants and specific topics covered, this research points to common experiences: premarital sex largely sanctioned by peers but not adults, fear of pregnancy, limited knowledge of contraceptive methods, misinformation that certain common pharmaceutical products (e.g., decaris) prevent pregnancy, barriers to accessing contraceptives from health facilities and pharmacies, shame and stigma.

A few differences did emerge. Urban participants cited cost as a barrier to contraception, whereas rural participants did not. Contraceptives are provided free of charge in rural health zones supported by ASSP. Similarly, only female participants in the urban areas mentioned the judgmental attitude of health personal as a barrier to contraception use, whereas both males and females in rural areas did. Rural participants perceived contraceptive use as a female's domain, whereas urban participants did not discuss this topic.

We acknowledge several limitations of the research. The FGD guides covered slightly different topics and the focus group participants differed in age in the urban and rural areas. Findings from FGD cannot be generalized to the larger population. The selection of "strong" versus "weak" health zones based on FP performance used to select the communities in the larger study may have limited relevance to SRH among young people. The process of transcribing audiotapes from the local language in French, then producing quotations in English may distort the original meaning.

Our findings are consistent with other studies from the DRC. The 2013–2014 DHS showed that men and women want large families of 7 and 6 children respectively [1]. The DHS study also demonstrates that awareness of contraception is high [1]. The recent PMA2020 report for Kinshasa shows a gap between the average onset of sexual activity (17.3 years), and the first use of contraception (20.5 years) [24]. The DHS reported that 27% of 15–19 years old women have begun child bearing [1]. Another quantitative survey showed that the majority (54%) of unmarried sexually active youth did not use contraception because they were not married [25]. A qualitative study in the DRC among women aged 15–35 years revealed that women frequently used deworming or anti-malarial medicines after

sex as a form of emergency contraception [26]. Similar to young people in our study, qualitative research from Eastern DRC among adults yielded highly similar results to the current study on SRH themes [27]. Adults also shared similar concerns and experiences related to shame and stigma associated with using contraception [12, 13, 27].

Our findings are also similar to SRH results reported elsewhere in sub-Saharan Africa. A study in Zimbabwe found that adolescents feared pregnancy and its potential social, financial, educational and health impact [28]. A systematic review conducted to explore the limits of modern contraceptive use found that lack of knowledge hindered use [29]. In Ethiopia, a study found that among health workers with an unfavorable attitude towards providing FP to adolescents, some indicated setting up penal rules and regulations against adolescents that practice premarital sex [30]. Attitudes of health care providers discouraged young men and women from seeking care [30–32]. Similar to our findings, stigma and shame discouraged Tanzanian adolescents from seeking reproductive health care [33].

Prior to 2015, SRH programming in the DRC was very limited, even in Kinshasa. Only 20 of 516 health zones nationwide offered any type of SRH service for young people. As of 2017, however, 120 health zones have funding for SRH programming [20]. The PNSA coordinated the development of a National Strategic Plan for the Health and Wellbeing of Adolescents and Youth 2016–2020, which provides a vision for future programming and has attracted external donor funding to this largely neglected area [34]. As shown in this study, the needs for information and services are great in both urban and rural areas. Yet in a country with widespread resistance only a few years ago, SRH programming is gaining increasing acceptance among political decision-makers, community opinion leaders, and other gatekeepers.

Conclusion

Although the DRC has achieved gains in acceptance in SRH programming, our findings signal a pressing need for information and services for young people in both urban and rural areas. The widespread acceptance of premarital sex among adolescents, the limited knowledge of contraception methods, and misinformation that certain pharmaceutical products prevent pregnancy increase their risk for pregnancy and STIs. The findings also suggest that fear of pregnancy, the judgmental attitude of health providers, and fear of side effects are major concerns among adolescents and young people within the urban and rural areas. Addressing the SRH needs of adolescents and young people can have lifelong protective benefits. As DRC continues to expand its implementation of SRH programming, it is vital to address the persistent needs and challenges of adolescents and young people for access to modern contraception and other SRH services.

Abbreviations

ASSP: Accès au Soins de Santé Primaire; DHS: Demographic and Health Survey; DRC: Democratic Republic of Congo; FGD: Focus group discussion; FP: Family planning; HIV: Human immunodeficiency virus; PMA2020: Performance Monitoring and Accountability 2020; PNSA: Programme National de Santé de L'Adolescent (National Program of Youth and Adolescent Health); SRH: Sexual and reproductive health; STI: Sexually transmitted infections

Acknowledgements

The authors would like to thank the Bill and Melinda Gates Foundation for support of the urban study (grant number 2015-OPP1117997); and the United Kingdom Department for International Development (DFID) for funding the rural data collection (grant number IMA-DFID/ASSP102012-1/Tulane).

Funding

The research received funding from the Bill and Melinda Gates Foundation for the urban study (grant number 2015-OPP1117997); and from the United Kingdom Department for International Development (DFID) for the rural area (grant number IMA-DFID/ASSP102012-1/Tulane).

Authors' contributions

MM and JTB designed the study and developed the study tools and recruitment strategy. MM and PGN coordinated data collection, supervised transcription of the audiotapes and translation to French, and analyzed the data. MM and JTB contributed to the interpretation of the findings. JTB and FW wrote the manuscript and all authors reviewed and approved the publication for publication. All authors read and approved the final manuscript.

Competing interests

The authors declare that they have no competing interests.

Author details

[1]Programme National de Santé de la Reproduction (National Program for Reproductive Health) and Programme National de Santé de l'Adolescent (National Program for Adolescent Health), Ministry of Health, Avenue des Cliniques n 43/cliniques kinoises, Commune de la Gombe, Kinshasa, Democratic Republic of Congo. [2]L'Institut Supérieur de Dévéloppement Rural, Avenue des Cliniques n 43/cliniques kinoises, Commune de la Gombe, Kinshasa, Democratic Republic of Congo. [3]Department of Global Community Health and Behavioral Sciences, Tulane University School Public Health and Tropical Medicine, 1440 Canal Street, New Orleans, LA 70112, USA. [4]Department of Global Health Management and Policy, Tulane University School Public Health and Tropical Medicine, 1440 Canal Street, New Orleans, LA 70112, USA.

References

1. Ministère du Plan et Suivi de la Mise en oeuvre de la Révolution de la Modernité (MPSMRM/Congo); Ministère de la Santé Publique (MSP/Congo); ICF International. Enquête Démographique et de Santé en République Démocratique du Congo 2013–2014. Rockville: 2014.
2. Population Reference Bureau (PRB): 2016 World Population Data Sheet. 2016. http://www.worldpopdata.org. Accessed 1 Apr 2017.
3. United Nations Development Programme, (UNDP): Human Development Report 2016: Human Development for everyone. 2016. http://hdr.undp.org/en. Accessed 15 Jan 2018.
4. Darroch JE, Woog V, Bankole A, Ashford L: Adding it up: costs and benefits of meeting the contraceptive needs of adolescents. 2016.
5. MacQuarrie K, Mallick L, Allen C. Sexual and Reproductive Health in Early and Later Adolescence: DHS Data on Youth Age 10–19; 2017. p. 45.
6. Mulumeoderhwa M. 'A girl who gets pregnant or spends the night with a man is no longer a girl': forced marriage in the eastern Democratic Republic of Congo. Sexuality & Culture. 2016;20(4):1042–62.
7. United Nations, Department of Economic and Social Affairs: World Fertility Patterns 2015 - Data Booklet (ST/ESA/SER.A/370). 2015.
8. Cavazos-Rehg PA, Krauss MJ, Spitznagel EL, Bommarito K, Madden T, Olsen MA, Subramaniam H, Peipert JF, Bierut LJ. Maternal age and risk of labor and delivery complications. Maternal Child Health J. 2015;19(6):1202–11.
9. Edilberto L, Mengjia L. Adolescent pregnancy: a review of the evidence. New York: United Nations Population Fund; 2013.
10. LeGrand TK, Mbacké CS. Teenage pregnancy and child health in the urban Sahel. Stud Fam Plan. 1993;1:137–49.
11. Shahabuddin A, Nöstlinger C, Delvaux T, Sarker M, Bardají A, De Brouwere V, Broerse JE. What influences adolescent girls' decision-making regarding contraceptive methods use and childbearing? A qualitative exploratory study in Rangpur District, Bangladesh. PLoS One. 2016;11(6):e0157664.
12. Muanda MF, Ndongo GP, Messina LJ, Bertrand JT. Barriers to modern contraceptive use in rural areas in DRC. Culture, Health & Sexuality. 2017;19:1–13.
13. Muanda M, Ndongo PG, Taub LD, Bertrand JT. Barriers to modern contraceptive use in Kinshasa, DRC. PLoS One. 2016;11(12):e0167560.
14. Erulkar AS, Onoka CJ, Phiri A. What is youth-friendly? Adolescents' preferences for reproductive health services in Kenya and Zimbabwe. Afr J Reprod Health. 2005;1:51–8.
15. Radovich E, Dennis ML, Wong KL, Ali M, Lynch CA, Cleland J, Owolabi O, Lyons-Amos M, Benova L. Who meets the contraceptive needs of young women in sub-Saharan Africa? J Adolesc Health. 2017;62(3):273–80.
16. Biddlecom AE, Singh S, Munthali A. Adolescents' views of and preferences for sexual and reproductive health services in Burkina Faso, Ghana, Malawi and Uganda. Afr J Reprod Health. 2007;11(3):99–110.
17. Amuyunzu-Nyamongo M, Biddlecom AE, Ouedraogo C, Woog V. Qualitative evidence on adolescents' views of sexual and reproductive health in sub-Saharan Africa. Occasional Report. 2005;16. The Alan Guttmacher Institute.
18. Romaniuk A. Persistence of high fertility in tropical Africa: the case of the Democratic Republic of the Congo. Popul Dev Rev. 2011;37(1):1–28.
19. Izale K, Govender I, Fina JL, Tumbo J: Factors that influence contraceptive use amongst women in Vanga health district, Democratic Republic of Congo. African journal of primary health care & family medicine 2014, 6(1):1–7.
20. Kwete D, Binanga A, Mukaba T, Nemuandjare T, Mbadu MF, Kyungu MT, Sutton P, Bertrand JT: Family planning in the Democratic Republic of the Congo: encouraging momentum, Formidable Challenges. 2018. Manuscript Submitted for Publication.
21. Muanda M, des cas É. Analyse de l'offre et de la demande de la Planification Familiale dans les zones de santé appuyées par le projet ASSP (Accès au Soins de Santé Primaire) en RDC. République Démocratique Du Congo: Ministère de la Santé Publique; 2016.
22. USAID. Evidence to action (E2A): sexual and reproductive life stages Framework 2017. https://www.e2aproject.org/news-item/e2a-newsletter-october-november-2017/. Accessed 15 Jan 2018.
23. Muanda M. Rapport: Analyse Des Obstacles a L'Utilisation De La Contraception Moderne Dans La Ville De Kinshasa, RDC. République Démocratique Du Congo: Ministère de la Santé Publique; 2015.
24. Performance Monitoring and Accountability 2020 (PMA2020) project: PMA2016/KINSHASA-R5: family planning brief. 2017. Baltimore: Kinshasa School of Public Health, Tulane University School of Public Health and Tropical Medicine, Bill & Melinda Gates Institute for Population and Reproductive Health, Johns Hopkins Bloomberg School of Public Health. https://pma2020.org/reports/pma2016kinshasa-r5. Accessed 1 Apr 2017.
25. Kayembe P, Dikamba N, Anglewicz P. PMA 2020 sur les Jeunes de 15 à 24 ans. Proceedings of the Table Ronde Sur La Santé des Adolescents, Faire

Attitudes toward sexual and reproductive health among adolescents and young people in urban...

79

Progresser La Santé Des Adolescents Et Des Jeunes En RDC. Kinshasa, DRC: Role De La Planification Familiale; 2015. Accessed 1 Apr 2017

26. Hernandez JH, Muanda M, Garcia M, Matawa G. Awareness and perceptions of emergency contraceptive pills among women in Kinshasa, Democratic Republic of the Congo. Int Perspect Sex Reprod Health. 2017;43(3):121–30.

27. Warren N, Alvarez C, Makambo MT, Johnson-Agbakwu C, Glass N. "Before the war we had it all": family planning among couples in a post-conflict setting. Health Care Women Int. 2017;38(8):796-812.

28. Chikovore J, Nystrom L, Lindmark G, Ahlberg BM. "How can I gain skills if I Don't practice?" the dynamics of prohibitive silence against pre-marital pregnancy and sex in Zimbabwe. PLoS One. 2013;8(1):e53058.

29. Williamson LM, Parkes A, Wight D, Petticrew M, Hart GJ. Limits to modern contraceptive use among young women in developing countries: a systematic review of qualitative research. Reprod Health. 2009;6(1):3.

30. Tilahun M, Mengistie B, Egata G, Reda AA. Health workers' attitudes toward sexual and reproductive health services for unmarried adolescents in Ethiopia. Reprod Health. 2012;9(1):19.

31. Aaro LE, Flisher AJ, Kaaya S, Onya H, Fuglesang M, Klepp KI, Schaalma H. Promoting sexual and reproductive health in early adolescence in South Africa and Tanzania: development of a theory- and evidence-based intervention Programme. Scand J Public Health. 2006;34(2):150–8.

32. Geary RS, Gómez-Olivé FX, Kahn K, Tollman S, Norris SA. Barriers to and facilitators of the provision of a youth-friendly health services programme in rural South Africa. BMC Health Serv Res. 2014;14(1):259.

33. Hokororo A, Kihunrwa AF, Kalluvya S, Changalucha J, Fitzgerald DW, Downs JA. Barriers to access reproductive health care for pregnant adolescent girls: a qualitative study in Tanzania. Acta Paediatr. 2015;104(12):1291–7.

34. MSP/PNSA: Plan Stratégique National de la Santé et du Bien-être des Adolescents et des Jeunes 2016–2020. 2016.

7

Decision-making preceding induced abortion: a qualitative study of women's experiences in Kisumu, Kenya

Ulrika Rehnström Loi[1][*][iD], Matilda Lindgren[1], Elisabeth Faxelid[1], Monica Oguttu[2,3] and Marie Klingberg-Allvin[4,5]

Abstract

Background: Unwanted pregnancies and unsafe abortions are prevalent in regions where women and adolescent girls have unmet contraceptive needs. Globally, about 25 million unsafe abortions take place every year. In countries with restrictive abortion laws, safe abortion care is not always accessible. In Kenya, the high unwanted pregnancy rate resulting in unsafe abortions is a serious public health issue. Gaps exist in knowledge regarding women's decision-making processes in relation to induced abortions in Kenya. Decision-making is a fundamental factor for consideration when planning and implementing contraceptive services. This study explored decision-making processes preceding induced abortion among women with unwanted pregnancy in Kisumu, Kenya.

Methods: Individual face-to-face in-depth interviews were conducted with nine women aged 19–32 years old. Women who had experienced induced abortion were recruited after receiving post-abortion care at the Jaramogi Oginga Odinga Teaching and Referral Hospital (JOOTRH) or Kisumu East District Hospital (KDH) in Kisumu, Kenya. In total, 15 in-depth interviews using open-ended questions were conducted. All interviews were tape-recorded, transcribed and coded manually using inductive content analysis.

Results: Respondents described their own experiences regarding decision-making preceding induced abortion. This study shows that the main reasons for induced abortion were socio-economic stress and a lack of support from the male partner. In addition, deviance from family expectations and gender-based norms highly influenced the decision to have an abortion among the interviewed women. The principal decision maker was often the male partner who pressed for the termination of the pregnancy indirectly by declining his financial or social responsibilities or directly by demanding termination. In some cases, the male partner controlled decision-making by arranging an unsafe abortion without the woman's consent. Strategic choices regarding whom to confide in were employed as protection against abortion stigma. This contributed to a culture of silence around abortion and unwanted pregnancy, a factor that made women more vulnerable to complications.

Conclusions: The findings suggest that financial, social and gender-based dependencies influence women's agency and perceived options in decision-making regarding abortion.

Keywords: Abortion, Decision-making, Qualitative methodology, In-depth interviews, Kenya

* Correspondence: ulrika.rehnstrom.loi@ki.se
[1]Department of Public Health Sciences/IHCAR, Karolinska Institutet, SE-171 77 Stockholm, Sweden
Full list of author information is available at the end of the article

Plain English summary

Unwanted pregnancies and pregnancy termination are common in countries where women who want to prevent or delay childbearing have limited access to contraceptives. Around 25 million unsafe abortions take place worldwide each year. Recent evidence shows that nearly half a million induced abortions take place in Kenya every year. In this study, we used in-depth interviews to explore the decision-making processes preceding induced abortion among women with unwanted pregnancies in Kisumu, Kenya.

This study shows that the interviewed women decided to terminate their pregnancies for the following reasons: poverty, poor timing of the pregnancy and absence of support from male partners. The main decision maker was usually the male partner who pressed for the termination of the pregnancy indirectly by declining his financial or social responsibilities or directly by forcing his partner to terminate the pregnancy. In some cases, the male partner arranged an unsafe abortion without the woman's knowledge or consent. Participants were affected by social stigma and carefully selected whom to talk to about the abortion. This strategy was used as protection against humiliation and shame. This contributed to a culture of silence around abortion and unwanted pregnancy, a factor that made women vulnerable to complications.

Background

Where women and adolescent girls have unmet contraceptive needs, unwanted pregnancies and unsafe abortions are common. About 25 million unsafe abortions (45% of all induced abortions) occur globally, most of them (97%) in low resource settings [1]. Despite the availability of safe and effective interventions, unsafe abortions still contribute to maternal morbidity and mortality [2]. The majority of maternal deaths due to unsafe abortions occur in low-income settings where women experience low social status combined with legal and social restrictions to sexual and reproductive rights [3]. Women tend to opt for unsafe abortions where safe abortion services are not acceptable, accessible or affordable [4]. The number of unsafe abortions tends to be higher among poor women because women with strong social or economic resources are more likely to access safe abortions, regardless of the legal context [5].

The World Health Organization (WHO) defines unsafe abortion as *"the termination of an unwanted pregnancy by persons lacking the necessary skills, or in an environment lacking minimal medical standards, or both"* [6], while also emphasising the impact of the social and legal context on abortion safety [7]. A recent study showed the disparity in abortion safety between low- and high-resource settings, indicating that in high-resource settings almost all abortions were safe, while only one in four abortions in Africa were safe [1].

The 2030 Agenda for Sustainable Development renewed the commitments by 193 Member States of the United Nations to reduce global maternal mortality through universal access to sexual and reproductive health (SRH) services, education and information. Moreover, sexual and reproductive health and rights (SRHR), ensuring the ability to make decisions about one's contraceptive and own health, is core to the post-2015 goals because of its remarkable potential to contribute to sustainable development [8].

Contraceptives allow women/couples to decide if and when to become pregnant. Modern contraceptives play an important role in reducing maternal deaths by preventing unwanted pregnancies and prolonging birth intervals [9]. Contraceptives are, however, underutilised in many low-resource settings [10, 11], largely as a result of limited availability of a range of contraceptive methods, including to modern long-acting reversible contraceptive methods [11], and social stigma surrounding young women's contraceptive use [12].

Women's decision-making preceding an induced abortion is influenced by factors at different levels [13, 14]. Individual-level factors include marital status, education level, economic independency and whether the woman was a victim of rape or incest [15]. Interpersonal factors such as parental and partner support have also been found to influence decision-making [15], as have societal determinants like religion and social stigma and norms [13]. Relevant organisational factors include access to sexuality education [15] and the availability of facilities providing abortion services [14].

The Kenyan context

The majority of the population in Kenya is Christian (83%), with 48% identifying as Protestant and 24% as Roman Catholic [16]. Kenyan women are economically dependent on men, and Kenyan cultures are largely patriarchal [17]. Marriage occurs comparatively early; among women aged 25–49 the median age at first marriage was 20.2 years. About 53% of married women of reproductive age use a modern contraceptive method. Among married women aged 15–49 years, 18% have unmet contraceptive need, which contributes to a high total fertility rate (3.9 births per woman) [18].

A recent national study estimated that about 464,000 induced abortions occur in Kenya annually, with a national abortion rate of 48 abortions per 1000 women of reproductive age (15–49 years) [19]. This figure is above the rate for all of sub-Saharan Africa (SSA), which is 31 abortions per 1000 women of reproductive age [20]. It is estimated that the induced abortion rate in Kenya is highest in the Rift Valley region and the combined Nyanza and Western regions [19].

Until 2010, abortion was only legally allowed to save the life of a pregnant woman. However, in 2010 a revised constitution was adopted permiting abortion when "*in the opinion of a trained health professional, there is need for emergency treatment, or the life or health of the mother is in danger, or if permitted by any other written law*" [21]. Thus far, the implementation of the constitution has been slow, and both knowledge and practice may differ throughout the country. A lack of transparency and clarity with regard to the circumstances in which abortion is legal contributes to Kenya's high maternal mortality ratio (MMR) [22]. The MMR in Kenya has remained almost constant since 1990. According to the 2014 Kenya Demographic Health Survey, the MMR is 362 maternal deaths per 100,000 live births, and unsafe abortion is a major contributor [18]. Due to restrictive abortion legislation in Kenya [21], limited access to quality healthcare and stigma, most abortions occur outside authorised health care facilities and are classified as therefore considered unsafe [23].

Kenya is an important location to study women's decision-making preceding induced abortion given its high MMR, changing legal framework, social stigma surrounding unplanned pregnancies and the socioeconomic status of the majority of women in the country.

Nyanza province, in which Kisumu is the principal city, has one of the highest MMRs in Kenya [24], and the total fertility rate for this province is 4.3 children per woman, the fourth highest in the country [18].

Aim of the study

The aim of this study was to explore decision-making preceding induced abortion among women with unwanted pregnancies in Kisumu, western Kenya.

Methods
Study setting
The study was conducted at the Jaramogi Oginga Odinga Teaching and Referral Hospital (JOOTRH) and Kisumu East District Hospital (KDH) in Kisumu, western Kenya. Kisumu Medical and Education Trust (KMET), a non-governmental organisation, supported the collaboration with these two public hospitals in Kisumu. At the time of the study, the two facilities treated approximately 80 women per month for abortion-related complications.

Research team and reflexivity
The authors recognise the significance of reflexivity and transparency regarding researcher subjectivity in qualitative research. The research team consisted of five female researchers. The first author (URL) had prior relevant experience from an MSc in Public Health and as a PhD student in the researched subject. The second author (ML) is a social scientist (MSc student) with an interest in women's SRH. The third author (EF) is a professor in Reproductive and Perinatal Health Care with broad experience conducting quantitative and qualitative research in Kenya and other low-income countries. The fourth author (MO) is the Executive Director of KMET with vast SRH experience in the region. The final author (MKA) is a professor with a PhD in International Health who has extensive experience conducting research in low-resource settings using both quantitative and qualitative methods.

Conducting and transcribing the interviews was physically and emotionally exhausting. During data collection and interview transcription the researchers (ML and URL) had daily contact and discussed their personal experiences. The deep emotional experience of conducting these interviews allowed them to empathise with participants and was used during analysis.

Study design, sample selection and data collection
In total, 15 individual, in-depth interviews (IDIs) were conducted with nine women aged 19–32 years old. Follow-up interviews were conducted with six of the women. Purposive sampling was used to select women seeking care for abortion-related complications. The following inclusion criteria were used: 1) women over 18 years of age 2) who experienced an induced abortion, 3) received post-abortion care (PAC) at JOOTRH or KDH and 4) were willing to be interviewed.

Midwives at the two public hospitals in Kisumu identified possible interviewees between 1 January 2014 to 31 May 2014 by asking PAC-seeking women if they had tried to induce the abortion. All women who met the inclusion criteria and were asked to participate agreed to be interviewed. The respondents were informed about the study's aim and were assured of their confidentiality. Seven respondents were recruited from JOOTRH and two from KDH. Six women were interviewed face-to-face 7–10 days after receiving PAC, two were interviewed at the time of a three-month follow-up and one woman was approached while she was still admitted at the ward. In addition, a repeated interview was offered to all respondents approximately 2–5 weeks after the initial interview. Five of the respondents were interviewed face-to-face a second time, while one respondent was interviewed over the phone due to distance. Three respondents declined the request for a repeat interview. The reason for conducting follow-up interviews was to further enhance understanding and enrich the material as trust and affinity were built between researcher and informant.

The women were interviewed between February and April 2014 at JOOTRH and KDH by one of the authors

(ML) who has a master's degree in Gender Studies and conducted previous studies in Cultural Anthropology. She was trained in qualitative methodologies and at the time of the study was a postgraduate student in Global Health. The fact that the interviewer was not a clinician and a non-Kenyan might have encouraged respondents to speak to her more openly about a sensitive subject. During one interview the researcher used an interpreter to translate from Lou to English. The translator was an assistant from KMET. During the other interviews, the researcher was the only person in the room with the respondent. The interviews lasted on average 45 min.

A semi-structured interview schedule, using open-ended questions and suggestions for probing, was developed by the research team. The schedule was pilot tested and modified prior to initial data collection. The questions were framed to study women's decision-making preceding induced abortion, including the role played by their social networks.

Field notes were written directly after each interview to reflect on initial thoughts and reactions. With the written consent of the respondents, all interviews were tape-recorded and transcribed verbatim, including notations for nonverbal expressions, for analysis by the first and second authors (URL and ML) on an ongoing basis as data collection progressed. The interview with a translator was also transcribed in English. The research team met regularly to review progress and discuss interview techniques. Data collection continued until data saturation was reached [25]. Table 1 presents the characteristics of the respondents.

Data analysis

The data were analysed by the first and second authors (URL and ML) using inductive content analysis, including open coding, category development and abstraction [25, 26].

Inductive content analysis is a qualitative approach used to unconditionally analysing the data [27]. While analysis had already begun during interview transcription, open coding was conducted during the first reading of the transcripts. Thereafter, the transcripts were read through several times and coded manually. Meaning units were identified and transferred to Excel for classification into subcategories, generic categories and main categories. The process of analysis is presented in Fig. 1. Meaning units and categories were discussed and compared amongst all members of the research team in order to further improve the analysis and to maximise rigour [26].

Results

Inductive content analysis resulted in three main categories: 1) *Reasons for induced abortion*, 2) *A culture of silence* and 3) *Choosing abortion despite risks and limited information*. The results are presented according to these main categories together with their generic categories and citations from the interviews to clarify the findings. The abstraction process is illustrated in Fig. 2.

Reasons for induced abortion

The first main category, *Reasons for induced abortion*, is described through four generic categories: 1) *Financial inability to raise a child*, 2) *Social pressure associated with mistimed pregnancy*, 3) *Perceived lack of options* and 4) *Disagreement between partners and abortion without the woman's consent*.

Financial inability to raise a child

All women described their pregnancies as mistimed, unplanned or unwanted at the time of conception. A lack of financial stability or support were described by most

Table 1 Socio-demographic characteristics of respondents (R) at time of abortion

R (n = 9)	Age	No. of children	Relationship status	Occupation	Abortion method	Abortion provider	Other details
1	19	0	Partner	Selling vegetables	Surgical	Not sure	Tricked into abortion by her partner
2	20	0	Partner	University student	Medical	Chemist	Tricked into abortion by her partner
3	22	1	No relationship	University student	Medical	Physician at public hospital	Safe abortion
4	22	0	Partner	College student	Surgical	Chemist	Repeat abortion
5	25	0	Engaged	Primary school teacher	Medical	Physician at private clinic	Safe abortion
6	26	2	No relationship	Food preparation at hotel	Medical	Chemist	
7	29	1	No relationship	Unemployed	Medical	Physician at private clinic	HIV+
8	32	4	Married	Primary school teacher	Surgical	Chemist	HIV+ and pregnant with twins
9	32	4	Married	Unemployed	Overdose of malaria drugs	Self-administered	

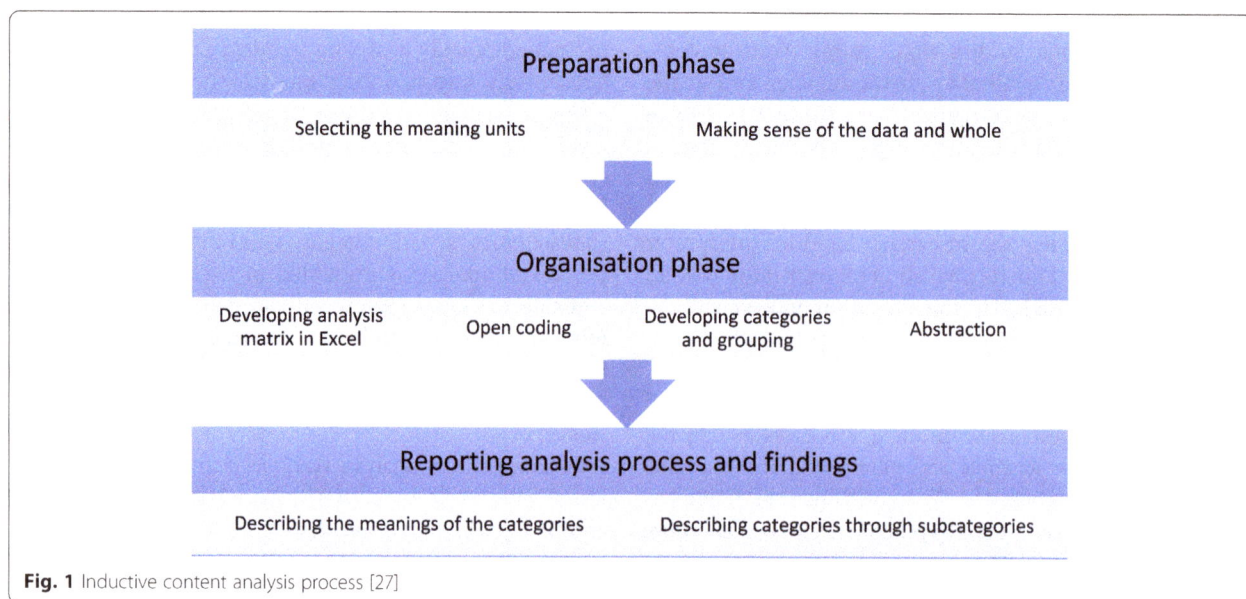

Fig. 1 Inductive content analysis process [27]

women as driving factors for the decision to terminate the pregnancy.

"I was financially unstable to sustain those children." (Respondent 8)

In some cases, the woman was the main provider of the household, and the pregnancy jeopardised the stability of her income. The pregnancy might diminish her employment opportunities, as an employer could decide to let a woman go once it was evident she was pregnant. Therefore, pregnancy termination provided the respondents with the potential for continued employment and secured economic independence.

"When [the pregnancy] is visible, you will be sacked. And when you are [alone] at home, who will support you? I have to work." (Respondent 6)

Women who were still students and living with their parents indicated that their parents would not financially support their costs of living and studies as well as the costs of raising an additional child.

The married respondents stressed that they had to prioritise resources and take care of the children they already had. All women with children mentioned the importance of providing an education for them. High school fees were frequently cited. The respondents stated they could not afford to educate an additional child. Several women specifically articulated their partner's unwillingness to financially support a child as the reason for terminating the pregnancy.

Furthermore, financial constraints were perceived as a barrier to safe abortion. Women frequently cited not

being able to afford to pay a professional to perform the abortion.

Social pressure associated with mistimed pregnancy
The unmarried respondents were concerned about the risk of negative views from family and community members if they continued the pregnancy at that particular time. Although engaged and employed, some women expected to be criticised and "talked about" by people in the community due to the mistimed pregnancy.

"Because [---] okay, people usually talk; in Kenya people will talk. Where you are staying, there are some people, those people like to gossip, people will definitely talk. [---] They'll say you are still in your mother's house [---] They won't be able to understand...and some will even criticise your relationship." (Respondent 5)

Others explained that having a child would end a harmonious relationship with their parents. Several young women living with their parents mentioned that they would not be welcome in their parents' house if they were pregnant.

"[---] she [mother] took me to the training [in hotel management and hospitality], she spend some money there, and then I didn't tell her [about the pregnancy] because she won't be happy because maybe she will then think that she had taken me to the training and spent money there, and then I will not be able to go and just sit at home [---] She would kick me out of the house, and maybe she would stop the training [---]." (Respondent 7)

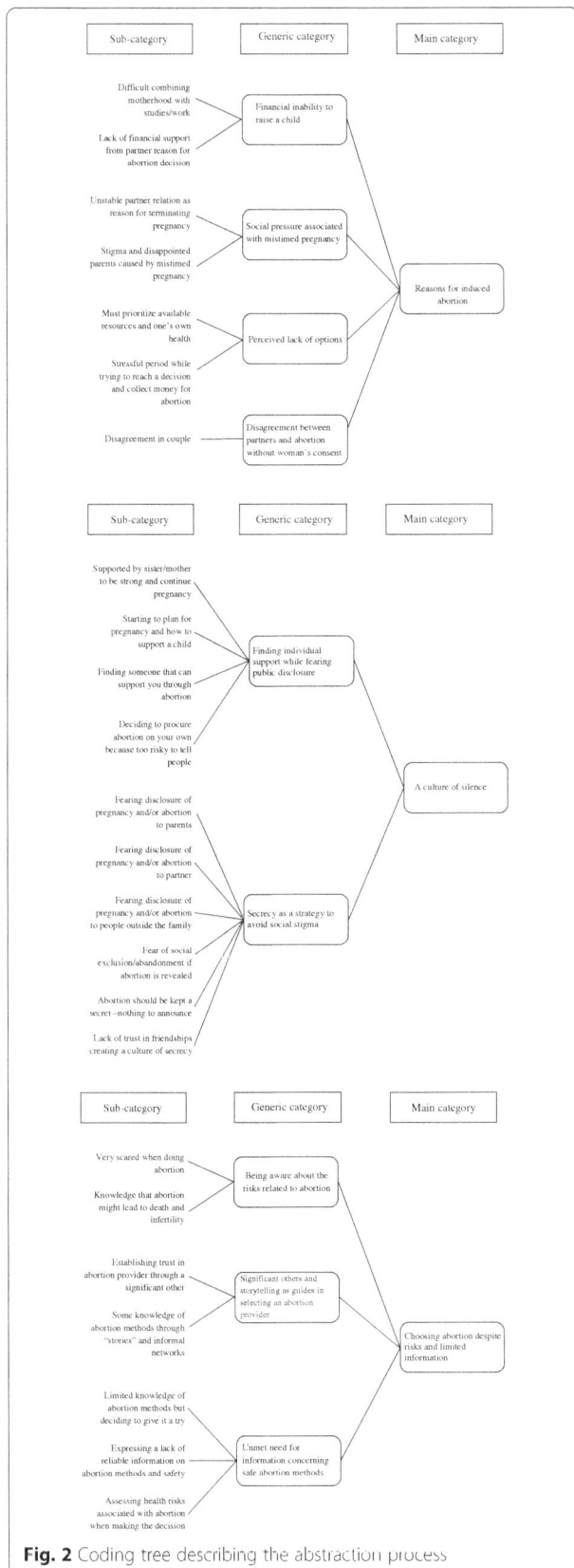

Fig. 2 Coding tree describing the abstraction process

The need for a supportive social network, including a stable partnership, emerged as fundamental to avoid severe conflicts in the decision-making process. Social networks could include actors providing either financial or couched support. Male partners had a significant direct or indirect influence on participants' decisions to opt for induced abortions. Several women expressed unstable partner relationships as a reason why they had chosen to have an abortion.

> "I already have two children, I am everything for these children... I am the mother and the father for these two children, so a third one would be too much problem. I just decided. I have to because that man never convinced me; I was not convinced at all that that man would provide anything." (Respondent 6)

Single women were afraid to raise a child alone.

> "So, I just thought that I have another kid and the father is not contributing with the school fees. Even my mother denied helping me. Yeah, for my kid and me also; so that's why I decided to do away with the abortion." (Respondent 7)

The social network was emphasised as central for single mothers. An additional child became an added burden, which could not be placed on family or friends.

Perceived lack of options

Some women expressed guilt and distress about lying to their partners and family about the pregnancy. Additionally, women expressed feelings such as heightened shame and self-blame because abortion was perceived as immoral and improper.

> "I felt bad because it was like murdering someone, but [---] I felt part of killing the kid because [---] I felt miserable for like a week [---] two weeks." (Respondent 2)

However, due to their economic, social or health circumstances, the termination of the pregnancy was considered the only available option.

> "I didn't have any option because I just knew that the situation I was in [HIV positive]; I was not able to [---] take care of this baby [---] according to the situation [HIV positive] now I was in." (Respondent 7)

While some women said that they decided on an abortion immediately upon realising they were pregnant, several respondents described experiencing a lot of stress and ambivalence in trying to decide what to do.

"I was still deciding what to do; I was still doubting. So many things run into my mind until I come with the decision to do [---] to [---] to [---] end the pregnancy. At that time [---] [I] even think I lost [---] [weight] cause [because of the] stress I have [---] having so many stress [---] losing weight cause of the stress." (Respondent 3)

Disagreement between partners and abortion without the woman's consent

Almost all women expressed some kind of disagreement with their partner in relation to the pregnancy. Some women articulated that they terminated the pregnancy without notifying their partner, fearing the possible consequences of anger, violence and divorce. On the other hand, a few women expressed their intention to abort and were discouraged and warned not to proceed by the partner. Participants articulated that their partners believed abortion was wrong and could cause complications and death. All single respondents decided not to reveal the pregnancy to their ex-partners. Although some of the respondents decided to terminate the pregnancy, others expressed that they were forced or even misled to terminate the pregnancy by their partners. When women were misled, their respective partners attempted to convince them to opt for an abortion. Although the women insisted on keeping the pregnancy, clandestine abortion providers supported the partners to induce abortion without the women's consent.

"He suggested for the abortion to be done, I told him no. [---] So he insisted, and he insisted. When he saw I'm not participating, he used a trick and told me that if you don't want then I want to advice you on how to be when you are pregnant and what drugs [to] use. [---] He injected me through a vein and told me it's to improve the appetite... [---] After injecting that drug I became unconscious. When I returned from my unconsciousness I found myself naked and I was bleeding." (Respondent 1)

This reveals that unsafe abortion in Kenya sometimes happens without the woman's consent. During the interview Respondent 1 disclosed she had reported her ex-partner to the police. While the women explained their partners' motives were based on social embarrassment and financial obligations, how the partners themselves would describe the situation and justify their actions is beyond the scope of this research.

A culture of silence

The main category *A culture of silence* is described through two generic categories: 1) *Finding individual support while fearing public disclosure* and 2) *Secrecy as a strategy to avoid social stigma.*

Finding individual support while fearing public disclosure

As seen under the first main category, several respondents described the time after they discovered they were pregnant as very stressful. While all of them feared public disclosure to some extent, they also expressed the need to tell someone about their condition. In many cases this person was a sister or a friend who had also been through an induced abortion. Most respondents were reluctant to tell their partners because they feared disagreement or abandonment. Among the women who informed their partners about the pregnancy, this confession commonly entailed asking for financial support. A majority of the non-married respondents also acknowledge that they were reluctant to tell their parents and preferred that their partner did not know about the pregnancy.

Respondents tended to keep the pregnancy to themselves for several weeks due to their fear of possible reactions. If the secret was shared, it had to be with a trustworthy person, usually a sister, as a tactic to avoid public disclosure. Furthermore, women feared receiving opposing advice, which could indicate that they had already made the decision to terminate the pregnancy and only sought affirmation.

"I was doubting what to do and on the other hand afraid of sharing with anybody. I believed if I share it with so many people some people will give me other advice, some will give me this; that's why I ended up sharing with my sister that I'm staying with because I trusted her." (Respondent 4)

Not infrequently, respondents indicated that they had chosen to state that the pregnancy had ended in a miscarriage instead of an induced abortion. Women made strategic choices regarding whom they confided in. While some women had the support of a sister or a female friend, others assessed the risk of telling someone to be so profound that they decided to keep the secret to themselves, which meant they had no one who could support them.

"I did not ask someone for advice because if you ask one they will start talking about it and everybody will know about it, so I was afraid to talk about it to someone [---] and maybe it will go back to my partner, and I didn't want that to happen. [---]." (Respondent 8)

Fear of negative consequences and death as a result of the abortion led some women to share their intention to terminate the pregnancy. Women expressed the desire to inform at least one person about the abortion; if there were negative consequences, someone would know where to look for the woman if she were not to return home.

Secrecy as a strategy to avoid social stigma

The majority of women expressed fear of rumours, social isolation and judgment if the abortion were revealed. Respondents believed that people in the community would perceive them as "killers". Additionally, they believed their peers would exclude them and avoid interacting with them. Social stigma and discrimination were expressed as segregation, as well as being perceived as a prostitute, labelled as a murderer, accused of being unfaithful and believed to be a poor candidate for marriage.

"In campus if you get pregnant and your boyfriend says I cannot take care of the baby, I'm not the father and stuff, they will start saying you are just like the others [---] maybe you have sex for money? Maybe you don't know the father of the kid? [---] So, they start calling you names like whore, slut [---] Someone says you are just a whore like anyone else, and after that everyone starts to isolate you [---]" (Respondent 2)

Fear of judgment and losing social respect created a culture of silence, where the harmful nature of rumours and negative responses fostered secrecy and silence surrounding abortion and a mistimed pregnancy. Women became afraid to share their decision to terminate the pregnancy with others, including friends, family and healthcare professionals due to a lack of trust and fear that their confidentiality would not be maintained. Induced abortions were secrets kept to avoid negative reactions.

Religious values and beliefs were apparent in all the interviews. Almost all women mentioned that abortion was a sin and not accepted by their church. Therefore, it was critical that other church members were not aware of the decision to terminate the pregnancy. A few respondents elaborated on this during follow-up interviews, clarifying the guilt, anxiety and angst they felt when attending church. They accused themselves of being sinners and struggled to ask for forgiveness from God.

"You see as a married women [---] you see [---] it seems like the woman is not even ready for the marriage [---] so something is wrong with her that cannot be explained, so they [the husbands] don't like it so easy, they see it as a sin, so there is no way I can tell about the abortion to him as I know the consequences can be bitter for me [---] when you do

such thing [abortion] since you are giving away God's blood, then you are trying to be like the Father. God gave you the child, and now you are removing it so it's a sin because you are competing with God." (Respondent 9)

Choosing abortion despite risks and limited information

The main category *Choosing abortion despite being aware of the risks* is explained through three generic categories: 1) *Being aware of the risks related to abortion*, 2) *Significant others and storytelling as guides for selecting an abortion provider* and 3) *Unmet need for information concerning safe abortion methods.*

Being aware of the risks related to abortion

The respondents generally described abortion as risky. All of them said they were aware of the health risks of having an abortion. Death, infertility, long-time infection, weakness and loss of body weight were commonly mentioned. Death was the most emphasised consequence and was frequently repeated. Women described having an induced abortion as gambling with life and death.

"I was [very] scared [---] because I know how dangerous it is. But I was like, okay – let it be, and if I'm going to die, so be it, that is how, that is my destiny now. [---] I had now decided; it's either death or survival. I was ready for anything." (Respondent 5)

All women highlighted abortion as an unsafe procedure in Kenya. The respondents were fully aware of the severity of abortion complications, and their decisions were framed with this knowledge in mind. Women considered the risk of giving birth to a child to be similarly high. Going through a pregnancy was also associated with health risks (including sickness during and after pregnancy), but abortion was framed as the preferred risk. However, some respondents were anxious about the future and did not want to be blamed for their decision to terminate the pregnancy.

Significant others and storytelling as guides in selecting an abortion provider

Evidence-based information regarding induced abortion was limited. Common information sources about induced abortion methods and procedures were informal social networks at high school and friends who had experience of abortion. Only a few respondents had consulted professional healthcare providers. Some women stated they knew about Marie Stopes, a reliable abortion provider; however, due to high transportation fees they opted for medical abortions using Misoprostol, which was provided by chemists.

"When I was in high school we used to have some cases [of abortion] so I had that knowledge from school, so I just decided to do it on my own. [---] I also knew about other methods, but I was afraid to use the others because I had not tried to do it before." (Respondent 9)

Unmet need for information concerning safe abortion methods

Respondent knowledge about safe abortion methods was low. Almost all women described induced abortions as very risky, even with the possible consequence of death. The general consensus was that no abortion is safe. Women tended to ask the local chemist about abortion drugs (Misoprostol) or quinine instead of reaching out to safe professional abortion providers due to a lack of accurate understanding of abortion legislation and safe abortion methods in Kenya.

"[Abortion is] when you take drugs [---] traditional herbals also terminate the pregnancy. Some people take juice, highly concentrated juice [---] only those once [are the abortion methods I know of]." (Respondent 6)

"I didn't know anything. I have a friend who went through it before [---], but she passed away two weeks after the abortion [---]." (Respondent 2)

Discussion

Similar to previous studies, this study reveals that the main reasons for induced abortion are socio-economic stresses and a lack of support from partners [28–31]. In cases where women informed their partners about the pregnancy, the principal decision maker was often the male partner who pressed for pregnancy termination indirectly by declining his financial or social responsibilities or directly by demanding the woman terminate the pregnancy. In some cases, the male partner misled the woman, overruling her decision to continue the pregnancy by arranging an unsafe abortion without her consent. A lack of financial security seemed to diminish participants' perceptions of available options. Furthermore, as mentioned above, gender-based power relations hindered women from actualising their decisions. Previous studies from Uganda and Ghana have disclosed similar findings where women's decision-making power regarding abortion was restricted by gender norms and power imbalances [30–32].

Similar to earlier studies, female friends or sisters were commonly referred to as important sources of information and moral support when undergoing an induced abortion. While sisters were believed to be trusted to keep knowledge about the abortion within the family, important knowledge-sharing also took place via female friends who had themselves been through an abortion. Together with sisters, these friends were regarded as trustworthy.

Regardless of relationship status, all respondents expressed concern about publicly disclosing the abortion, fearing negative remarks, the loss of social respect, isolation and divorce. Similar findings have been shown in Ethiopia, Sri Lanka and Kenya [33–35] and in further conceptualisations of abortion stigma, which entails shaming and discriminating against women and their families [36, 37]. Kumar et al. argue that abortion stigma builds on injustices and discrimination in society by depending on and appropriating existing power axes [36]. This study showed perceived stigma, referring to the perception that pregnancy termination will result in a woman being seen as inferior, to be very present in the participants' accounts [36]. Similar to Shellenberg et al.'s arguments, the fear of judgment effectively curtailed participants' willingness to disclose their abortion intention or experience [37]. Women handled these risks by making strategic choices regarding whom they confided in. A lack of trust and the fear of rumours confirm that other people's opinions are highly important to sustaining a positive social life. In many cases, lying, hiding and planning to escape were preferable to telling the truth.

A direct consequence of this secrecy is that it creates a culture of silence around mistimed pregnancies and abortion. Although it may protect women from social shame, hiding one's pregnancy and abortion makes women reluctant or scared to seek professional reproductive health information and care, which in turn makes them more vulnerable to complications, morbidities and mortality. This aligns with findings from a similar context showing that fear of stigma related to unintended pregnancy among young women, including the shame it brings to the family, as well as negative social sanctions, is a great driving force for unsafe abortion [33, 38]. The study also shows that fear of stigma delays care-seeking and consequently increases the risk of morbidity and mortality.

This study reveals that women encounter challenges in obtaining safe abortion information and services, regardless of the legal status of abortion in the country. A previous study from Kenya has similar findings [39].

Abortion-related social stigma preventing women's access to comprehensive SRH

Essential elements regarding abortion-related stigma found in this study should be reflected in the planning and implementation of SRH services in Kenya. Women who participated in this study repeatedly noted significant social stigma around induced abortion, which affected their decision-making regarding pregnancy termination. The abortion-related social stigma revealed in this study delayed and prevented the seeking of professional and safe PAC. Similarly, an earlier facility-based study from Kenya confirms the correlation between stigma and abortion-seeking behaviours among women seeking abortion care [40]. Young unmarried women faced both the stigma of pregnancy outside of marriage and abortion-related stigma. Previous research has shown comparable findings [41].

A recent systematic literature review critically analysed abortion stigma among healthcare providers in sub-Saharan Africa and Southeast Asia [42]. The findings demonstrate that healthcare providers have moral, social and gender-based reservations related to induced abortion. Furthermore, the study reveals that nurses and midwives often have pejorative attitudes towards women seeking abortion care and commonly reported an unwillingness to provide abortion care. As a consequence, nurses and midwives overlooked their responsibilities as caregivers and acknowledged that due to negative rapport between abortion provider and client, women seeking abortion care received inadequate care [42]. Because stigma is transmissible, it also deters healthcare providers who are prepared to provide abortion care from delivering these services. This stigmatisation enforces negative labels for the caregiver and may result in harmful professional consequences [43].

Abortion stigma is deep-rooted in government and political landscapes, organisations, communities and personal relationships [36]. The constant denial of a woman's right to freely decide on the number and spacing of her children directly influences maternal mortality [44]. Abortion-related stigma is a barrier to safe and accessible abortion care [43, 45]. Hence, decreasing social and cultural stigma around abortion among abortion providers would potentially strengthen women's access to quality reproductive healthcare and improve women's health by preventing future unintended pregnancies, as well as induced abortions and related complications.

Strengths and limitations

Despite the high prevalence of induced abortions in Kenya [19, 46], there is a shortage of qualitative research that analyses women's reasons for obtaining induced abortions in the country.

Studies on abortion in Kenya have primarily focused on incidence, clinical outcomes and stigma [19, 39, 47, 48]. The strengths of the present study are, first, that it focusses on women who terminated their pregnancies in the recent past and thus have fresh memories of the abortion experience. Second, the interviewer was nonclinical, from outside the Kenyan healthcare system and ensured participants' confidentiality. Third, the interviewer established a rapport with the participants, which facilitated insightful responses.

Finally, six respondents agreed to a repeated interview, which provided a unique opportunity to ask follow-up questions, probe for additional information and circle back to key questions to generate richer material.

A limitation of this study is that partners and other significant family members were not included as study subjects. Partners might have given different accounts of the decision-making process. The methodological challenges in gaining access to both partners' and parents' accounts first and foremost relate to privacy, as partners and parents were not necessarily informed of the pregnancy and/or abortion. Ethical concerns prevented the recruitment of partners via the participants as this would require the women's consent, which, in turn, could influence the sample. Similarly, ethical concerns prevented the inclusion of women under 18 years of age in the study and by coincidence there were no women over the age of 32 years interviewed. It could be argued that adolescent women and older women would have responded differently about decision-making preceding induced abortion. Even though research among underage women is difficult to conduct, young women are by far the most affected by severe complications due to unsafe abortions [47]. More research is therefore needed to understand underlying social attitudes towards young women who have undergone induced abortions.

Furthermore, contraceptive failure and change of pregnancy intention during pregnancy were not included in this study, which could be perceived as a limitation.

The impact of HIV status on decision-making in relation to induced abortion has been demonstrated in other studies [49, 50]. This sample included two women who reported themselves as HIV positive, which also influenced their decisions to have induced abortions (along with financial reasons). However, analysis of this relationship should be based on a larger sample.

The results from this qualitative study are the reports of PAC-seeking women in Kenya during in-depth interviews.

Conclusions

A lack of financial independence, a lack of social support, deviance from family expectations and gender-based norms influenced abortion decision-making among women with unwanted pregnancies. Strategic choices regarding whom to confide in were employed as protection against abortion stigma. This, however, contributed to a culture of silence around abortion and mistimed pregnancy. Silence and stigma act as driving forces for unsafe abortions and put women in situations where an unsafe abortion can occur without their consent. Unwanted pregnancies can also be stressful for men, and interventions targeting unsafe abortions must take both sexes into consideration and address the problem of forced abortions as a reproductive health issue.

Abbreviations

HIV: Human Immunodeficiency Virus; IDI: In-depth interview; JOOTRH: Jaramogi Oginga Odinga Teaching and Referral Hospital; KDH : Kisumu East District Hospital; KMET: Kisumu Medical and Education Trust; MMR: Maternal mortality ratio; PAC: Post-abortion care; SRH: Sexual and reproductive health; SRHR : Sexual and reproductive health and rights; SSA: Sub-Saharan Africa; WHO: World Health Organization

Acknowledgements

The authors wish to express their sincere appreciation to the women who took part in this study and to the directors of JOOTRH and KDH for granting permission to collect data. In addition, special recognition goes to the staff of KMET for their assistance during data collection in Kisumu. This article represents the opinions of the named authors and not the necessarily the views of their institutions or organisations.

Funding

The Swedish International Development Agency (Sida) funded the study by providing a Minor Field Study grant to ML. The Doctoral School in Health Care Sciences at Karolinska Institutet provided a PhD grant to URL. The funders had no role in the study planning, implementation or analysis, the decision to publish or the preparation of the manuscript.

Authors' contributions

MKA and EF conceived the presented study and developed the study design with contributions from URL. ML conducted all face-to-face interviews with support from URL. URL and ML led the content analysis with input from all authors. All authors discussed the results. URL wrote the first draft of the article. All authors commented on and approved the final manuscript. The research team included MO, a Kenyan and senior professional as co-author as she was involved in the study's planning, supported data collection and also contributed to the improvement of the manuscript.

Ethics approval and consent to participate

Ethical approval was granted by the Regional Ethics Appeals Board in Stockholm (Reference number 2013/902–31/1) and the JOOTRH Ethics and Review Committee in Kisumu (Reference number ERC 42/13). Verbal and written consent were sought and received from all respondents. Information about the confidentiality and safe storage of the data was provided both orally and in writing. The participants were informed that they could withdraw their participation at any time without consequence. Confidentiality was protected as the interviews were conducted in a private room where conversations could not be overheard, and only researchers involved in the study had access to the interview material. Participants were given small financial compensation to cover transportation costs and the potential loss of income; the amount was low enough to not jeopardise the voluntary nature of participation. The study area was not included in the presentation of sociodemographic information to protect the anonymity of the respondents. After conducting the first two interviews, the research team perceived that some women may require professional support. Therefore, the author who conducted the interviews (ML) arranged for such care by KMET.

Competing interests

The authors declare that they have no competing interests.

Author details

[1]Department of Public Health Sciences/IHCAR, Karolinska Institutet, SE-171 77 Stockholm, Sweden. [2]College of Health Sciences, School of Nursing Sciences, University of Nairobi, Nairobi, Kenya. [3]Kisumu Medical Education Trust (KMET), Kisumu, Kenya. [4]Department of Women's and Children's Health, Karolinska Institutet, SE-171 77 Stockholm, Sweden. [5]School of Education, Health and Social Studies, Dalarna University, Högskolegatan 2, 791 31 Falun, Sweden.

References

1. Ganatra B, Gerdts C, Rossier C, Johnson BR, Jr., Tuncalp O, Assifi A, et al. Global, regional, and subregional classification of abortions by safety, 2010-14: estimates from a Bayesian hierarchical model. Lancet 2017;390(10110):2372–2381.
2. Darroch J, Audam S, Biddlecom A, Kopplin G, Riley T, Singh S, et al. Adding it up: investing in contraception and maternal and newborn health. 2017. https://www.guttmacher.org/fact-sheet/adding-it-up-contraception-mnh-2017. Accessed 16 June 2018.
3. World Health Organization. Packages of interventions for family planning, safe abortion care, maternal, newborn and child health. Geneva: World Health Organization; 2010.
4. World Health Organization. Safe abortion: technical and policy guidance for health systems. Geneva: World Health Organization; 2012.
5. Singh S, Wulf D, Hussain R, Bankole A, Sedgh G. Abortion worldwide: a decade of uneven progress. New York: Guttmacher Institute; 2009.
6. World Health Organization. World Health Organization information sheet in unsafe abortion incidence and mortality global and regional levels in 2008 and trends during 1990–2008. Geneva: World Health Organization; 2012.
7. Ganatra B, Tunçalp Ö, Johnston HB, Johnson BR, Gülmezoglu AM, Temmerman M. From concept to measurement: operationalizing WHO's definition of unsafe abortion. Bull World Health Organ. 2014;92(3):155.
8. United Nations. Global Sustainable Development Report. New York: Department of Economic and Social Affairs; 2016. p. 2016.
9. Petruney T, Wilson LC, Stanback J, Cates W Jr. Family planning and the post-2015 development agenda. Bull World Health Organ. 2014;92(8):548–548A.
10. Tsui AO, McDonald-Mosley R, Burke AE. Family planning and the burden of unintended pregnancies. Epidemiol Rev. 2010;32:152–74.
11. Sedgh G, Hussain R. Reasons for contraceptive nonuse among women having unmet need for contraception in developing countries. Stud Fam Plann. 2014;45(2):151-69.
12. Hakansson M, Oguttu M, Gemzell-Danielsson K, Makenzius M. Human rights versus societal norms: a mixed methods study among healthcare providers on social stigma related to adolescent abortion and contraceptive use in Kisumu. Kenya BMJ Glob Health. 2018;3(2):e000608.
13. Alhassan AY, Abdul-Rahim A, Akaabre PB. Knowledge, awareness and perceptions of females on clandestine abortion in Kintampo north municipality. Eur Sci J. 2016:95–112.
14. Frederico M, Michielsen K, Arnaldo C, Decat P. Factors influencing abortion decision-making processes among young women. Int J Environ Res Public Health. 2018;15(2).
15. Gbagbo FY, Amo-Adjei J, Laar A. Decision-making for induced abortion in the Accra metropolis. Ghana Afr J Reprod Health. 2015;19(2):34–42.
16. Kenya National Bureau of Statistics (KNBS). The 2009 Kenya population and housing census. Kenya National Bureau of statistics (KNBS). https://www.knbs.or.ke/category/census-2009-summary-of-results/. Accessed 15 June 2018.
17. Mutongu ZB, Women's Participation in Community-Based Organizations' Development as a Strategy for Poverty Reduction in Kenya. https://www.cbeinternational.org/sites/default/files/Women%27s_Muntongu.pdf. Accessed 18 June 2018.
18. Kenya National Bureau of Statistics. Kenya Demographic and Health Survey 2014. Rockville, MD, USA: Kenya National Bureau of Statistics. https://dhsprogram.com/pubs/pdf/fr308/fr308.pdf. Accessed 18 June 2018.
19. Mohamed SF, Izugbara C, Moore AM, Mutua M, Kimani-Murage EW, Ziraba AK, et al. The estimated incidence of induced abortion in Kenya: a cross-sectional study. BMC Pregnancy Childbirth. 2015;15:185.
20. Sedgh G, Singh S, Shah IH, Ahman E, Henshaw SK, Bankole A. Induced abortion: incidence and trends worldwide from 1995 to 2008. Lancet. 2012; 379(9816):625–32.
21. Government of Kenya. The Constitution of Kenya. Revised Edition. Nairobi, Kenya: National Council for Law Reporting (NCLR). 2010. http://www.wipo.int/edocs/lexdocs/laws/en/ke/ke019en.pdf. Accessed 18 June 2018.
22. Hussain. R. In: Brief: unintended pregnancy and abortion in Kenya. New York: Guttmacher Institute. p. 2012.

23. Ziraba AK, Izugbara C, Levandowski BA, Gebreselassie H, Mutua M, Mohamed SF, et al. Unsafe abortion in Kenya: a cross-sectional study of abortion complication severity and associated factors. BMC Pregnancy Childbirth. 2015;15:34.

24. National Council for Population and Development (NCPD) and UNFPA Kenya Country Office. Kenya Population Situation Analysis. Nairobi: NCPD and UNFPA; 2013.

25. Polit DF, Beck CT. Nursing research: generating and assessing evidence for nursing practice. Tenth edition. Philadelphia: Wolters Kluwer Health; 2017.

26. Vaismoradi M, Turunen H, Bondas T. Content analysis and thematic analysis: implications for conducting a qualitative descriptive study. Nurs Health Sci. 2013;15(3):398–405.

27. Elo S, Kyngas H. The qualitative content analysis process. J Adv Nurs. 2008; 62(1):107–15.

28. Arambepola C, Rajapaksa LC. Decision making on unsafe abortions in Sri Lanka: a case-control study. Reprod Health. 2014;11:91.

29. Maina BW, Mutua MM, Sidze EM. Factors associated with repeat induced abortion in Kenya. BMC Public Health. 2015;15:1048.

30. Schwandt HM, Creanga AA, Adanu RM, Danso KA, Agbenyega T, Hindin MJ. Pathways to unsafe abortion in Ghana: the role of male partners, women and health care providers. Contraception. 2013;88(4):509–17.

31. Chae S, Desai S, Crowell M, Sedgh G. Reasons why women have induced abortions: a synthesis of findings from 14 countries. Contraception. 2017; 96(4):233–41.

32. Cleeve A, Faxelid E, Nalwadda G, Klingberg-Allvin M. Abortion as agentive action: reproductive agency among young women seeking post-abortion care in Uganda. Cult Health Sex. 2017;19(11):1286–300.

33. Osur J, Orago A, Mwanzo I, Bukusi E. Social networks and decision making for clandestine unsafe abortions: evidence from Kenya. Afr J Reprod Health. 2015;19(1):34–43.

34. Kebede MT, Hilden PK, Middelthon AL. The tale of the hearts: deciding on abortion in Ethiopia. Cult Health Sex. 2012;14(4):393–405.

35. Olsson P, Wijewardena K. Unmarried women's decisions on pregnancy termination: qualitative interviews in Colombo, Sri Lanka. Sex Reprod Healthc. 2010;1(4):135–41.

36. Marlow HM, Wamugi S, Yegon E, Fetters T, Wanaswa L, Msipa-Ndebele S. Women's perceptions about abortion in their communities: perspectives from western Kenya. Reprod Health Matters. 2014;22(43):149–58.

37. Kumar A, Hessini L, Mitchell EM. Conceptualising abortion stigma. Cult Health Sex. 2009;11(6):625–39.

38. Shellenberg KM, Moore AM, Bankole A, Juarez F, Omideyi AK, Palomino N, et al. Social stigma and disclosure about induced abortion: results from an exploratory study. Glob Public Health. 2011;6(Suppl 1):S111–25.

39. Rossier C. Abortion: an open secret? Abortion and social network involvement in Burkina Faso. Reprod Health Matters. 2007;15(30):230–8.

40. Yegon EK, Kabanya PM, Echoka E, Osur J. Understanding abortion-related stigma and incidence of unsafe abortion: experiences from community members in Machakos and trans Nzoia counties Kenya. Pan Afr Med J. 2016;24:258.

41. Yegon E, Mwaniki P, Echoka E, Osur J. Correlates of individual-level stigma and unsafe abortions among women seeking abortion care in trans Nzoia and Machakos counties, Kenya. Annals of Tropical Medicine and Public Health. 2016;9(4):226–34.

42. Gipson JD, Hirz AE, Avila JL. Perceptions and practices of illegal abortion among urban young adults in the Philippines: a qualitative study. Stud Fam Plan. 2011;42(4):261–72.

43. Rehnstrom Loi U, Gemzell-Danielsson K, Faxelid E, Klingberg-Allvin M. Health care providers' perceptions of and attitudes towards induced abortions in sub-Saharan Africa and Southeast Asia: a systematic literature review of qualitative and quantitative data. BMC Public Health. 2015;15:139.

44. Hessini L. A learning agenda for abortion stigma: recommendations from the Bellagio expert group meeting. Women Health. 2014;54(7):617–21.

45. Dunn JT, Lesyna K, Zaret A. The role of human rights litigation in improving access to reproductive health care and achieving reductions in maternal mortality. BMC Pregnancy Childbirth. 2017;17(Suppl 2):367.

46. World Health Organization. Unsafe abortion: global and regional estimates of the incidence of unsafe abortion and associated mortality in 2008. In: Sixth edition; 2011.

47. Ministry of Health Kenya. Incidence and complications of unsafe abortion in Kenya: Key findings of a national study. 2013. https://www.guttmacher.org/sites/default/files/report_pdf/abortion-in-kenya.pdf. Accessed 18 June 2018.

48. Mutua MM, Maina BW, Achia TO, Izugbara CO. Factors associated with delays in seeking post abortion care among women in Kenya. BMC Pregnancy Childbirth. 2015;15:241.

49. Orner P, de Bruyn M, Cooper D. "it hurts, but I don't have a choice, I'm not working and I'm sick": decisions and experiences regarding abortion of women living with HIV in Cape Town, South Africa. Cult Health Sex. 2011; 13(7):781–95.

50. Chi BK, Hanh NT, Rasch V, Gammeltoft T. Induced abortion among HIV-positive women in northern Vietnam: exploring reproductive dilemmas. Cult Health Sex. 2010;12(Suppl 1):S41–54.

8

Use of menstrual cups among school girls: longitudinal observations nested in a randomised controlled feasibility study in rural western Kenya

Anna Maria van Eijk[1][*] ⓘ, Kayla F. Laserson[2,3], Elizabeth Nyothach[2], Kelvin Oruko[2], Jackton Omoto[4], Linda Mason[1], Kelly Alexander[1], Clifford Oduor[2], Aisha Mohammed[5], Alie Eleveld[6], Isaac Ngere[7], David Obor[2], John Vulule[2][^] and Penelope A. Phillips-Howard[1]

Abstract

Background: A menstrual cup can be a good solution for menstrual hygiene management in economically challenged settings. As part of a pilot study we assessed uptake and maintenance of cup use among young school girls in Kenya.

Methods: A total of 192 girls between 14 to 16 years were enrolled in 10 schools in Nyanza Province, Western Kenya; these schools were assigned menstrual cups as part of the cluster-randomized pilot study. Girls were provided with menstrual cups in addition to training and guidance on use, puberty education, and instructions for menstrual hygiene. During repeated individual visits with nurses, girls reported use of the menstrual cup and nurses recorded colour change of the cup.

Results: Girls were able to keep their cups in good condition, with only 12 cups (6.3%) lost (dropped in toilet, lost or destroyed). Verbally reported cup use increased from 84% in the first 3 months ($n = 143$) to 96% after 9 months ($n = 74$). Colour change of the cup, as 'uptake' indicator of use, was detected in 70.8% of 192 participants, with a median time of 5 months (range 1–14 months). Uptake differed by school and was significantly higher among girls who experienced menarche within the past year (adjusted risk ratio 1.29, 95% CI 1.04–1.60), and was faster among girls enrolled in the second study year (hazard ratio 3.93, 95% CI 2.09–7.38). The kappa score comparing self-report and cup colour observation was 0.044 ($p = 0.028$), indicating that agreement was only slightly higher than by random chance.

Conclusions: Objective evidence through cup colour change suggests school girls in rural Africa can use menstrual cups, with uptake improving with peer group education and over time.

Keywords: Schoolgirls, Menstrual cup, Menstrual hygiene management, Silicone, Mooncup, Adolescents, Sexual and reproductive health, Africa, Kenya

* Correspondence: Anna.vanEijk@lstmed.ac.uk
^Deceased
[1]Department of Clinical Sciences, Liverpool School of Tropical Medicine (LSTM) Pembroke Place, Liverpool L3 5AQ, UK
Full list of author information is available at the end of the article

Plain English summary

Girls in developing countries with few means to take care of themselves can find it hard to attend school during menstruation. The menstrual cup can be a good solution for dealing with menstruation in areas where alternatives such as sanitary pads are expensive or scarce. However, people have been concerned if the menstrual cup is acceptable for young girls in these settings. As part of a larger study looking into the use of menstrual items in rural Africa, school girls were given menstrual cups. They got puberty education and training on how to use them and keep them in good condition. They visited a nurse regularly; during these visits they talked about cup use and the cup was inspected for damage and colour change, a potentially more objective measure of cup use. Generally, girls were able to maintain their cups in good condition, with only 12 cups lost. More girls used the cup over time, showing that it takes a while to get used to the cup. There was low agreement between what girls said they did (use the cup) and if the cup had a colour change (looked like it was being used). Peer education helped girls get used to the cups, and cups of girls enrolled in the second study year showed colour change much faster.

Background

Menstrual hygiene management (MHM) for school-aged girls in low and middle income countries can be challenging when they have limited funds for, and access to, high quality hygiene products and poor sanitary conditions to deal with menstruation [1]. Use of inferior products, such as unhygienic cloths or prolonged use of a material before changing, can cause skin irritation, restriction in movement, and concerns about leaking and odour in school [2, 3]. Inadequate MHM has been associated with an increased risk of urogenital infections [4, 5]. Inability to deal with the blood flow reportedly can lead to absenteeism at school or the workplace, although data are difficult to interpret [2, 6–9]. Qualitative studies note girls' stigma if menstrual blood leaks at school, resulting in an inability to focus on lessons and withdrawal from school activities [2, 3, 10]; these studies also suggest that lack of options for MHM leads to school absenteeism and drop-out [2, 10, 11]. Both qualitative and quantitative studies indicate that girls value modern menstrual products [2, 3, 12–14], such as branded sanitary pads; in some settings transactional sex is used to obtain these products from boys and men [2, 5, 12]. Improved MHM may thus be considered an essential component among a variety of interventions to strengthen girls' sexual and reproductive health, can reduce their sexual exposures, and increase their chance of reaching their potential in school [1].

An alternative to sanitary pads is the menstrual cup, which has received attention in relatively small-scale studies in high income [15–18], and low and middle income countries, including among schoolgirls [5, 19–22]. Made of high grade medical grade silicone, rubber, latex or elastomer, these bell-shaped receptacles collect menstrual flow when inserted into the vaginal canal, and can be emptied and reinserted with a need to boil the cup only at the end of a cycle [23, 24]. Cups have the advantage of reuse, and can potentially last up to 10 years. First introduced in the 1930's, there are now ~ 100 brands available worldwide – marketed as an eco-friendly and cost-saving approach to menstrual care [23]. Cups have been shown to be safe with no incumbent infection risk among European [15, 16] and North American women [17]. Preliminary studies of acceptability in low and middle income countries suggest cups are a potential option for girls as well as women [19, 20, 25]. Studies to date have reported outcomes based on women and girls' self-reported cup use, but have not physically evaluated actual cup use or their robustness for sustained use in impoverished settings where environmental hazards (extreme temperatures, household pests) may reduce shelf-life [7]. A systematic review of MHM products recommended more rigorous ascertainment of cup use before large scale trials are conducted to determine cost-effectiveness [26].

As part of a pilot study examining the feasibility and safety of menstrual cup use on outcomes such as school attrition, and sexual and reproductive infections among primary schoolgirls who have reached menarche in rural western Kenya, [5, 24] our previous qualitative study demonstrated girls' reported cup use and acceptance [22]. In the current quantitative study, we utilise colour change of the cups as a more objective measure of uptake and use by girls, and compare this against girls' reported use, and examine factors that appear to influence the time taken for girls' to start using the cup [5].

Methods

Setting

The study was carried out in Gem District, Siaya County, nested within a wider health and demographic surveillance system (HDSS), which follows a population of ~ 230,000 individuals, described elsewhere [27]. Gem covers a rural area of 300 km^2, with its southernmost point ~ 12 km from Lake Victoria. The population are mostly members of the Luo ethnic group, and are mainly subsistence farmers [28]. Siaya is an impoverished area [29]: while the wider (former Nyanza) Province has a literacy rate of 70%, compared to the national average of 62%, school surveys estimate four out of 10 child learners miss school daily in Siaya County [30]. The gender equity occurring in primary school falls during adolescence, with a quarter more boys than girls attending secondary school by 18 years of age [31, 32]. The public health burden is typical of rural African communities [27]; past mortality among adolescents and young adults has been largely ascribed to communicable diseases and injuries [33], and maternal mortality among females

[34]. Gender-based violence is one of the highest in Kenya, with 22% of women reporting to have ever experienced sexual violence (compared to 14% for the whole country) [35].

The menstrual solutions study

The research presented is part of a menstrual feasibility study, a single-site, three-arm, open cluster randomized controlled 'proof of concept' pilot study [5]. In brief, 30 of 62 primary schools in the area included in a water, sanitation and hygiene (WASH) survey, were selected based on minimum WASH criteria [36]. The 30 primary schools were randomized into three groups; menstrual cups, sanitary pads, or usual practice. Girls from these schools were eligible to participate if aged 14–16 years, if they lived in the study area, received parental consent, assented, experienced three or more menses, and had no reported disability precluding participation. The study examined the acceptability, use, and safety of menstrual products, and social and schooling experiences of girls followed over one academic year. This paper focuses exclusively on girls' experience of the menstrual cup in the 10 schools randomly allocated to the cup group. Findings on main outcomes [5], focus group discussions [22], the laboratory confirmed safety of the cups, examining *Staphylococcus aureus* infection, toxic shock syndrome toxin-1, and cup contamination [24], and water, hygiene, and sanitation associated with MHM in the schools [36–38], have been published elsewhere.

The menstrual cup

Eligible girls in the menstrual cup schools were provided with one Mooncup® size B for nulliparous women (Additional file 1: Figure S1). This brand was selected because it has been tested in the UK [15, 16] and internationally [16, 25], is produced to ISO 13485:2003 standards (a regulated quality management system requiring that the service provided by an organisation "consistently meet[s] customer and regulatory requirements applicable to medical devices and related services"), and is registered by the U.S. Food and Drug Agency of Medicines (FDA; Registration Number 3009117944). The white colour of the cup when new, changing to light brown after use, allowed for physical observation of use. According to the manufacturer, when inserted into the vaginal canal the cup collects ~ 30 ml of menstrual blood, lasting 4–8 h depending on flow before emptying is required [39]. While a variety of menstrual cups are available for sale through distributors in Kenya, none were available or marketed at the time in the rural study area.

Safety precautions

Participants, families, communities, schools, and health facilities received written information in English and the local language about the Menstrual Solutions Study, the menstrual cup, symptoms of toxic shock syndrome, and contact information for the research team and local village community health worker. Guidance on toxic shock syndrome was provided in the information sheets, and contact details given should girls experience any symptoms. At each school, girls elected a favoured teacher to be the study focal point to strengthen communication between research nurses, schools, participants, and the research team. Research study nurses were each allocated a cluster of 3–4 study schools comprising at least one school from each intervention arm, and were responsible for monitoring the health and wellbeing of study participants within these schools. Soapy water for handwashing was made available for all participating schools. Other safety assessments over time are reported elsewhere [40].

Participant training

All participating girls received a puberty and hygiene classroom lesson from the school-allocated study nurse. For girls in the cup arm, this included an anatomical and practical base for cup-specific training. Study nurses were first provided with menstrual cups for their own use, and had a training session with the study gynaecologist, and with the menstrual hygiene WASH expert. Nurses then gave classroom training on cup use and safety to girls in the 10 cup-allocated schools. Training included how to fold and insert the cup, how to remove and empty it, how to keep it clean and boil at the end of each cycle, and how to store it to prevent loss or damage. Nurses reinforced use and safety messages, and requested girls communicate directly with them if they had any problems. Written materials were provided in addition to classroom demonstrations. A rolling enrolment of participants took place across two study years, between August 15, 2012 and August 27, 2013 with menstrual cups provided shortly after enrolment. Nurse assessment visits of participants occurred between October 2012 and November 2013. Early feedback from informal discussions with participating girls and focal point teachers indicated girls were reluctant to start using their cup. As a consequence, peer-to-peer classroom training was conducted by Luo 'champion' secondary schoolgirls from a school in a contiguous area, who had received cups from a charity in the previous 6 years and demonstrated expertise with use, in all cup schools in October 2012.

Monitoring cup use

Study nurse clinical assessments of each participant privately but within the school campus were planned for a minimum of once per term per girl, with nurses visiting their schools on average once per week. However, it was not possible to conduct these at predetermined intervals due to logistical issues, such as schools not wanting girls to be assessed on certain days as well as girls being absent or too busy with school lessons or activities on the days that nurses visited. Nurses had face-to-face discussions with individual girls about the use of their assigned menstrual product to ascertain use, hygiene requirements, and any problems encountered. Girls in the menstrual cup arm were asked specific questions on their cup use, if they dropped it, shared use with another person, and how they cleaned their cup. Girls were requested to bring in their cup (barring current use) for physical examination at each screening visit, whereby aspects of the cup were documented by the reporting nurse, including colour change, tail length, damage, detritus and smell (Additional file 1: Table S1).

Outcome measures and data analysis

All survey data were captured through field netbook entries. After cleaning, data were imported, transformed and analysed using Stata (version 14). Data were merged with girls' family socio-economic status, derived from multiple component analysis recorded in their household, with 5 quintiles of poorest to least poor, dichotomised into poorest (quintile 1–2), and less poor (3–5), and girls with missing data were included as a third category [5]. Evidence of cup use was defined by observed change in colour of the cup from clear/white to yellow/brown at nurse assessment. Additional physical observed evidence of use was a trimmed stem of the cup (see Additional file 1: Figure S1), which could demonstrate that girls had adapted the cup for their own size. Further evidence was girls' self-reported use to a study nurse during the assessment. Total follow up time for each participant was calculated as the date of cup receipt to the date of the final nurse assessment visit, or the date of reported loss of cup or cup replacement. Characteristics of girls who verbally reported cup use or not were compared using generalized estimating equations with a logit link, and exchangeable correlation [41]. Characteristics of girls with cups showing colour change were compared with girls whose cups did not change over the study period using Pearson's χ^2 test and Fishers Exact test if small numbers, and generalized linear regression with a log link and binomial distribution [42]; covariates examined included age, socio-economic status, class, years since menarche at time of cup receipt, total follow up time and number of assessment visits. Models were adjusted for clustering by school. The Mann-Whitney test was used to compare the follow up time among girls with and without a cup colour change. Non-parametric survival analysis was conducted using Kaplan-Meier survival analysis to plot time to event (first visit with colour change of the menstrual cup or first verbal report of cup use); the log-rank test was used to compare the plots. Cox regression was additionally conducted to examine

differences in time to colour change by the covariates mentioned above with school as cluster variable. To evaluate the relationship between verbal responses on cup use with the observed changes in the cup, a variable was created which showed the verbal response at the time of first report of cup colour change if this occurred, and the verbal response at the last nurse assessment visit if the colour change did not occur. We used the kappa score to compare self-report and cup colour observation; if there would be complete agreement this score would be 1, whereas for no agreement other than what would be expected by chance, the score would approximate 0. A p-value of < 0.05 was considered statistically significant.

Ethical considerations

The Menstrual Solution Study was granted ethical approval from the Scientific and Ethical Review Boards of the Kenya Medical Research Institute and the Ethics Committee of the Liverpool School of Tropical Medicine, and was considered CDC "non-engaged" by the Center for Global Health of the U.S. Centers for Disease Control and Prevention. Parents provided written informed consent and girls gave their written informed assent; participants were informed they had the right to withdraw at any time.

Results

Characteristics of the study population

Among the 267 girls in the 10 schools allocated to the menstrual cup arm, 60 were excluded because they did not meet the eligibility criteria for the study, and 7 girls did not want to participate (after they received a cup) [5]. Among the 207 participating girls who received a cup, 192 presented their cups for viability checks at least once, and comprised the study population for this nested sub-study. The majority of girls were in class 7 at the time of enrolment (56.3%, Table 1), with a mean age of 14.6 years. Twelve percent of girls were in households with the poorest two quintiles. Most girls (87.2%) had started their menstruation before reaching 15 years; the mean duration of menses was 3.7 days (standard deviation 1.7) and only 10% had menses longer than 5 days. About one in five girls said their menses was heavy, and the majority of girls (62.0%) reported cramps when menstruating. Before enrolment in the study, 88% reported they had (ever) used commercial sanitary pads.

Follow up of participants

Participants were followed up for a median of 10.9 months (IQR 6.1–12.5), with a median of four (range 1–12) cup assessment visits. Ten percent of participants were seen once only by the study nurse. Three quarters (74.5%) of girls had their first nurse visit within 3 months after the receipt of the cup. The median

Table 1 Characteristics of study participants, Menstrual Solutions Pilot study, Western Kenya, 2012–2013

Characteristic at enrolment	Number (%), N = 192
Class at time of enrolment	
5	14 (7.3)
6	47 (24.5)
7	108 (56.3)
8	23 (12.0)
Age at enrolment, years	
14	93 (48.4)
15	80 (41.7)
16	19 (9.9)
Mean age (sd), years	14.6 (0.7)
Socio-economic status household of girls[a]	
Poorest 2 SES quintiles	22 (11.5)
Higher 3 SES quintiles	138 (71.9)
No information	32 (16.7)
Age at menarche in years[b]	
Mean age at menarche (sd)	13.5 (1.0) n = 188
< 13	20 (10.6)
13	63 (33.5)
14	81 (43.1)
15	24 (12.8)
Mean days of bleeding (sd)	3.7, sd 1.4, range 2–14
Days of bleeding	
≤ 5	172 (89.6)
6–7	18 (9.4)
> 7	2 (1.0)
Amount of bleeding	
Heavy	40 (20.8)
Medium	96 (50.0)
Light	56 (29.2)
Cramps when menstruating	Any: 119 (62.0)
Mild cramps	59 (30.7)
Moderate cramps	30 (15.6)
Severe cramps	30 (15.6)
Material used for menstruation before enrolment	
Used some pads	169 (88.0)
Used cloths	21 (10.9)
Used other items	2 (1.0)

Abbreviations: *sd* standard deviation
[a]The socio-economic status of the household was calculated using a weighted average from multiple correspondence analyses (MCA), whereby indicators were generated from biennial household surveys in the Health and Demographic Surveillance System [5]
[b]Unknown for 4 girls

duration of physical cup observation follow-up was 7.4 months, ranging from 1 to 14 months, slightly shorter than the median participation in the study. Twenty-eight participants stopped observations before the end of the study and the reasons included pregnancy (14), marriage (1), migration (7), withdrawal (1), and 'other' (5).

Self-reported menstrual cup use, problems with use and maintenance

During the nurses assessment visits, 83.9% of 143 girls screened within 3 months stated they had used the cup, and this increased to 96.0% after 9 months (Additional file 1: Figure S2). Problems with cup use as reported to the nurses, such as with insertion or emptying, decreased from 21% among girls in first 3 months of provision, to 3% after 9 months (Fig. 1) whereas most girls reported good habits with regard to hygiene (Additional file 1: Figure S3). A list of complaints and issues reported to the nurses can be found in the Additional file 1: Table S2. None of the girls reported sharing the cup with other girls or women. When exploring factors associated with a verbal report of cup use among all study visits (Additional file 1: Table S3), girls were more likely to self-report cup use if they had started their menstruation in the previous year compared to girls who had menstruated for more than a year (RR 2.03, 1.04–3.94, $p = 0.04$, adjusted for school), and less at a visit in the first 3 months (0.38 0.19–0.79, $p = 0.010$ compared to a visit after 9 months). Self-report of cup use varied significantly by school (Additional file 1: Table S3).

Observed cup viability

During the follow up visits to the study nurse, only minor defects were detected on cups which did not result in the need for cup replacement (Additional file 1: Figure S3). Two girls required new cups due to extensive damage (one eaten by rat and one burnt during too long boiling). Thirteen girls within this cohort followed required a new cup during the study because they had dropped the cup in the toilet or pit latrine (7), or somewhere else (3), or leaking occurred (3: replaced with a bigger cup).

Cup colour change

A colour change of the cup was recorded after observation by nurses for 136 of 192 participants (70.8%); the median time to first colour change was 5 months (range 0.3–13.8 months, mean 5.6 months, standard deviation 3.3), with cups of 34 girls (25%) having colour change within 3 months, 44 (32.4%) within 4–6 months, 35 (25.7%) within 7–9 months and 23 (16.9%) after 9 months. Girls without a cup colour change were more likely to have left the study prematurely (26.8% vs. 9.6%, $p = 0.002$). The median total follow-up time for girls with a cup colour change was 8.9 months (range 1–13.8),

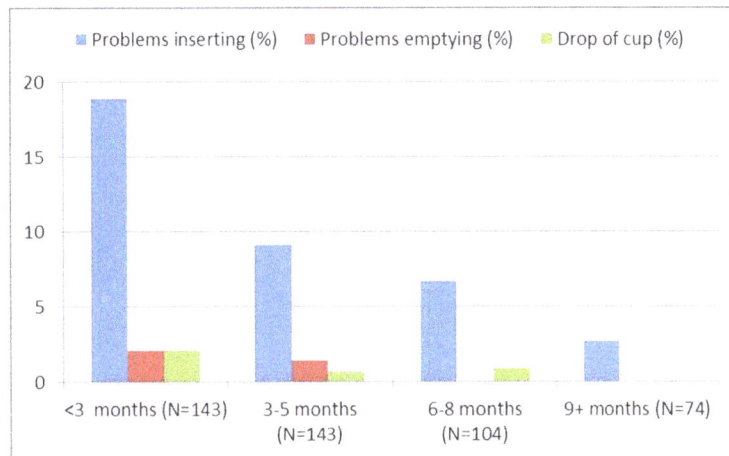

Fig. 1 Menstrual cup problems over time, Western Kenya, 2012–2013

whereas this was 4.1 (range 1.1–13.8) among the 56 girls without colour change of the cup (Mann-Whitney test $p < 0.001$). Girls without a cup colour change were more likely to become pregnant (6/56 vs. 3/136, $p = 0.04$ Fisher exact test), more likely to migrate (4/56 vs. 3/136, $p = 0.22$ Fisher exact test) and more likely to drop out (4/56 vs. 1/136, $p = 0.05$ Fisher exact test); there was no difference by enrolment year. A significantly shorter follow up time among girls without a cup colour change remained after excluding girls who left the study prematurely.

The uptake of cup use as assessed by colour change of the cup differed significantly by school (Additional file 1: Figure S4, chi-square test $p < 0.001$) and was significantly more common among girls who started menstruation recently at the time of enrolment (< 1 year, 84.3%) compared to girls who menstruated for a longer time (≥1 year, 66.0%, chi-square test $p = 0.013$). This remained significant in multivariate analysis when adjusted for number of follow up visits and duration of follow up (adjusted risk ratio 1.29, 95% CI 1.04–1.60, $p = 0.023$) (Additional file 1: Table S4 for full analysis). Time to cup colour change was significantly associated with year of enrolment with a faster colour change among girls who were enrolled in the second study year (hazard ratio 3.93, 2.09–7.38, $p < 0.001$, Table 2).

Observed cup colour change and self-reported cup use

There was a discrepancy between reported cup use and observed cup use from colour change of the cup or physical change such as the cup stem being cut for comfort, with reported use much higher than any of the other measures (Additional file 1: Figure S2 & S4). Self-reported use was at least once by 187 out of the 192 girls (97.4%) and increased faster than a colour change of the cup (70.8% in total, Fig. 2). Among the 136 girls with a cup colour change, 131 (96.3%) said they used the

cup at the visit that the colour change was noted; however, 89.3% of girls whose cup did not changed colour (50/56) said they used it as well ($p = 0.06$). The girls with a self-report of cup use but without a cup colour change were not significantly different by age, school class or socio-economic profiles compared to girls with a cup with colour change, but were less likely to be in their first year of menstruation (Additional file 1: Table S5). The kappa score comparing self-report and cup colour observation was 0.044, which indicates that the agreement was only slightly higher than by random chance.

Discussion
Main findings

Among 192 young school-going girls in Kenya (mean age 14.6 years) provided with menstrual cups in addition to training and guidance on use, puberty education and instructions for MHM, colour change of the cup as an indicator of use was detected in 70.8%. Verbal reports of cup use did not correspond well with colour changes of the cup; verbally reported cup use increased from 84% in the first 3 months ($n = 143$) to 96% after 9 months ($n = 74$) whereas cup colour change was detected among 22% and 74% in the same time periods, respectively. Time to cup colour change was faster among girls enrolled in the second year of the study (hazard ratio 3.93, 95% CI 2.09–7.38) who might have had a greater amount of peer support. Uptake differed by school and was higher among girls who experienced menarche more recently (adjusted OR 1.29, 95% CI 1.04–1.60). Girls were able to keep their cups in good condition, with only 12 cups (6.3%) lost (dropped in toilet, lost or destroyed).

Interpretation

Few studies have evaluated the potential use of an insertable menstrual product among schoolgirls in an economically

Table 2 Factors affecting time to colour change of the menstrual cup, as observed during visits to the study nurse, Western Kenya, 2012–2013

Variable	n	Univariate Hazard ratio, 95% CI[a]	p-value	Multivariate Hazard ratio, 95% CI[a]	p-value
Class at time of enrolment					
5 or 6	61	0.73, 0.57–0.94	0.013	NS	
7 or 8	131	Reference			
Age at enrolment (years)					
14	93	Reference		NS	
15	80	1.17, 0.88–1.56	0.268		
16	19	3.81, 1.59–9.14	0.003		
Socio-economic status household of girls					
Poorest 2 quintiles	22	1.12, 0.73–1.72	0.589	Not included	
Higher 3 SES quintiles	138	0.90, 0.70–1.15	0.410		
No information	32	Reference			
Material used for menstruation before enrolment					
Used some pads	169	Reference		Not included	
Cloths/other	23	0.92, 0.48–1.73	0.788		
Time since menarche at enrolment					
< 1 year	51	1.01, 0.63–1.62	0.958	Not included	
≥ 1 year	141	Reference			
Enrolment year					
2012	126	Reference		Reference	
2013	66	3.93, 2.09–7.38	< 0.001	3.93, 2.09–7.38	< 0.001
Enrolled before/after peer education[b]					
Before peer education	102	Reference		NS	
After peer education	90	2.77, 1.25–6.13	0.012		

CI confidence interval, NS not significant in multivariate model
Note: a hazard ratio > 1 indicates a shorter duration to cup colour change
[a]School included as cluster variable
[b]Peer-to-peer classroom training conducted by 'champion' secondary schoolgirls from a school in a contiguous area in October 2012

impoverished setting. The current study presents unique objective evidence depicting a conservative estimate of actual use, based on biologically-plausible physical changes to the menstrual cup acquired over time, and compares this against girls' self-reported cup use. These data show that cup uptake was gradual, with initial resistance, as reported in other studies [43–45], requiring intervention through mentorship. Our research team sought advice from Luo girls in a secondary school in Siaya County, who were experienced menstrual cup users (courtesy of long-term charity provision). Their assistance as champions for peer-to-peer training of our study girls helped to initiate cup use; this was only significant as a variable in univariate but not in the multivariate Cox regression model and not in any other model. The importance of the peer group may be indirectly postulated by the difference seen in uptake (verbal and by cup colour change) by school, and illustrate the strong social component, including peers and teachers. The faster uptake among girls enrolled later in the study may be a

consequence of the presence of peers familiar with cup use; the importance of peers was also observed in study among school girls in Nepal and Uganda [21, 45]. Presence of study nurses, strong research communications, and goodwill among the schools and community to examine this unmet need for schoolgirls may have strengthened resolve to participate. During the follow-up in this study, we detected no evidence of health or hygiene risks associated with menstrual cup use, similar to previous studies [15–17, 40].

Verbal self-reported responses showed higher and faster uptake compared with a more objective measure using colour change as an approximation of use. While menstrual flow may have an effect on time to cup colour change, we note manufacturers indicate cups' colour will change from white to light brown following use; however, such a colour change may not occur with coloured cups. Cup colour change was used here as a binary variable; there was no evidence of a gradual darkening of the cup over increased use, thus we were unable to

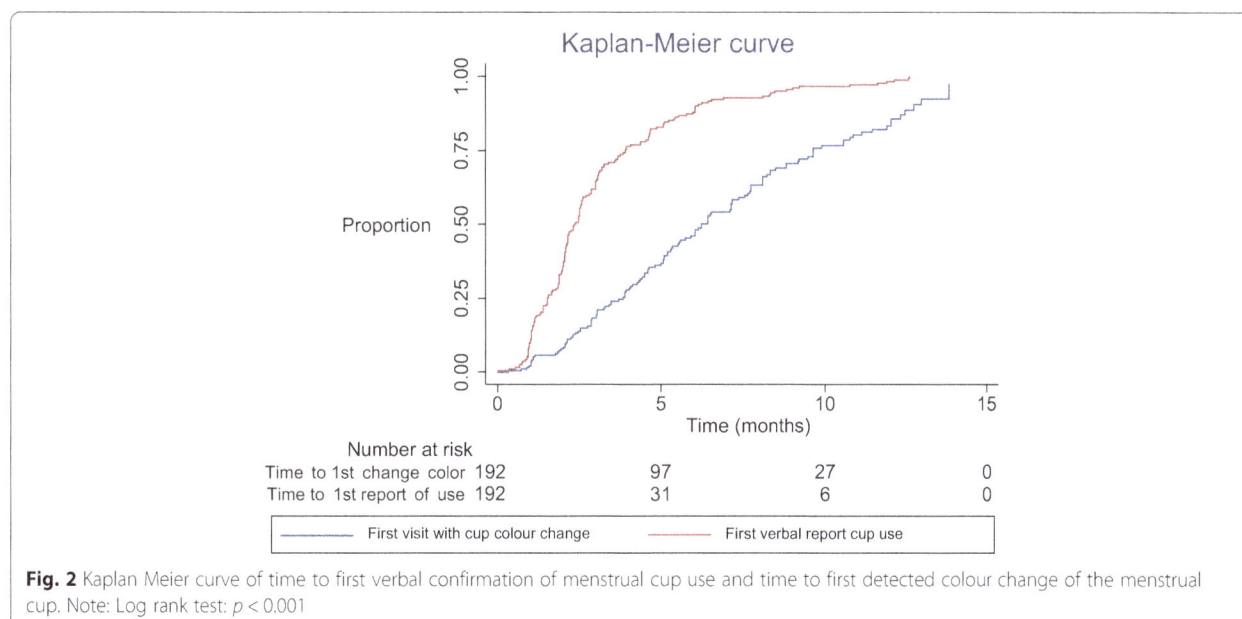

Fig. 2 Kaplan Meier curve of time to first verbal confirmation of menstrual cup use and time to first detected colour change of the menstrual cup. Note: Log rank test: $p < 0.001$

analyse as a 'dose-response'. Our results suggest programs and research screening on use should be cautious when relying on self-reported use only to assess the impact of cups on recipients' lives. This is especially important for trials using menstrual cups where, in absence of a more objective measure, the impact is under-estimated because 'cup users' are over-estimated. For example, in a per-protocol analysis of the data of the feasibility pilot [5], the greatest impact of cups on sexually transmitted infections and bacterial vaginosis was after girls had been provided the cups for 9 months or longer. Among girls with discoloured cups the measured outcomes of dropout and sexually transmitted infections (combined outcome) were halved (relative risk [RR] 0.48; 95% confidence limits 0.25–0.91) if they had the cup for 9 months, compared with controls; while for girls with no cup colour change having the cup for at least 9 months there was no difference from controls (RR 1.42; 0.48–4.18) [5]. This significant outcome difference adds credibility to cup-colour change as a predictor of cup use. In addition, from our and other studies introducing menstrual cups, it is clear that cup provision alone (without supportive training) is inadequate to 'pull' girls and women over the threshold to actual use, and that peer and other ongoing support is critical, especially in the early months following provision [21, 44].

Strengths and limitations

We used colour change of the cup as an indicator of use but there are no scientific directions on the gradation of cup discoloration with use over time from the manufacturer, or guidelines. While some biases may occur with heavy or light menstrual flow, we consider this measure

as more objective than self-reported use or observation of the trimming of the tail of the cup, supported by differences in 'impact' effects depending on observed cup colour change. Discoloration has been described for menstrual cups and diaphragms, without decrease of effectiveness or life span, and has been ascribed to effects of local vaginal conditions [46, 47]. It is possible that vaginal infections may affect colour change; we asked girls for symptoms but there was no agreement between reported symptoms and infections identified. No girls complained to nurses that they could not use the menstrual cup due to any ongoing symptoms. Colour change was reported for some girls very soon after receipt of the cup, so a noticeable colour change may occur early. Colour change of the cup during use can be reverted when it is put for a couple of hours in sunlight [47]; however, the school girls were instructed to carefully put their cup away in a pouch in between menses after boiling, to avoid theft or loss, and their verbal reports indicated they hid the cup to prevent others using it. In addition, girls and women are often embarrassed to leave menstrual materials in the open, and usually they are cleaned, dried and stored out of view, despite guidelines for e.g. cloths to dry in sunlight [8]. We note girls were not informed we would use cup colour change as an indicator of use. We cannot exclude that girls treated the cup in other ways that may have reverted the colour, but we are not aware of such methods. It is possible some girls may have stopped using the cup after colour change; however, other studies have shown once use is initiated, girls and women report continued use [17, 21]. The cups were distributed to girls as they were enrolled, reducing follow up time to a short duration for a few girls who were recruited late. The nurses' assessments of some girls (due to their absence, or school events) were less regular. This may have led to an under-estimation of the duration required until the cup colour changed, and may have contributed marginally to a conservative estimate of 'actual' use. Strengths of this study include the establishment of a longitudinal monitoring system and the systematic recording of multiple indicators of use, and detailed personal characteristics.

It may also be questioned if some girls did not use the cup at all, but allowed others, e.g. a sibling or friend to use it instead, creating the colour change; and we noted 2.6% of girls screened presented nurses with a cup that showed a colour change while their self-reports stated they did not use it. As the cup size was for girls, sharing with adult women would have been minimal due to potential leakage, but we acknowledge some sharing with siblings may have taken place. However, in focus group discussions participants feared cup use by another person may spread infection, and that they hid their cup [22]. During the nurse assessments, all girls denied sharing the cup with others.

Conclusion

Our data provide objective physical evidence that schoolgirls, including young girls recently transitioning through menarche, are able and willing to embrace use of an insertable menstrual solution to manage their monthly periods in a rural African setting. Preliminary uptake was slow and peer support and mentoring was required; it may take up to 6 months before confidence to use is established. Comparison between self-reports and physical evidence suggests self-reported use likely over-inflates use. We found no evidence of high risk of damage or loss of product, and hygiene standards were reportedly maintained. Examination of safety when used for a longer duration, the barriers that result in a slow uptake and evaluations of the cost-benefit of menstrual cups over other products on health, wellbeing and schooling outcomes may help define menstrual cups' potential role for managing girls' and women's menstrual needs in low and middle income countries. Menstrual cups have an upfront cost and may be scarce in impoverished areas. Some charities have developed cup distribution programs. However, efforts will be required to develop more sustainable marketing strategies to enable girls and women to access cups in such areas, with schemes for subsidies or pay-over-time in addition to peer-support development, especially for the first months, to enhance the uptake; to strengthen such activities and further research a cup coalition has been formed following a summit in January 2018 [48].

Additional file

Additional file 1: Figure S1. Image of mooncup. **Figure S2.** Use of menstrual cup by self-report, colour change, or presence of clipped tail per study year quarter, Western Kenya, 2012-2013. **Figure S3.** Observed and reported menstrual cup hygiene among school girls, western Kenya. **Figure S4.** Menstrual cup use by verbal report at first report of cup colour change or at last nurse visit if no colour change, and as assessed by cup colour change by school, Western Kenya, 2012-2013. **Table S1.** Monitoring of menstrual cup use. **Table S2.** Examples of complaints and issues reported to the nurses on menstrual cup use by school girls, Western Kenya. **Table S3.** Factors associated with a verbal report of cup use during the study period among school girls in Western Kenya. **Table S4.** Factors associated with the presence of cup colour change during the study period among school girls in Western Kenya. **Table S5.** Factors associated with self-report of menstrual cup use among school girls with no cup colour change compared to self-report of cup use among school.

Acknowledgements

We thank the head teachers, school staff, girls and their parents in the study schools for their participation in this study. Field and office staff, including the study research nurses, are warmly thanked for their conscientiousness and hard work. We appreciate the administrative support provided by Jiwanti Kabuka of HDSS KEMRI/CDC in Kenya, and Alison Reynolds of LSTM, Liverpool. The HDSS is part of the INDEPTH Network. We thank Mooncup Ltd. for provision of menstrual cups at a discounted price.

Funding

This study is part of the proof of concept feasibility study on menstrual solutions for schoolgirls funded by the UK Medical Research Council/ Department for International Development / Wellcome Trust Project Protect (G1100677/1). Funders had no role in study design, data collection and analysis, decision to publish, or preparation of the manuscript.

Disclaimer

The findings and conclusions in this report are those of the authors and do not necessarily represent the official position of the Centers for Disease Control and Prevention.

Authors' contributions

PPH, LM, KFL, and AMvE conceptualized and drafted the paper; EN, KO, KA oversaw data gathering and quality assurance; AmvE, PPH, CO, and DO processed and analysed the data; PPH, LM, KA, JV, AM, JO, KFL, and IN provided scientific leadership in developing the Ms. Study research activities; KA provided technical advice on menstrual cups, and JO, AMvE and AM advised on reproduce health. All authors have reviewed the manuscript.

Competing interest

The authors declare that they have no competing interests.

Author details

[1]Department of Clinical Sciences, Liverpool School of Tropical Medicine (LSTM) Pembroke Place, Liverpool L3 5AQ, UK. [2]Centre for Global Health Research, Kenya Medical Research Institute (KEMRI), Kisumu, Kenya. [3]Division of Global Health Protection, Center for Global Health, Centers for Disease Control and Prevention (CDC), Atlanta, USA. [4]Department of Obstetrics and Gynaecology, Siaya District Hospital, Ministry of Health, Siaya, Kenya. [5]Division of Reproductive Health, Ministry of Health, Nairobi, Kenya. [6]Safe Water and AIDS Project, Kisumu, Kenya. [7]Ministry of Health, Siaya County, Kenya.

References

1. Sommer M, Caruso BA, Sahin M, Calderon T, Cavill S, Mahon T, Phillips-Howard PA. A time for global action: addressing Girls menstrual hygiene management needs in schools. PLoS Med. 2016;13:e1001962.
2. Mason L, Nyothach E, Alexander K, Odhiambo FO, Eleveld A, Vulule J, Rheingans R, Laserson KF, Mohammed A, Phillips-Howard PA. We keep it secret so no one should know - a qualitative study to explore young school girls attitudes and experiences with menstruation in rural western Kenya. PLoS One. 2013;8:e79132.
3. McMahon SA, Winch PJ, Caruso BA, Obure AF, Ogutu EA, Ochari IA, Rheingans RD. The girl with her period is the one to hang her head reflections on menstrual management among schoolgirls in rural Kenya. BMC Int Health Hum Rights. 2011;11:7.
4. Das P, Baker KK, Dutta A, Swain T, Sahoo S, Das BS, Panda B, Nayak A, Bara M, Bilung B, et al. Menstrual hygiene practices, WASH access and the risk of urogenital infection in women from Odisha, India. PLoS One. 2015;10:e0130777.
5. Phillips-Howard PA, Nyothach E, Ter Kuile FO, Omoto J, Wang D, Zeh C, Onyango C, Mason L, Alexander KT, Odhiambo FO, et al. Menstrual cups and sanitary pads to reduce school attrition, and sexually transmitted and reproductive tract infections: a cluster randomised controlled feasibility study in rural western Kenya. BMJ Open. 2016;6:e013229.
6. Tegegne TK, Sisay MM. Menstrual hygiene management and school absenteeism among female adolescent students in Northeast Ethiopia. BMC Public Health. 2014;14:1118.
7. Phillips-Howard PA, Caruso B, Torondel B, Zulaika G, Sahin M, Sommer M. Menstrual hygiene management among adolescent schoolgirls in low- and middle-income countries: research priorities. Glob Health Action. 2016;9:33032.
8. van Eijk AM, Sivakami M, Thakkar MB, Bauman A, Laserson KF, Coates S, Phillips-Howard PA. Menstrual hygiene management among adolescent girls in India: a systematic review and meta-analysis. BMJ Open. 2016;6:e010290.
9. Ronitzsch S. Dropping out of school because of menstruation? An analysis of factors of success for menstrual hygiene management-projects in low and lower-middle income countries. Marburg: Philipps-University; 2015.
10. Sommer M. Where the education system and women's bodies collide: the social and health impact of girls' experiences of menstruation and schooling in Tanzania. J Adolesc. 2010;33:521–9.
11. Sommer M, Sahin M. Overcoming the taboo: advancing the global agenda for menstrual hygiene management for schoolgirls. Am J Public Health. 2013;103:1556–9.
12. Phillips-Howard P, Olilo G, Burmen B, Otieno F, Odongo F, Odour C, Nyothach E, Amek N, Zielinski-Gutierrez E, Odhiambo F, et al. Menstrual needs and associations with sexual and reproductive risks in rural Kenyan females: a cross-sectional behavioural survey linked with HIV prevalence. J Women's Health. 2015;24:801–11.
13. Montgomery P, Ryus CR, Dolan CS, Dopson S, Scott LM. Sanitary pad interventions for girls' education in Ghana: a pilot study. PLoS One. 2012;7:e48274.
14. Crofts T, Fisher WA. Menstrual hygiene in Ugandan schools and investigation of low-cost sanitary pads. J Water Sanit Hyg Dev. 2012;2:50–8.
15. Stewart K, Powell M, Greer R. An alternative to conventional sanitary protection: would women use a menstrual cup? J Obstet Gynaecol. 2009;29:49–52.
16. Stewart K, Greer R, Powell M. Women's experience of using the Mooncup. J Obstet Gynaecol. 2010;30:285–7.
17. Howard C, Rose CL, Trouton K, Stamm H, Marentette D, Kirkpatrick N, Karalic S, Fernandez R, Paget J. FLOW (finding lasting options for women): multicentre randomized controlled trial comparing tampons with menstrual cups. Can Fam Physician. 2011;57:e208–15.
18. North B, Oldham M. Preclinical, clinical, and over-the-counter Postmarketing experience with a new vaginal cup: menstrual collection. J Women's Health. 2011;20
19. Averbach S, Sahin-Hodoglugil N, Musara P, Chipato T, van der Straten A. Duet for menstrual protection: a feasibility study in Zimbabwe. Contraception. 2009;79:463–8.
20. Beksinska ME, Smit J, Greener R, Todd CS, Lee ML, Maphumulo V, Hoffman V. Acceptability and performance of the menstrual cup in South Africa: a randomized crossover trial comparing the menstrual cup to tampons or sanitary pads. J Women's Health. 2015;24:151–8.
21. Oster E, Thornton R. Determinants of technology adoption: peer effects in menstrual cup up-take. J Eur Econ Assoc. 2012;10:1263–93.
22. Mason L, Laserson K, Oruko K, Nyothach E, Alexander K, Odhiambo F, Eleveld A, Isiye E, Ngere I, Omoto J, et al. Adolescent schoolgirls' experiences of menstrual cups and pads in rural western Kenya: a qualitative study. Waterlines. 2015;34:15–30.
23. Menstrual Cup Master List. 2016. Available at: https://menstrualcups.wordpress.com/menstrual-cup-master-list/. Accessed 29 Jan 2018.
24. Juma J, Nyothach E, Laserson KF, Oduor C, Arita L, Ouma C, Oruko K, Omoto J, Mason L, Alexander KT, et al. Examining the safety of menstrual cups among rural primary school girls in western Kenya: observational studies nested in a randomised controlled feasibility study. BMJ Open. 2017;7:e015429.
25. Oster E, Thornton R: Determinants of Technology Adoption: Private Value and Peer Effects in Menstrual Cup Take-Up NBER Working Paper No 14828; 2009.
26. Sumpter C, Torondel B. A systematic review of the health and social effects of menstrual hygiene management. PLoS One. 2013;8:e62004.
27. Odhiambo FO, Laserson KF, Sewe M, Hamel MJ, Feikin DR, Adazu K, Ogwang S, Obor D, Amek N, Bayoh N, et al. Profile: the KEMRI/CDC health and demographic surveillance system–western Kenya. Int J Epidemiol. 2012;41:977–87.
28. Cohen D, Atieno-Odhiambo E. Siaya: the historical anthropology of an African landscape. London: James Currey, Ltd; 1989.
29. Meltzer MI, Terlouw DJ, Kolczak MS, Odhacha A, ter Kuile FO, Vulule JM, Alaii JA, Nahlen BL, Hawley WA, Phillips-Howard PA. The household-level economics of using permethrin-treated bed nets to prevent malaria in children less than five years of age. Am J Trop Med Hyg. 2003;68:149–60.
30. UWESO. Are Our Children Learning? Annual Learning Assessment Report 2011. 2012. Available at: http://www.uwezo.net/publications/reports/. Accessed 30 Jan 2018.
31. Mensch BS, Clark WH, Lloyd CB, Erulkar AS. Premarital sex, schoolgirl pregnancy, and school quality in rural Kenya. Stud Fam Plan. 2001;32:285–301.
32. Mensch BS, Lloyd CB. Gender differences in the schooling experiences of adolescents in low-income countries: the case of Kenya. Stud Fam Plan. 1998;29:167–84.
33. Phillips-Howard PA, Odhiambo FO, Hamel M, Adazu K, Ackers M, van Eijk AM, Orimba V, Hoog AV, Beynon C, Vulule J, et al. Mortality trends from 2003 to 2009 among adolescents and young adults in rural western Kenya using a health and demographic surveillance system. PLoS One. 2012;7:e47017.
34. Desai M, Phillips-Howard PA, Odhiambo FO, Katana A, Ouma P, Hamel MJ, Omoto J, Macharia S, van Eijk A, Ogwang S, et al. An analysis of pregnancy-related mortality in the KEMRI/CDC health and demographic surveillance system in western Kenya. PLoS One. 2013;8:e68733.
35. Kenya National Bureau of Statistics. ICF International: Kenya Demographic and Health Survey 2014. Nairobi: Kenya National Bureau of Statistics (KNBS) and ICF Macro. p. 2015.
36. Alexander K, Oduor C, Nyothach E, Laserson K, Amek N, Eleveld A, Mason L, Rheingans R, Beynon C, Mohammed A, et al. Water, sanitation and hygiene conditions in Kenyan rural schools: are schools meeting the needs of menstruating girls? Water. 2014;6:1453–66.
37. Nyothach E, Alexander KT, Oduor C, Mason L, Oruko K, Odhiambo FO, Vulule J, Laserson KF, Phillips-Howard PA. Handwashing for menstrual hygiene management among primary schoolgirls in rural western Kenya. Waterlines. 2015;34:279–95.
38. Oduor C, Alexander KT, Oruko K, Nyothach E, Mason L, Odhiambo FO, Vulule J, Laserson KF, Phillips-Howard PA. Schoolgirls' experiences of changing and disposal of menstrual hygiene items and inferences for Wash in schools. Waterlines. 2015;34:397–411.
39. Mooncup. Advice and Facts. 2011. Available at: http://www.mooncup.co.uk/advice-centre/faqs.html. Accessed 30 Jan 2018.
40. Juma J, Nyothach E, Laserson KF, Oduor C, Arita L, Ouma C, Oruko K, Omoto J, Mason L, Alexander K, et al. Examining the safety of menstrual cups among rural primary school girls in western Kenya: observational studies nested in a randomised controlled feasibility study. BMJ Open. 2017;7(4):e015429.
41. Hanley JA, Negassa A, Edwardes MD, Forrester JE. Statistical analysis of correlated data using generalized estimating equations: an orientation. Am J Epidemiol. 2003;157:364–75.
42. Cummings P. Methods for estimating adjusted risk ratios. Stata J. 2009;9:175–96.
43. African Population and Health Research Center: Attitudes towards, and acceptability of, menstrual cups as a method for managing menstruation: experiences of women and school girls in Nairobi, Kenya. Nairobi, Kenya; 2010.
44. Tellier M, Hyttel M, Gad M: Assessing acceptability and hygienic safety of menstrual cups as a menstrual management method for vulnerable young women in Uganda red cross Society's life planning skills project. 2012.
45. Hyttel M, Thomsen CF, Luff B, Storrusten H, Nyakato VN, Tellier M. Drivers and challenges to use of menstrual cups among schoolgirls in rural Uganda: a qualitative study. Waterlines. 2017;36:109–24.

9

Implementation project of the non-pneumatic anti-shock garment and m-communication to enhance maternal health care in rural Tanzania

Godfrey Mbaruku[1^], Michelle Skaer Therrien[2], Robert Tillya[1], Selemani Mbuyita[1*] ⬤, Zacharia Mtema[1], Iddajovana Kinyonge[1], Ritha Godfrey[1], Silas Temu[1] and Suellen Miller[2]

Abstract

Background: Obstetric hemorrhage (OH) remains one of the leading causes of maternal mortality, particularly in rural Africa. Tanzania has a high maternal mortality ratio, and approximately 80% of the population accesses health care lower level facilities, unable to provide Comprehensive Emergency Obstetric Care (CEmOC). The non-pneumatic anti-shock garment (NASG) has been demonstrated to reduce mortality as it buys time for women in shock to be transported to or to overcome delays at referral facilities.

Methods: This report describes one component of an ongoing maternal health improvement project, Empower, implemented in 280 facilities in four regions in rural Tanzania. The NASG along with a Closed User Group (CUG) mobile phone network were implemented within the overall EmOC project. Simulation trainings, repeated trainings, and close hands-on supportive supervision via site visits and via the CUG network were the training/learning methods. Data collection was conducted via the CUG network, with a limited data collection form, which also included free text options for project improvement. One-to-one interviews were also conducted. Outcome Indicators included appropriate use of NASG for women with hypovolemic shock We also compared baseline case fatality rates (CFR) from OH with endline CFRs.
Data were analyzed using cohort study Risk Ratio (RR). Qualitative data analysis was conducted by content analysis.

Results: Of the 1713 women with OH, 419 (24.5%) met project hypovolemic shock criteria, the NASG was applied to 70.8% ($n = 297$), indicating high acceptability and utilization. CFR at baseline (1.70) compared to CFR at endline (0.76) showed a temporal association of a 67% reduced risk for women during the project period (RR: 0.33, 95% CI = .19, .60). Qualitative feedback was used to make course corrections during the project to enhance training and implementation.

Conclusions: This implementation project with 280 facilities and over 1000 providers supported via CUG demonstrated that NASG can have high uptake and appropriate use for hypovolemic shock secondary to OH. With the proper implementation strategies, NASG utilization can be high and should be associated with decreased mortality among mothers at risk of death from obstetric hemorrhage.

* Correspondence: smbuyita@gmail.com
^Deceased
[1]Ifakara Health Institute, Dar es Salaam, Tanzania
Full list of author information is available at the end of the article

Plain English summary

Obstetric hemorrhage (OH), defined as excessive bleeding during pregnancy, childbirth, or the first 24 h after childbirth, remains a leading cause of death for women, particularly in rural Africa. OH can lead to shock, a state in which the body's vital organs lack enough oxygen, which leads to organ failure and death. In Tanzania women die from bleeding and shock due to long distances from emergency health services, Comprehensive Emergency Obstetric Care (CEmOC). One way this problem has been addressed is with the use of a lightweight, cost-efficient compression garment, the non-pneumatic anti-shock garment (NASG), which stabilizes women who have lost excessive blood, allowing them to survive delays in travelling to or receiving care at CEmOC facilities. Until now, there have been questions if NASGs can be implemented effectively in rural areas.

This study introduced the NASG at 280 health facilities in rural Tanzania along with a Closed User Group (CUG) mobile phone network. A CUG network is a service from a cellular phone company which allows phone calls to be made at no charge to other phones on the same network.

Data was collected on 1713 women with OH, and 24.5% (419) of these women had signs of shock. The NASG was applied to ~ 71%% (n = 297) of women with shock, showing high uptake and appropriate use. The rate of women dying from OH during the study at facilities, called the case fatality rate (CFR), was reduced during the study period.

Background

Obstetric hemorrhage (OH) is one of the leading causes of maternal deaths, accounting for 33.9% of maternal deaths in Africa to 13.4% of maternal deaths in developed countries, with the majority of deaths occurring in low resource settings (LRCs) [1, 2]. Deaths due to hemorrhage are highly preventable if managed appropriately, but deaths frequently occur in rural areas far from comprehensive emergency obstetric care (CEmOC) centers able to provide surgery and blood transfusions, the definitive treatments for severe hemorrhage with hypovolemic shock [3, 4]. One first aid management tool for hypovolemic shock secondary to obstetric hemorrhage is the non-pneumatic anti-shock garment (NASG). This low-technology, easy to apply, circumferential pressure device, is made of stretchy compression neoprene and closes tightly with Velcro, reversing shock, restoring vital signs, and decreasing blood loss in the pelvis and uterus [5]. This first aid device buys valuable time, to enable transfer from rural and lower level facilities, and during the often-long delays for blood transfusions or surgeries that can occur, even in tertiary and university teaching hospitals in LRCs.

Morbidity and mortality outcomes using the NASG have been positively compared to outcomes with standard treatment of shock/hemorrhage in women with a variety of OH etiologies, and the NASG was found to be effective in decreasing blood loss by over 50% [6–9]. A systematic review including 5 studies and 1247 women [10] with OH /shock found a decreased mortality of 48% (Relative Risk (RR) 0.52 (95% Confidence interval (CI) 0.36 to 0.77) at referral, tertiary-level facilities. A Cluster Randomized Clinical Trial (CRCT) was conducted in Zimbabwe and Zambia [9] to determine if early application of the NASG at the primary health facility level improved outcomes compared to later application at the referral facilities. The reduction in mortality was clinically significant at 55%, but there was an inadequate sample of women in hypovolemic shock (actual sample size, n = 880 vs. the predicted n = 2400) necessary to have adequate power to determine statistical significance [11].

The NASG is currently recommended by the International Federation of Gynecologists and Obstetricians (FIGO) [12] and the World Health Organization (WHO) [13] and can be found in PPH guidelines and manuals, such as WHO (Managing Complications 2nd edition) [14], Global Library of Women's Medicine (GLOWM) PPH Recommendations [15], and JHPIEGO's Helping Mothers Survive Bleeding After Birth [16], as well as in JHPIEGO's 2018, 5-year report "Survive and Thrive" [17]. A healthcare technology assessment performed for WHO [18] resulted in a positive recommendation for including the NASG in Emergency Maternal and Obstetric Care (EMOC) management. In 2015 the UN Commission on Life-Saving Commodities for Women and Children (UNCoLSC), the Clinton Health Access Initiative, Inc. (CHAI), the Safe Motherhood Program at the University of California, San Francisco (UCSF), and the Blue Fuzion Group entered into an agreement to decrease costs of the NASG by 75% in order to enhance NASG scale up in LMICs [19].

Despite these global recommendations and endorsements and despite pilot implementation and scale up projects conducted in India [20, 21], Nigeria [22], Ethiopia [23, 24], Niger [25], Timor Leste [26], and Colombia [27], there have been fewer publications on how the NASG is accepted and used by clinicians and health systems [26, 28–31].

The publications/reports that have measured utilization reported a range from 14% to 47% in Nigeria and Timor Leste [26, 28, 30]. While not published, a few presentations on a two-phase evaluation of a national PPH project in Niger, which introduced misoprostol, uterine balloon tamponade (UBT), and NASG as a PPH prevention and treatment package, reported extremely low rates of use and raised the issue of a need for strategic planning around the use of the new technologies, NASG (and UBT) [32–34].

This paper will focus on utilization rates, provider acceptability, barriers to utilization, and those elements of training and supportive supervision in-person and via use of a Closed User Group (CUG) phone system, which fostered higher, appropriate rates of NASG use in a large maternal health implementation project in rural Tanzania.

Methods

The 2010 Demographic and Health Survey revealed that in 5 years, Tanzania reduced maternal mortality from 578 to 454 maternal deaths per 100,000 live births [35, 36]. While emergency obstetric care (EmOC) is available at regional hospitals, a recent study of 22,243 live births in rural districts of Tanzania found that only 29% of deliveries occurred in a hospital [3].

This project was a component of the Empower II Project conducted by the Ifakara Health Institute (IHI), which implements Maternal, Newborn and Child Health (MNCH) interventions in real world settings to produce learning for improvements and scale up. Empower I lasted from July 2007 to June 2012 and Empower II launched in March 2013. Collectively, Empower works in four rural regions of Tanzania and targets a total population of 3,919,342 of which 813,092 are women of reproductive age. The NASG/CUG component described

below was conducted from November 2014 to June 2016. Members of the University of California, San Francisco (UCSF) Safe Motherhood Program served as consultants for the NASG portion of the project.

This project component addressed challenges around prompt management of OH and around OH referral between facilities through the introduction of the NASG (LifeWrap-NASG, Hong Kong) along with a Closed User Group (CUG) mobile phone network for public dispensaries, health centers, and three public referral hospitals, as well as three private referral hospitals in the eight districts of Geita, Nyang'hwale, Kalambo, Sumbawanga, Singida, Ikungi, Shinyanga, and Kahama (Fig. 1 for a map of the regions). A total of 280 facilities were enrolled: 17 Comprehensive Emergency Obstetric Care (CEmOC) facilities and 263 Basic Emergency Obstetric Care (BEmOC) facilities (17 health centers and 246 dispensaries). To qualify as a CEmOC referral facility, a site needed to have an operating theater and the capacity to perform a blood transfusion. BEmOC level health centers served a population of 50,000 people and provide inpatient care. Dispensaries provided the lowest level of care, serving a population of 10,000 people, and offering delivery beds and outpatient services. While dispensaries were intended to provide BEmOC care, not every dispensary was completely able to do so (the majority were

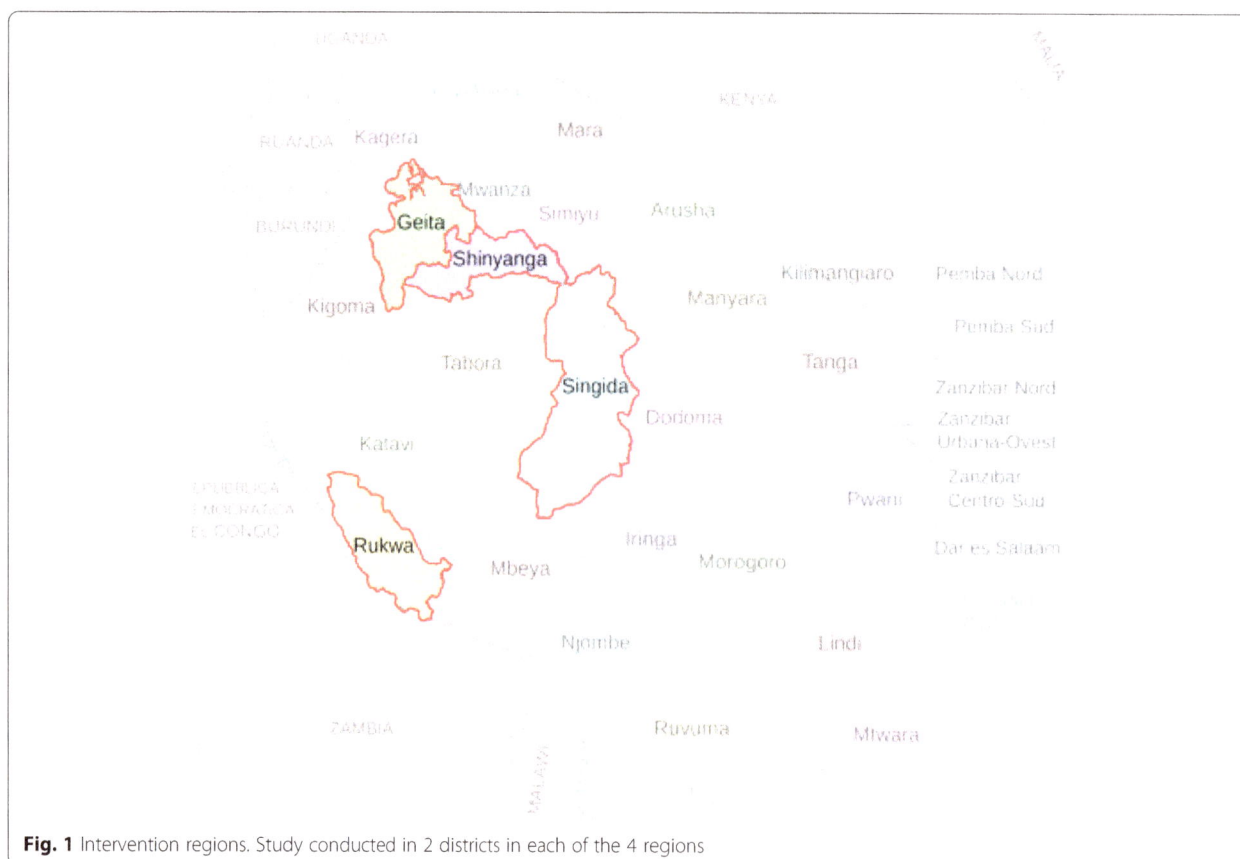

Fig. 1 Intervention regions. Study conducted in 2 districts in each of the 4 regions

not able to perform these signal functions: parenteral anticonvulsants, removal of retained product, and assisted instrumental delivery).

In addition to the NASG, the project introduced mobile phones on a CUG network. Five hundred eight cell phones were supplied, three per CEmOC facility, 2 per BEmOC facility, and four for each of the 8 Council Health Management Teams (CHMT) with phone service from the Airtel telecommunications company. Phones on a CUG network may call other phones within the network without airtime fees, so that health workers could communicate about patients, call for an ambulance, and contact IHI project staff for information and support.

The study trained participants to use the NASG for pregnant and postpartum women with hypovolemic shock secondary to obstetric hemorrhage of any etiology: ectopic pregnancy, molar pregnancy, complications of abortion, retained placenta, placenta previa, uterine atony, uterine rupture, and genital trauma. Women were classified as having hypovolemic shock if they had any amount of bleeding combined with either a systolic blood pressure of ≤80 mmHg or altered consciousness. Women were included whether the hemorrhage began at home, at the facility, or at another site.

Training

Three phases of training were conducted: a Training of Trainers (TOT) in October 2014, a series of Phase 1 trainings for CEmOC facilities was conducted in November 2014, and a series of Phase 2 training for BEmOC facilities was conducted in February 2015. Sessions specific to the NASG were 1.5–2 days in length and taught a curriculum developed by the UCSF Safe Motherhood Program [curriculum and training videos in English and a video of training in Swahili are available at: http://www.safemotherhood.ucsf.edu/resources/videos/, the NASG/CUG content was incorporated into scheduled Empower Emergency Obstetric Care (EmOC) trainings.

At the TOT 19 trainers were certified to support ongoing cascade trainings as well as project supervision. Only trainers who were able to pass a skills test and had a written exam score of ≥ 70% were certified to train for the project. Phase 1 consisted of four trainings, one per region at CEmOC facilities. Each facility sent four to five CEmOC providers, who were trained in clinical management of women with hypovolemic shock with the NASG and how to train other facility staff in NASG use. A phased approach was used, beginning project implementation only at district hospitals and other CEmOC health facilities for the first 3 months of the program (December 2014 – February 2015), before moving to Phase 2 training and introduction of NASGs to lower level facilities that referred patients to these CEmOC facilities.

Phase 2 consisted of 16 trainings in Swahili for BEmOC health center and dispensaries, four trainings per region. The trainings were conducted in March–April 2015, BEmOC facilities sent two staff members to represent each dispensary and 3–4 staff for each health center. These trainings were integrated with another scheduled Empower training on maternal health service provision. A total of 863 staff were trained in Phase 1 and Phase 2 by IHI, UCSF, and TOT trainers, including surgeons, obstetricians, medical officers, midwives, clinical assistants, registered nurses, clinical officers, medical attendants, anesthetists, anesthesiologists, and enrolled nurses.

At the start of Phase 2 meetings were held with IHI project staff, district medical officers, and hospital administrators to review the logistics for implementation, as well as to hear their experiences and challenges during the initial 3 months.

In December 2015, 20 ambulances were equipped with NASGs (one per ambulance) and 21 drivers received training on applying and transporting women with NASGs. As an additional training tool for all levels of facilities, four-minute low resolution (7 MB) and high resolution (11 MB) videos that instructed on NASG application for average, short, large, and unconscious patients were uploaded to the CUG phones during supervision to be used to refresh trained staff or train new staff.

All phases of the training included multiple simulations for a variety of shock and hemorrhage situations (how to transport, placing on conscious and unconscious women, removing when a woman is stable and remains stable, replacing if a woman goes back into shock, etc.). Simulations have been documented to improve retention and team work [37, 38]. We also held unexpected "emergency simulations" during lunch and break times, when participants did not expect to be performing a simulation. An actor playing the husband would carry in an "unconscious and dying," severely shocked patient/actress and participants had to quickly form a team and demonstrate how they would apply the NASG, manage the hemorrhage and shock of the unconscious and dying actress, and make a referral/transport if necessary.

At the trainings facility staff were informed that they would be receiving the CUG network phones, which became property of the Regional Medical Office. Those who accepted the CUG phones on behalf of the facility signed a contract outlining obligations for maintenance and use, as well as conditions in case of loss or damage. During the Phase 2 training, an introduction to the electronic data collection forms was presented. CEmOC facilities were given onsite training for the electronic forms when their CUG phones were distributed.

Phones distributed for use with the CUG network were Java-enabled Nokia phones. The closed user group was a subscription service through the Airtel company, which provided SIM cards for mobile phones to make calls at no cost to other phones on the network. The CUG phones were also programmed with a data entry system created on OpenXdata. Data was transmitted from the phones via General Packet Radio Service (GPRS) using an http protocol to send data to a local server running a MySQL database for storage and management. The data could be accessed remotely using a secure web-based platform located at: http://maternal.esurveillance.or.tz/.

Entry Criteria/Enrollment: Women were included in the study if they presented with or developed hypovolemic shock secondary to OH at any participating facility. Staff were instructed to apply the NASG for women presenting with signs of obstetric hemorrhage and hypovolemic shock, whether the patient would be referred out or managed on site.

Hemorrhage Management: All facilities had received training on EmOC through the Empower project. Evidence-based guidelines for PPH management included prophylaxis with uterotonics, treatment for PPH with uterotonics, Intravenous fluids, and referral/transport of women who continued to bleed despite uterotonic treatment.

Outcome Indicators: As this was an implementation project, the main outcomes were increased and appropriate use of NASG and CUG network. We set project targets for improvement at 75% increase from the baseline of 0, since both technologies had never been used before. Process indicators included: percentage of facilities with an NASG available and locatable in < 10 min, percentage of health facilities in compliance with established NASG disinfection protocols, percentage of facilities with a CUG network phone available, percentage of facilities able to show a charged CUG network, percentage of facilities that conducted regular training drills, and percentage of phones lost. We also compared baseline case fatality rates (CFR) from OH with endline CFR and predicted a decrease of 25%.

Data collection

From July –August 2014, IHI staff traveled to each of the 280 sites to collect baseline data. This consisted of reviewing all available hard copy registries to determine the CFR, looking at cases of reported OH and number of deaths attributed to OH for the 12 months from July 1, 2013 – June 30, 2014, the facility-based numbers were compared to the official Regional Reports. Baseline data were also gathered on availability of electricity, presence of cell phones for referrals, and transportation availability for all sites. The number of annual deliveries was gathered from district reporting.

Paper-based data collection on NASG use at the CEmOC facilities occurred from Dec 2014-March 2015, however as not all sites had begun NASG implementation, this data was used for training purposes only and not included in the analysis. CUG network phones were rolled out to all facilities during March–April 2015 during the Phase 2 BEmOC trainings. Both paper forms and electronic data entry forms were written in Swahili.

Facility staff were instructed to complete a case report for each woman with signs of obstetric hemorrhage. This data was recorded on a hard copy register for each site, and later entered into the electronic OpenXdata data entry form on the CUG phone and submitted to the central server by designated health care providers who had been trained for each facility. When there were discrepancies in the electronic records, data was verified against the paper-based register, and if additional verification was required, against other maternity and gynecology registries. In addition, sites sent month-end reports summarizing the number of deliveries, the number of obstetric hemorrhages, and the number of maternal deaths. This data was used to ensure 1) that all facilities were sending data on a regular basis 2) that the total number of OH reported was equal to the number of detailed OH case reports received. In cases of discrepancies or when the month-end report had not been submitted, the project team called facility staff using the CUG network to request the reports.

In addition to the patient data, the data form contained a free text comment field which allowed the provider to supply any additional information. Other fields allowed providers to give the reason they did not use uterotonics, the NASG, or the CUG phone for each patient if applicable.

Besides the quantitative electronic data on patient outcomes, we used a supervision tool to record the process indicators described above to ensure that the NASGs and CUG phones were at the facility and in working condition. These forms were completed by project staff during three rounds of supervision, with all 280 sites visited during each of the three rounds. The final forms were completed during the April–May 2016 supervision as an endline measure.

On-site supervision was conducted three times throughout the 15 months: from July – August 2015, December 2015 – January 2016, April – May 2016. Each site received three visits by project staff, at which time they were asked to demonstrate their skills, electronic reports were verified against paper records, and troubleshooting was performed for the phones. The physical condition of the NASGs and phones were verified and recorded on the supervision forms along with the number of staff trained, the number of staff not yet trained, and the frequency of drills.

Qualitative data collection

Feedback was sought to further enhance training and use of CUG and NASG. In addition to the patient data, the data forms contained the free text comment field noted above, which allowed the provider to supply any additional information. Qualitative informal interviews were conducted with facility staff during all three rounds of routine supervisory visits for sites, focusing on sites with apparent overuse (use on women not meeting criteria) or with lower numbers of uses than predicted.

For 2 weeks in July 2015, formal interviews were conducted with 19 facility staff, 15 of them working at the dispensary level, about their experiences with NASG. Thirteen of the staff had been trained, but not yet had a patient that required application of the NASG. Questions focused on ease of use, reasons for overuse or non-use, suggestions for improving training, and NASG acceptability. Due to the timing during the earlier stage of the project, most of the interviews focused on providers' confidence and theoretical concerns following their training, as few providers had prior experience.

Data analysis Quantitative data analysis was conducted using R (R Core Team (2017). R: A language and environment for statistical computing. R Foundation for Statistical Computing, Vienna, Austria. URL https://www.R-project.org/) and Stata 12.1 (StataCorp. 2011. *Stata Statistical Software: Release 12*. College Station, TX: StataCorp LP). Cohort study Risk Ratio (RR) methods within Stata were used to compute relative risk and Chi-Square statistics for the association of the use of the NASG with case fatality rates. Qualitative data analysis was conducted by seeking themes within the various responses to open-ended fields and to the structured one to one interviews.

Results

One thousand seven-hundred thirteen women with obstetric hemorrhage from any etiology were observed during the 15-month data collection period, with reporting from 276 facilities (98.6%). Estimated median blood loss was 500 mL ($n = 1672$, 97.6%), range 0 ml–3500 ml). Only 5.4% ($n = 92$) of women were missing blood pressure recordings and 5.6% ($n = 96$) were missing pulse, but consciousness level was recorded for all women. Blood loss estimates were missing for 3.0% ($n = 51$) of women. Additionally, 1.4% of facilities (4 dispensaries) failed to send any reports (monthly totals or individual cases).

Table 1 compares conditions between women who had OH ($n = 1713$), but did not receive the NASG ($n = 1256$), and those women who had OH and did receive the NASG ($n = 457$). The majority of the women who received the NASG had lower SBPs and were more likely to have altered level of consciousness. Of the 1713 women with OH, 419 (24.5%) met project hypovolemic shock criteria. Table 2

Table 1 Characteristics of all women with Obstetric Hemorrhage ($n = 1713$), those who received the Non-pneumatic Anti-Shock Garment ($n = 297$), and those who did not receive the Non-pneumatic Anti-Shock Garment ($n = 122$)

Variables	Women with NASG applied n (%)	Women without NASG applied n (%)	Total Frequency ($n = 1713$)
Systolic blood pressure			
≤ 80	183 (73.2)	67 (26.8)	250 (100)
81–90	113 (47.7)	124 (52.3)	237 (100)
> 90	147 (13.0)	987 (87.0)	1134 (100)
Missing	14 (15.2)	78 (84.8)	92 (100)
Consciousness level			
Normal	230 (16.4)	1176 (83.6)	1406 (100)
Confused/ unconscious	227 (73.9)	80 (26.1)	307 (100)

compares only those women who met study criteria of hypovolemic shock secondary to OH ($n = 419$), and shows worsening conditions and rates of use for different etiologies among those who received the NASG ($n = 297$) and women who did not receive the NASG ($n = 122$). As shown in Fig. 2, the NASG was applied to 70.8% ($n = 297$) of these women. Of the subgroup of 225 women (53.7%) experiencing shock who were transported to higher level care, 85.8% ($n = 193$) had the NASG applied before transfer, exceeding project targets of 75%. Of these 225 women transferred, 164 (72.8%) had referral communication using the CUG network.

A comparison of CFR at baseline (1.70) to CFR at the end of the project (0.76) showed a 67% reduced risk for women during the project ([RR: 0.33, 95% CI = .19, .60], not shown).

Supplemental qualitative data was voluntarily added by providers for 66.4% ($n = 1138$) of the hemorrhage cases in the free text comment field of the data screen: This field was frequently used to send positive feedback regarding the program such as:

"NASG helped, patient came to normal 120/60." (Was 70/40).

"NASG has helped the patient keep well".

"Died and back, NASG saves lives."

Nasg inaokoa maisha ya akina mama "NASG saves mother's lives."

Mgonjwa alishukuru sana watoa huduma vazi lilimuokoa "The patient thanked the service providers who had saved her".

Challenges were also reported, mainly when ambulances or other transport were called, but did not arrive for referrals, resolving missing data on hard copy records with electronic records, and additional support requests for training or referrals.

Interview data theme analysis showed the following categories of obstacles and opportunities in the early days of the implementation project: perceived training needs,

Table 2 Characteristics of women who met study criteria of hypovolemic shock secondary to obstetric hemorrhage (n = 419) who received non-pneumatic anti-shock garment (n = 297) and women with hypovolemic shock who met criteria, but did not receive non-pneumatic anti-shock garment (n = 122)

Variables	Women with NASG applied n (%)	Women without NASG use n (%)	Total frequency n = 419 n (%)
Referred to higher care			
Yes	193 (85.8)	32 (14.2)	225 (100)
No, managed at facility	104 (53.6)	90 (46.4)	194 (100)
NASG applied			
Yes	297 (100)	0 (0)	297 (71)
No	0 (0)	122 (100)	122 (29)
Etiology			
Complications of abortion	46 (41.8)	64 (58.2)	110 (100)
Uterine atony	65 (84.4)	12 (15.6)	77 (100)
Retained placenta	50 (79.4)	13 (20.6)	63 (100)
Placenta previa	33 (78.6)	9 (21.4)	42 (100)
Placental abruption	30 (85.7)	5 (14.3)	35 (100)
Ruptured uterus	25 (73.5)	9 (26.5)	34 (100)
Lacerations	23 (88.5)	3 (11.5)	26 (100)
Ectopic pregnancy	4 (66.7)	2 (33.3)	6 (100)
DIC	5 (83.3)	1 (16.7)	6 (100)
Other	16 (80.0)	4 (20.0)	20 (100)
Systolic blood pressure			
≤ 80	183 (73.2)	67 (26.8)	250 (100)
81–90	52 (76.5)	16 (23.5)	68 (100)
> 90	56 (59.6)	38 (40.4)	94 (100)
Missing	6 (85.7)	1 (14.3)	7 (100)
Consciousness status			
Normal	70 (62.5)	42 (37.5)	112 (100)
Confused	148 (75.5)	48 (24.5)	196 (100)
Unconscious	79 (71.2)	32 (28.8)	111 (100)

limitations to cascade training, desire for experience, and transportation difficulties [39]. From these early interviews, we learned how to improve the training and implementation of the project. Due to low patient volume at the dispensaries, these providers expressed fears that they anticipated not being proficient enough to apply the NASG correctly. There was a belief expressed that perhaps practice should occur on live patients in a hospital environment, rather than in a controlled simulation of the training center.

Process indicators

Data collected during endline supervision are reported in Table 3. At endline, 280 facilities (100%) had an NASG

and 271 (96.8%) had all their NASGs disinfected, laundered, folded, and stored in an area where they were not exposed to potential damage by pests. The only indicator where facilities did not exceed targeted outcomes, was that only 43% reported conducting regular training drills.

Discussion

This large scale implementation project in rural Tanzania demonstrated that appropriate utilization rates of 71% of women in hypovolemic shock could be achieved, even in lower level health care facilities. Positive contributing factors included adequate, frequent training and supportive supervision to use the NASG, clear definitions and parameters of hypovolemic shock, rapid and responsible access from project management and clinicians via the CUG, and intensive follow up for every death that occurred and for cases of non-use with women who met eligibility criteria. Although there was some use on women who did not meet the hypovolemic shock criteria, none of these women suffered side effects or morbidities/mortalities. The study also showed a temporal association of a 67% decrease in CFR in the study facilities at the project endline.

Alongside the near universal use of NASG for critically ill women with obstetric hemorrhage reported from one high-level facility in Cali, Colombia [27], this project demonstrated high utility among providers in very different settings and among different types of providers in rural Tanzania. Likewise, in Tamil Nadu State in India, the NASG has almost universal application at all levels of health care facilities, including on all 108 Emergency Management and Research Institute ambulances throughout the state [40]. In Timor Leste among ambulances and lower level facilities, there was uptake of NASG, including use on 40/86 PPH cases in only a 10-month period. The Colombia, Tamil Nadu, Timor Leste results, and this report contradict a finding of low utilisation from an evaluation of a national implementation project in Niger, in which misoprostol, UBT, and NASG were introduced. Of the 59 maternal deaths reviewed, only 4 women received the NASG [33].

However, the protocol for that project instructed that the NASG should not be applied for every woman with PPH. Rather, a sequenced approach was used, patients were given prophylactic misoprostol, then, if a hemorrhage occurred, the woman was treated with misoprostol. If the woman continued bleeding, a UBT was inserted. If the above treatments did not stop the bleeding, then NASG would be applied [26]. The low percentage of uses reported might indicate that the first two steps (miso and UBT) avoided some of the need for the NASG. However, limitations around primary data collection make it difficult to determine. In conversation with a national trainer from Health and Development International (HDI), the implementing organization working with the MOH in Niger (Zeidou A 2018, oral communication 14 August 2018), we learned that the Niger project did not keep

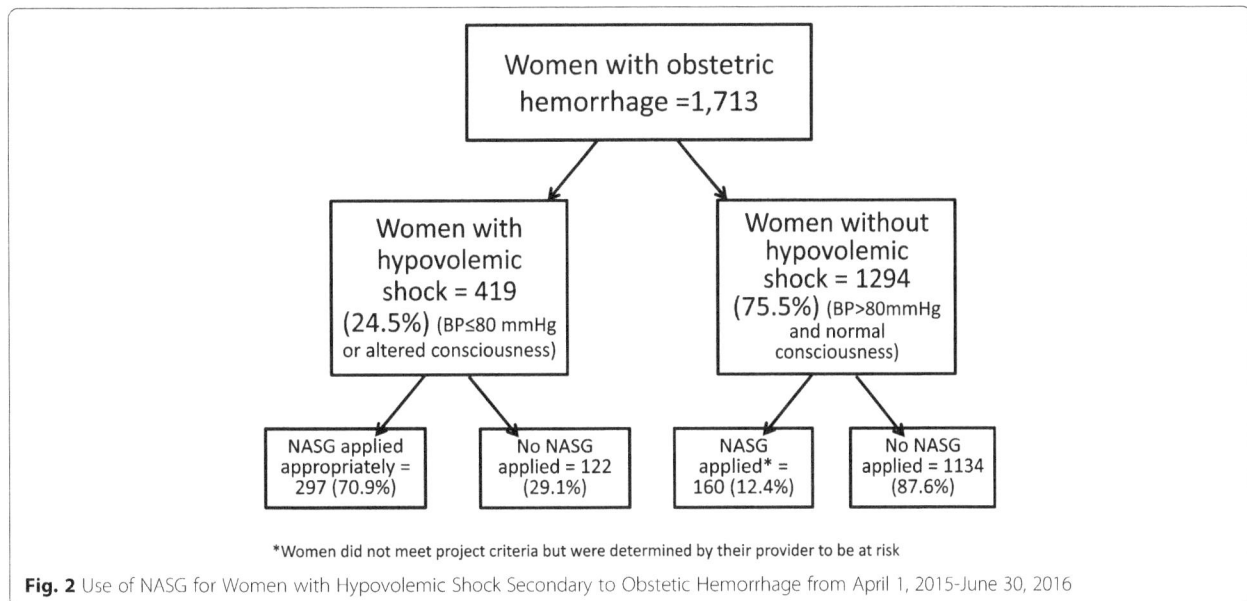

Fig. 2 Use of NASG for Women with Hypovolemic Shock Secondary to Obstetic Hemorrhage from April 1, 2015-June 30, 2016

its own data throughout the project; they attempted to do so in 2015, but following low (approximately 5%) reporting they were asked by government partners to halt and transition to the use of official government regional reporting. Beginning in 2016 they only utilized MOH reporting. For these reasons, the evaluation team conducted its own data collection, by reviewing the case records on only 59 (35%) of the 171 reported deaths. Finding a use of NASG on only 7% of the women included in the mortality review, may not reflect low use of NASG. It might, instead, be more interesting to see the numbers/percentages of use on women with severe hemorrhage/hypovolemic shock who did not die. Since that data is not available, it seems improbable that this low rate of NASG can be generalizable to the other women in this project or to any other project. While we agree that hypovolemic shock secondary to OH is a rare event, it is still possible to demonstrate adequate use with more reliable data.

It is also possible that differentials between other reports and the Niger report could be due to different approaches to training in the Empower project (frequent doses, higher use of simulations and practice), supportive supervision, close follow-up of cases, or use of primary concurrently collected data as seen in Tanzania and Timor Leste. Lower utilization rates, < 35% of PPH cases, found in two Nigerian states, Ibadan [30] and Ondo [28], may also reflect these differences in training, supply chain, exchange and return plans, political support, policy support, regulations over who can use NASGs (not allowing midwives, the front line workers, to use NASGs) [30]. They might also reflect examining rates of use against all OH cases, rather than only the severe cases with hypovolemic shock.

However, even the projects reporting lower than expected use can impart important lessons about project implementation of new technologies. We note in our study and in others a preference for onsite training with real OH cases, more hands-on skills sessions, and that the rarity of severe PPH may result in loss of skills' competencies. We noted this in our first round of qualitative interviews [39]. The Tanzania project seemed to have reduced some of these problems, first in the initial planning and then through course corrections responding to feedback; instituting a phased approach with adequate

Table 3 Endline supervision of facility process indicators $N = 280$ FACILITIES

Indicator	Baseline	Endline	Target
Percentage of facilities that have a NASG available and can locate it in less than 10 min ($n = 280$)	0 0%	280 100%	210 75%
Percentage of higher level health facilities in compliance with established NASG disinfection protocols ($n = 280$)	0 0%	272 97.1%	210 75%
Percentage of facilities able to produce a charged functional CUG network mobile phone within 15 min	0 0%	274 97.9%	210 75%
Percentage of facilities that conduct regular training /drills on NASG and CUG protocols ($n = 280$)	0 0%	120 42.8%	210 75%
Percentage of phones lost ($n = 590$)	0 0%	35 6%	59 10%

time during training for hands-on skills practice and team work; time to learn lessons and make course corrections before widespread implementation; continuous real-time review of hemorrhage case reports to determine whether the NASG was being used appropriately on women with hypovolemic shock, with follow-up conducted by CUG for facilities/individual staff that had problems with compliance in use of the NASG or reporting data; ability to contact project staff over the CUG system when challenges or questions arose; ability of district staff who were certified during the TOT to provide supervision and retraining during their routine quarterly site visits; encouragement of skills practicum sessions at the facility level to overcome rarity of severe PPH cases; and the ability for facility staff to view training videos on the CUG phones.

In Tanzania the utilization by already trained providers of a new emergency obstetric first-aid device for severe hemorrhage cases, which often cause high anxiety and fear, involves a difficult behavior change [41–43]. The Empower providers have been dealing with severe hemorrhage and maternal mortality, often for years, and often with horrible outcomes. Intensive hands-on simulation training during the project may have helped overcome this obstacle. Having the videos on their phones may have also decreased anxiety as newly trained health care workers had a readily available model to show application and management. These providers were already highly motivated by participation in Empower I and II, already updated on PPH management, EMOC, and improving referrals.

In some reports which recommend more hands-on training, they also suggest that the training might be costly. In this project, except for the two original TOTs, training for NASG/CUG was incorporated into ongoing EmOC training. Another question about costs, involve the CUG system and its sustainability. While we did not do a formal cost analysis, Regional Tanzanian government officials managing health services already had a budget equal to $175 USD per month to cover communications costs for four officials in a single region. This is equal to the monthly cost for the entire CUG network which covered all the health facilities in one district, as well as the District Medical Officers, who also received phones as part of the project. There are also comments about the "high costs" of the NASG. For this project, the initial purchase price was $55.00/per NASG. As the NASG can be washed and re-used multiple times, this results in a highly cost-effective management tool [19, 44, 45].

Limitations

While not a limitation to an implementation project, limitations to this project's generalizability should be noted. This was not a randomized clinical trial, we compared endline process indicators results to baseline rates of 0 at baseline where there were no NASGs or CUGs available. We did

encounter some difficulties with data collection on paper forms and with referrals on the providers' own cell phones, this resulted in the switch to the CUG phone network and electronic data collection. The temporal differences since baseline, such as participation in Empower trainings could also have improved the providers' EmOC skills; there may have been an increase in the number of women who received appropriate prophylaxis and/or treatment uterotonics during the intervention period as compared to the baseline period. Included in limitations were limitations to the training, particularly during the first few months, however, we did collect qualitative data on obstacles, and were able to respond and make course corrections in the training to emphasize even more simulations, practicums, and hands-on experiences. Total reporting was from 98.6% of all facilities, with all non-reporting facilities being dispensaries. Reports were received from all referral sites. The facilities that were unable to send reports had low network coverage or other technical obstacles, including being too close to the Zambian border to connect to a Tanzanian network. We attempted to overcome these difficulties by retrieving hard copy forms, sending a local project technician to troubleshoot the phones, or by having facility staff travel to an area with service in order to send monthly reports; however 4 facilities did not succeed in sending reports and were excluded from analysis. The emphasis was placed on ensuring all the referral facilities had complete reporting. There are methodological limitations with comparing CFR at baseline to CFR at endline, including the fact that other factors besides the NASG that could have affected the CFR outcomes during the project period. We will conduct further analyses on this data to investigate this association.

Strengths

However, there are many strengths to this project. First this was a real-world implementation project in rural facilities with a high need for overcoming delays in distance and in lack of definitive shock treatment at lower levels. There were high numbers of facilities (280) across a number of levels of a health care system. There were high response rates among facilities participating in the project, in the trainings, and in reporting. Embedding the NASG/CUG components into overall EmOC training was a strength, and also improved cost-effectiveness vs. holding a separate, stand-alone training. Management referrals and follow up with the CUG was a big strength, which contributed not only to the high response rates and validation of statistics, but also to case referral follow up. Evidence-based training in management of OH in the Empower II Project, followed, in our trainings, with clear objective clinical parameters of hypovolemic shock secondary to OH (not just an unreliable blood loss estimation), enabled the providers to appropriately apply NASGs to those women who really needed them.

Another method of ascertaining accuracy in utilization was the careful follow-up of mortalities and non-use through continuous review of incoming OH reports and month-end reporting accompanied with follow-up by CUG phone if reports were not received, if the facilities reported fewer than anticipated OH cases, or if case management appeared inconsistent with protocols for appropriate NASG use. If phone calls did not work to improve both reporting or use, the issue was escalated to facility management and ultimately district level management for in-person follow-up by a senior trainer. While these are not necessary in all implementation studies, this rigor did allow the project to demonstrate that high utilization is possible. At the end of the project, the region of Singida had generated sufficient government support to enable the region to independently scale up to the three districts that had not been included in the project, using their regional trainers and purchasing the necessary NASGs. For sustainability, the intensive follow up and data collection could be eliminated, but the simulation training and emphasis on supportive supervision could be more affordably sustained.

Conclusion

Despite few existing reports on real world use of the NASG within rural health care settings, this study of 276 reporting facilities and over 1000 providers supported via CUG demonstrated that NASG can have high uptake with appropriate use for hypovolemic shock secondary to OH. A phased introduction, practical hands-on training, supportive supervision as needed through the CUG network, real-time monitoring of OH case reports, and ability to watch training videos on the phones seem to be keys to acceptability and utilization. Incorporating NASG/CUG training into already established EmOC training and implementations also enhanced program success. It is clear by comparison to projects with fewer or lower quality and/or stand-alone training, supervision, communication, and referrals that a one-time training followed by distribution of the NASG to clinics and facilities might result in low utilization. Adding NASG training to pre-service curricula may further enhance uptake for new nurses, midwives, doctors, and other skilled maternal health care workers, who will arrive at their new posts already possessing skills and confidence in NASG application, management, and removal. With the proper implementation strategies, NASG utilization can be high and should be associated with decreased mortality among mothers at risk of death from obstetric hemorrhage.

Funding

This work was funded by the ELMA Foundation and Comic Relief. The funders had no role in the study design, data collection and analysis, decision to publish, or preparation of the manuscript.

Authors' contributions

SM, SM, RT, IK, MST, ZM, RG, GM participated in the design of the intervention and data collection protocols and tools, ZM, MST, RT, IK, ST oversaw data collection, MST performed the data analysis, SM, MST, and GM contributed to the writing of the manuscript. All authors read and approved the final manuscript.

Competing interests

The University of California San Francisco collects a royalty for the use of the name, LifeWrap which is one brand of non-pneumatic antishock garment and was the brand used in this project.

Author details

[1]Ifakara Health Institute, Dar es Salaam, Tanzania. [2]University of California, San Francisco, School of Medicine, Department of Obstetrics, Gynecology, and Reproductive Sciences, Safe Motherhood Program, California, USA.

References

1. Say L, Chou D, Gemmill A, Tunçalp Ö, Moller A-B, Daniels J, et al. Global causes of maternal death: a WHO systematic analysis. Lancet Glob Heal 2014;2(6):e323–e333. Available from: http://www.thelancet.com/article/S2214109X1470227X/fulltext. [cited 2014 Jul 15]
2. Ronsmans C, Graham WJ. Maternal mortality: who, when, where, and why. Lancet 2006;368(9542):1189–1200. Available from: http://www.ncbi.nlm.nih.gov/pubmed/17011946 [cited 2014 Jul 10]
3. Hanson C, Cox J, Mbaruku G, Manzi F, Gabrysch S, Schellenberg D, et al. Maternal mortality and distance to facility-based obstetric care in rural southern Tanzania: a secondary analysis of cross-sectional census data in 226 000 households. Lancet Glob Heal 2015;3(7):e387–e395. Available from: http://linkinghub.elsevier.com/retrieve/pii/S2214109X15000480. [cited 2018 Aug 15]
4. Berg CJ, Harper MA, Atkinson SM, Bell EA, Brown HL, Hage ML, et al. Preventability of Pregnancy-Related Deaths. Obstet Gynecol 2005;106(6):1228–1234. Available from: http://content.wkhealth.com/linkback/openurl?sid=WKPTLP:landingpage&an=00006250-200512000-00004. [cited 2018 Aug 15]
5. Stenson A, Miller S, Lester F. The Mechanisms of Action of the Non-pneumatic Anti-Shock Garment. In: Arulkumaran S, Karoshi M, Keith L, Lalonde A, editors. A Comprehensive Textbook of Postpartum Hemorrhage: An Essential Clinical Reference for Effective Management 2nd Ed. 2nd ed. London: Sapiens Publishing; 2012. p. 331–40.
6. Miller S, Fathalla MMF, Youssif MM, Turan J, Camlin C, Al-Hussaini TK, et al. A comparative study of the non-pneumatic anti-shock garment for the treatment of obstetric hemorrhage in Egypt. Int J Gynecol Obstet 2010;109(1):20–24. Available from: http://www.ncbi.nlm.nih.gov/pubmed/20096836. [cited 2018 Aug 15]
7. Miller S, Fathalla MM, Ojengbede OA, Camlin C, Mourad-Youssif M, Morhason-Bello IO, et al. Obstetric hemorrhage and shock management: using the low technology Non-Pneumatic Anti-Shock Garment in Nigerian and Egyptian tertiary care facilities. BMC Pregnancy Childbirth 2010;10(1):64. Available from: http://www.ncbi.nlm.nih.gov/pubmed/20955600. [cited 2018 Aug 15]
8. Turan J, Ojengbede O, Fathalla M, Mourad-Youssif M, Morhason-Bello IO, Nsima D, et al. Positive Effects of the Non-pneumatic Anti-shock Garment on Delays in Accessing Care for Postpartum and Postabortion Hemorrhage in Egypt and Nigeria. J Women's Heal 2011;20(1):91–98. Available from: http://www.ncbi.nlm.nih.gov/pubmed/21190486. [cited 2018 Aug 15]
9. Miller S, Bergel EF, El Ayadi AM, Gibbons L, Butrick EA, Magwali T, et al. Non-Pneumatic Anti-Shock Garment (NASG), a First-Aid Device to Decrease Maternal Mortality from Obstetric Hemorrhage: A Cluster Randomized Trial. Abdel-Aleem H, editor. PLoS One 2013;8(10):e76477. Available from: http://dx.plos.org/10.1371/journal.pone.0076477. [cited 2017 Feb 13]

10. Pileggi-Castro C, Nogueira-Pileggi V, Tunçalp Ö, Oladapo OT, Vogel JP, Souza JP. Non-pneumatic anti-shock garment for improving maternal survival following severe postpartum haemorrhage: a systematic review. Reprod Health 2015;12(1):28. Available from: http://www.ncbi.nlm.nih.gov/pubmed/25889868. [cited 2018 Aug 15]

11. El Ayadi AM, Butrick E, Geissler J, Miller S. Combined analysis of the non-pneumatic anti-shock garment on mortality from hypovolemic shock secondary to obstetric hemorrhage. BMC Pregnancy Childbirth 2013;13:208. Available from: http://www.pubmedcentral.nih.gov/articlerender.fcgi?artid=3834872&tool=pmcentrez&rendertype=abstract. [cited 2015 Aug 23]

12. Lalonde A, International Federation of Gynecology and Obstetrics. Prevention and treatment of postpartum hemorrhage in low-resource settings. Int J Gynecol Obstet 2012;117(2):108–118. Available from: http://www.ncbi.nlm.nih.gov/pubmed/22502595. [cited 2018 Aug 17]

13. World Health Organization. WHO recommendations for the prevention and treatment of postpartum haemorrhage. Geneva: World Health Organization; 2012. Available from: http://www.who.int/reproductivehealth/publications/maternal_perinatal_health/9789241548502/en/. [cited 2015 Aug 23]

14. World Health Organization, UNICEF, United Nations Population Fund (UNFPA). Managing complications in pregnancy and childbirth: a guide for midwives and doctors. 2nd ed. Geneva: World Health Organization; 2017.

15. Karoshi M, Keith L, Arulkumaran S, Lalonde A. Postpartum hemorrhage: Guidelines for Immediate Action, Wall Chart. Global Library of Women's Medicine. 2012.

16. JHPIEGO. Helping Mothers Survive Bleeding After Birth: Providers Guide: Jhpiego Corporation; 2015. p. 48. http://resources.jhpiego.org/resources/helping-mothers-survive-bleeding-after-birth-complete-training-package-english-african.

17. Survive & Thrive. Guiding the way forward: Survive & Thrive 5-year Report (2012-2017). 2018. https://surviveandthrive.org/about/Documents/Survive%20%20Trive%205%20year%20report%20FINAL.pdf.

18. Chhaya VA, Sharma JK, Ameel M, Sundararaman T. Healthcare Technology Assessment for Non-Pneumatic Anti Shock Garment for Obstetric Shock Prevention. [http://www.who.int/medical_devices/global_forum/E02.pdf]

19. United Nations Commission on Life Saving Commodities. UN Commission on Life Saving Commodities 2014 Progress Report. Geneva; 2015. http://www.who.int/woman_child_accountability/ierg/reports/UNCOLSC_submission_iERG_2015.pdf.

20. Satia JK, Jayantilal K, Misra M, Arora R, Neogi S. Innovations in maternal health : case studies from India. New Delhi: Sage Publications; 2014.

21. Mankikar S, Nanda R, Miller S. NASG reduces mortality in Indian women with PPH. Int J Gynecol Obstet. 2012;119(S3):S413.

22. Sloan NL, Storey A, Fasawe O, Yakubu J, McCrystal K, Wiwa O, et al. Advancing Survival in Nigeria: A Pre-post Evaluation of an Integrated Maternal and Neonatal Health Program. Matern Child Health J 2018;22(7):986–997. Available from: http://www.ncbi.nlm.nih.gov/pubmed/29427018. [cited 2018 Aug 27]

23. Demeke Z. Non-Pneumatic Anti-Shock Garment pilot in Ethiopia to reduce maternal mortality secondary to obstetric hemorrhage. CHAI Ethiopia. Presented at the Global Maternal Health Conference 2013 January, 2013.

24. Gebrehiwot Y. Use of the Non-Pneumatic Anti-shock Garment (NASG) to Reduce Maternal Mortality in Ethiopia. Ethiopia: Tewodros Emiru; 2013.

25. Zeidou A. Lutte contre la mortalite maternal: Experience du Niger. Lome, Togo: Presentation at Togo Ministry of Health Postpartum Hemorrhage Technical Meeting; 2017.

26. John Snow Inc. Timor Leste Health Improvement Project Final Report. 2015. https://www.jsi.com/JSIInternet/Inc/Common/_download_pub.cfm?id=18016&lid=3.

27. Escobar MF, Füchtner CE, Carvajal JA, Nieto AJ, Messa A, Escobar SS, et al. Experience in the use of non-pneumatic anti-shock garment (NASG) in the management of postpartum haemorrhage with hypovolemic shock in the Fundación Valle Del Lili, Cali, Colombia. Reprod Health 2017;14(1):58. Available from: http://www.ncbi.nlm.nih.gov/pubmed/28499381. [cited 2018 Aug 14]

28. Ohaeri B, Ogbeye GB. Assessment of Utilisation of Non-Pneumatic Anti Shock Garment (NASG) in the Control of Post-Partum Haemorrhage among Midwives in Selected Hospitals in Ondo-State, Nigeria [Internet]. Vol. 10,

International Journal of Caring Sciences. [cited 2018 Aug 17]. Available from: www.internationaljournalofcaringsciences.org

29. Sharma J, Negandhi P, Das AM, Sethy G, Neogi SB. Using nonpneumatic anti-shock garment for postpartum hemorrhage management and referral at the public health facilities: A pilot study in two districts of Bihar. Indian J Public Health 2016;60(4):316–322. Available from: http://www.ncbi.nlm.nih.gov/pubmed/27976656. [cited 2018 Aug 13]

30. Kolade OA, Tijani A, Oloyede Oladeji M, Bayo Lawal A. Midwives' Knowledge and Utilization of Anti-Shock Garment In Prevention of Postpartum Haemorrhage Shock at the University College Hospital, Ibadan Nigeria. IOSR J Nurs Health Sci. 2014;3:9–16.

31. Jordan K, Butrick E, Yamey G, Miller S. Barriers and Facilitators to Scaling Up the Non-Pneumatic Anti-Shock Garment for Treating Obstetric Hemorrhage: A Qualitative Study. Roy JK, editor. PLoS One 2016;11(3):e0150739. Available from: http://dx.plos.org/10.1371/journal.pone.0150739. [cited 2018 Aug 15]

32. Sheldon W, Tarnagada M. National Scale-up of Niger's PPH Initiative: Lessons learned from introducing new strategies into services. Presented Dec 5-6, 2017. Gynuity Postpartum Hemorrhage Meeting. 2017.

33. Dabash R. Misoprostol for PPH Prevention and Treatment: Learning from Senegal, Niger and Pakistan. Washington, DC: Postpartum Hemorrhage Community of Practice Annual Meeting; 2018.

34. Reproductive Health Supplies Coalition. Integrating misoprostol for PPH management in national programs: What we have learned from research evaluation? Presented Oct 10-14, 2016. 2016.

35. National Bureau of Statistics Tanzania, ORC Macro. Tanzania Demographic and Health Survey 2004-05. Dar es Salaam, Tanzania: NBS/Tanzania and ORC Macro; 2005.

36. National Bureau of Statistics, ICF Macro. Tanzania Demographic and Health Survey 2010. Dar es Salaam, Tanzania: NBS/Tanzania and ICF Macro; 2011. cited 2018 Aug 26]. Available from: https://dhsprogram.com/publications/publication-FR243-DHS-Final-Reports.cfm

37. Fritz J, Walker DM, Cohen S, Angeles G, Lamadrid-Figueroa H. Can a simulation-based training program impact the use of evidence based routine practices at birth? Results of a hospital-based cluster randomized trial in Mexico. van Wouwe JP, editor. PLoS One 2017;12(3):e0172623. Available from: http://dx.plos.org/10.1371/journal.pone.0172623. [cited 2018 Aug 15]

38. Merién AER, van de Ven J, Mol BW, Houterman S, Oei SG. Multidisciplinary Team Training in a Simulation Setting for Acute Obstetric Emergencies. Obstet Gynecol 2010;115(5):1021–1031. Available from: http://www.ncbi.nlm.nih.gov/pubmed/20410778. [cited 2018 Aug 15]

39. Onyewuenyi A. A Qualitative Approach to Understanding the Impact of Misuse and Misdiagnosis: Monitoring Use of the Non-Pneumatic Antishock Garment in Tanzania. San Francisco, CA: Seventh Annual CUGH Conference; 2016.

40. Neogi S, Mistra M. Innovative Approaches in Maternal and Newborn Care: Tamil Nadu Health System. In: Innovations in maternal health: Case studies from India. New Delhi: Sage Publications; 2014. p. 285–95.

41. Prochaska JO, Velicer WF, Rossi JS, Goldstein MG, Marcus BH, Rakowski W, et al. Stages of change and decisional balance for 12 problem behaviors. Health Psychol 1994;13(1):39–46. Available from: http://www.ncbi.nlm.nih.gov/pubmed/8168470. [cited 2018 Sep 1]

42. Rogers E. Diffusion of innovations. 3rd ed. New York: Free Press; 1983.

43. Althabe F, Buekens P, Bergel E, Belizán JM, Campbell MK, Moss N, et al. A Behavioral Intervention to Improve Obstetrical Care. N Engl J Med 2008; 358(18):1929–1940. Available from: http://www.ncbi.nlm.nih.gov/pubmed/18450604. [cited 2018 Sep 1]

44. Downing J, El Ayadi A, Miller S, Butrick E, Mkumba G, Magwali T, et al. Cost-effectiveness of the non-pneumatic anti-shock garment (NASG): evidence from a cluster randomized controlled trial in Zambia and Zimbabwe. BMC Health Serv Res 2015;15(1):37. Available from: http://www.ncbi.nlm.nih.gov/pubmed/25627322. [cited 2018 Aug 31]

45. Sutherland T, Downing J, Miller S, Bishai DM, Butrick E, Fathalla MMF, et al. Use of the Non-Pneumatic Anti-Shock Garment (NASG) for Life-Threatening Obstetric Hemorrhage: A Cost-Effectiveness Analysis in Egypt and Nigeria. Young RC, editor. PLoS One 2013;8(4):e62282. Available from: http://www.ncbi.nlm.nih.gov/pubmed/23646124. [cited 2018 Sep 1]

10

Acceptability and stakeholders perspectives on feasibility of using trained psychologists and health workers to deliver school-based sexual and reproductive health services to adolescents in urban Accra, Ghana

Philip Teg-Nefaah Tabong[1*], Ernest Tei Maya[2], Terence Adda-Balinia[3], Dela Kusi-Appouh[3], Harriet Birungi[4], Placide Tabsoba[3] and Philip Baba Adongo[1]

Abstract

Background: Adolescent sexual and reproductive health is recognized as a key developmental issue of international concern. However, adolescents' access to sexual and reproductive health (SRH) information and services is largely inadequate in sub-Saharan Africa. With increasing enrollment in schools, this could be an avenue to reach adolescents with SRH information and services. This study was therefore conducted to assess the acceptability and stakeholders' perspectives on the feasibility of using health workers and trained psychologists to provide school-based SRH services in Ghana.

Methods: Fourteen (14) focus group discussions (N = 136) were conducted; 8 among adolescents aged 12–17 years (4 boys, 4 girls groups), 4 among parents (2 males, 2 females groups) and two among mixed teacher groups. We also conducted 18 in-depth interviews with teachers, managers of schools, health workers, clinical psychologists, as well as adolescent SRH program managers in the Ghana Health Service, Ghana Education Service, UNICEF, UNESCO and National Population Council, Ghana. We audio-recorded all interviews and took field notes. Interviews were transcribed and transcripts imported into NVivo 11 for analysis using grounded theory approach to qualitative data analysis.

Results: Many respondents reported that it was challenging for parents and/or teachers to provide adolescents with SRH information. For this reason, they agreed that it was a good idea to have health workers and psychologists provide SRH information and services to adolescents in school. Although, there was general agreement about providing SRH services in school, many of the respondents disagreed with distribution of condoms in schools as they believed that availing condoms would encourage adolescents to experiment with sex. While majority of respondents thought it was acceptable to use psychologists and health workers to provide school-based sexual and reproductive health to adolescents, some teachers and education managers thought the implementation of such a program would oppose practical challenges. Key among the challenges were how to pay for the services that health workers and trained psychologists will render, and the availability of psychologists to cater for all schools.

(Continued on next page)

* Correspondence: philgh2001@yahoo.com
[1]Department of Social and Behavioural Sciences, School of Public Health, University of Ghana, Accra, Ghana
Full list of author information is available at the end of the article

(Continued from previous page)

Conclusion: Stakeholders believe it is feasible and acceptable to use trained psychologists and health workers to deliver school-based SRH information and services in the Ghanaian school context. However, provisions must be made to cater for financial and other logistical considerations in the implementation of school-based SRH programs.

Keywords: Sexual and reproductive health, Adolescents, Health workers, Psychologists, School-based adolescents health services, Feasibility, Acceptability, Ghana

Plain English summary

Adolescents face challenges accessing reproductive and sexual health services. The lack of access to these services make some adolescents engage in unhealthy sexual and reproductive health behavior. Globally, there has been a drive towards finding innovative ways to increase access to sexual and reproductive health services. With increasing enrollment of adolescents in school, it presents an opportunity to explore ways to use the school environment to increase access to sexual and reproductive health services. Many of the behaviors that adolescents put up are caused by psychological factors. This therefore calls for some level of expertise in psychology and health to be able to provide the needed assistance. We therefore conducted a study among teachers, students, managers of educational institutions, health care workers engaged in adolescent's sexual and reproductive health services and development partners on their views about using trained health workers and psychologists to deliver the service.

Our study found that students, teachers and various stakeholders believe the current strategies used to provide adolescents with sexual and reproductive health services were inadequate and therefore felt that it was better to use trained psychologists and health workers to deliver these services to adolescents in school. However, there was the need to do further consultation and put in measures to cater for logistical issues and incentives for the people to provide these services.

In conclusion, stakeholders in this study believe it was feasible and acceptable to use psychologists and health workers to deliver school-based sexual and reproductive health services.

Background

Adolescent sexual and reproductive health (ASRH) is recognized as a key developmental issue of global concern. While reproductive health information and service delivery have been identified as necessary programs for decades, availability of such programs for adolescents has only recently been more endorsed. The International Conference on Population and Development (ICPD) held in 1994 and the Fourth International Conference on Women held in 1995 endorsed the rights of young people to sexual and reproductive health (SRH) information and services [1]. Health and development

professionals and policy makers have built on this consensus to formulate and deliver needed programs that are specially designed to meet adolescents' developmental needs. Over the past decades, the framework of adolescent friendly health care has been used to better orient health services to the needs of young people. Initially described by the World Health Organization (WHO) and largely focused on primary health care in low-income countries, there is growing appreciation of the framework's potential to promote quality health care to adolescents in high-income countries within specialized health services [2].

Despite these commitments, SRH information and services remain largely inadequate in sub-Saharan Africa. Many adolescents face an early sexual debut and many face difficulties in obtaining SRH services [3–7]. Adolescents are also typically poorly informed about how to protect themselves from pregnancies and sexually transmitted infections (STIs), which threaten their health and survival [5, 7]. A nationwide survey in Ghana found that 14% of females aged 15–19 years had begun child bearing. Of these 14%; about 11% have had a life birth and 3% were pregnant at the time of the survey [8]. Contraceptive use are also low as another nationwide survey of 1037 adolescents shown an overall prevalence of 18.3% comprising 14.6% of modern methods and 3.7% of traditional methods [9]. Similarly, another study reported that unsafe sexual and unsafe abortion practices was common and viewed as normal [10].

Comprehensive Sexuality Education (CSE), which is defined as age-appropriate, culturally relevant, scientifically accurate, realistic, and nonjudgmental education about sexuality and relationships, offers an appropriate platform to provide adolescents with critical SRH information [11]. CSE has been reported to have significant impact in addressing the SRH needs of adolescents in other countries [12–14]. Reproductive health services incorporate a range of activities (e.g. health promotion, prevention, early diagnosis, treatment and care, rehabilitation). In Ghana, Population and Family Life Education (POP/FLE) a form of CSE was introduced into the basic education system of the Ghana Education Service (GES) between 1973 and 1979 on a pilot basis, re-activated in 1987 and again in 1994. Due to the lack of a comprehensive in-school approach to this the POP/FLE has been unable to achieve its goal as many adolescents have low knowledge on SRH [15–17].

Guidance and counselling services were established in 1976. The Ghana government came out with a policy, through a directive issued by the Ghana Education Service (GES), for the establishment of guidance and counselling in the nation's second cycle institutions [18]. The School Health Education Programme (SHEP) was also established in 1992 as a follow-up action on Ghana's commitment to the Jomtien World Declaration on Education for all and her ratification of the United Nations Convention of the Rights for the Child. It was established as a joint mandate to the Ministry of Education (MoE) and the Ministry of Health (MoH). The SHEP program was to facilitate the provision of health education to the door steps of school children, foster early detection of disability and to inculcate into them health promotion habits, attitudes and values. Despite all these interventions which are mostly handled by trained teachers, evidence from a study showed the desire of adolescents towards receiving accurate and more comprehensive reproductive and sexual health information and service in schools. An initial study conducted by Population Council under the Strengthening Evidence for Preventing Unintended Pregnancies (STEP UP) project in 2012 showed that 80% (both sexes) of the adolescents interviewed indicated the need for more information on reproductive health [19].

In developing countries parents, school teachers, mass media, social media and peers have been reported as the main sources of information on sexual and reproductive health [15, 20–22]. However, these channels have been reported to have challenges in meeting the informational needs and services of adolescents [15, 22, 23].

In Ghana, adolescents constitute about a quarter of the total population and their population is expected to continue to increase [24]. Despite this, many have been reported to have low and inaccurate knowledge about their sexual and reproductive health (SRH), [25–27]. A study among adolescents in Central Region of Ghana by Owusu, Blankson & Abane [20] showed that the major sources of information on SRH to adolescents were their friends (30%), radio/television (26%) and parents (13%) [20]. However, information adolescents receive from these sources have been reported in many instances to be inaccurate, not focused on adolescent needs and also limited in scope [15]. This lack of knowledge has led to high incidence of sexually transmitted infections (STIs) and unplanned pregnancy among adolescents in Ghana [28]. Beyond the lack of knowledge, access to reproductive health services such as contraceptives, treatment for STIs and safe abortion services have been a challenge in Ghana [8]. Socio-cultural barriers and lack of adolescent friendly SRH services leads to poor patronage of such services even when they are available [3, 29, 30].

Studies have also showed that the behavior during the period of adolescents are triggered by psychological factors [31, 32]. Many health compromising behaviors, such as unsafe sexual practices, use of tobacco, alcohol and other psychoactive substances, that begin during adolescence have profound consequences for their health and development and also long term wellbeing [2, 33, 34]. The use of nurses to provide ASRH services in schools and psychologists to provide counselling and psychological support to adolescents is believed to be essential in addressing the problem adolescent face. Nurses will also diagnose and treat STIs among adolescents and liaise with formal health facilities to provide comprehensive abortion services to reduce the negative effects of unsafe abortions as has been reported in a study [35–38]. Nonetheless, the use psychologists to provide school-based health services has not been reported in literature. Currently in Ghana psychologists are mainly employed in academia, industry, health facilities especially mental health facilities and the private sector. Although data is not readily available on the regional distribution of psychologists, records available at the Ghana Psychologist Council show there are about 116 clinical, 35 counselling and 10 educational psychologists [39]. Nonetheless, there are several trained psychologists who are not registered with the council and not practicing despite the fact that the Health Professionals Act, 2013, (Act 587 of 2013), Domestic Violence Act, 2007 and Mental Health Act 2012 requires members to be registered before they can be employed in the formal sector [40].

From our review of literature, no study has been conducted to assess the stakeholders' beliefs about the feasibility and acceptability of using trained psychologists and health workers to provide these services. The increase in enrollment in school in recent times makes the school environment presents an opportunity to reach students with CSE and SRH services. Thus, we conducted this study to assess the acceptability and stakeholders' perspectives about the feasibility of using health workers and trained psychologists to provide SRH services in schools in Ghana.

Methods

Study design

We conducted a qualitative study comprising of indepth interviews and focus group discussions (FGDs) with junior high school students, teachers, school managers and other stakeholders to assess their view on the feasibility of using psychologists and health professionals to deliver SRH information and services to in-school adolescents. We adopted grounded theory approach to qualitative research in this study. In grounded theory approach to qualitative research, the researcher undertakes a research and develops a theory or theoretical framework that is grounded on the data [41, 42]. The approach was used to identify the contextual issues and approaches to be adopted in Ghana.

Study area

The study was conducted in Nima in the Ayawaso sub-metropolis of the Accra Metropolitan Assembly. The Accra Metropolitan Assembly (AMA) has a total population of 1,665,086 representing 42% of the region's total population. Females constitute about 51.9% of the population [43]. The Metropolis, which is entirely urban (100%), has a fairly youthful population as about 42.6% of the population are children under 15 years [24]. Nima, the study site reflects the metropolitan structure as it serves as a hub for migrants. Forty-seven percent of residents are migrants; this proportion is the highest in the Greater Accra region [44]. Early marriage is common in the area [44]. There were 14 Junior High Schools in Nima with a total student population of 2492 aged between 12 and 17 years [45].

Recruiting of respondents

We recruited five categories of respondents into this study; students, parents, teachers, educational managers and representatives of development partners. The district education office supported the recruitment of students. We selected two out of the 14 junior high schools based on two main criteria: recorded high school dropout rates due to teenage pregnancy and presence of trained ASRH teachers. From the two selected schools, 79 adolescent students (39 females and 40 males) aged 12–17 years were recruited to participate in the study. We obtained the list of students who have not been absent from school over the term and students who have attended courses which included some SRH education. From this list, we selected the actual participants based on their willingness to participate. These students participated in age and sex-specific FGDs: female students aged 12–14 years; female students aged 15–17 years; male students aged 12–14 years; and male students aged 15–17 years.

We recruited parents of students in the two schools who regularly participated in school activities such as Parent Teacher Association (PTA) meetings. This was done to ensure that we selected parents who were engaged in school-related activities. Teachers and head teachers assisted the research team to purposively select parents who met this inclusion criterion. Purposive sampling was also employed to select key informants in education and health who were in-charge of adolescent SRH issues at various levels. We contacted Ghana Education

Service for contacts numbers of the managers who oversee adolescent reproductive health services in the Metropolis. We then reached out to them and booked an appointment for the interview. For representatives of development partner, the research team visited the various offices and the focal persons were informed about the study and a consent obtained before they were interviewed.

Data collection strategy
In-depth interviews

A semi-structured in-depth interview (IDI) guides was developed or the data collection. The same IDI guide was used in interviewing education managers, health workers, psychologists and development partners. The interview guide for these stakeholders focused on participants' views about school-based adolescent SRH services, how such services should be delivered, whether using trained psychologists and health workers to deliver these services was feasible, and the ranges of services that should be provided. Interviews were conducted in private and lasted between 45 and 60 min. All interviews were audio-recorded.

In all 18 key informants were selected and interviewed. In the educational sector, we recruited people such as basic education coordinators, school health coordinators, heads of basic schools, and teachers. We also interviewed key personnel in-charge of adolescents' SRH from the Ghana Health Service at sub-metropolis, metropolis and national levels. In addition we interviewed representatives from development partners whose activities include adolescent sexual and reproductive. Table 1 summarizes the number of different key informants who participated in the study.

Focus group discussions

Semi-structured FGDs were conducted to explore normative views about SRH information received while exploring the feasibility and acceptability of the proposed solution. Different FGD guides were designed for students, teachers and parents. The topic guides explored

Table 1 Summary of Key Informants

Category of Respondent	Number interviewed
Ghana Education Service Program Managers	5
Heads of Basic Educational Schools	3
Ghana Health Service ASRH Program Managers	4
Population Council Representative	1
Members of Ghana Psychologist Association	2
UNESCO Representative	1
Teachers	2
Total	18

adolescents' and parents' normative views on the following key broad areas: SRH information and services delivery preferences; viability and acceptability of providing in-school reproductive health services by health workers; delivering sexual and reproductive health care using psychologists and health workers at the school level. However, during the FGDs, inductive probing was conducted on emerging new areas. Two research assistants conducted the FGDs, one moderated the discussions while the second took detailed notes. The note taker took notes on the group dynamics and body language of participants as well as seating arrangements to supplement and guide the interpretation on the transcripts. All discussions were audio-recorded. Fourteen (14) separate group discussions were held: eight among adolescents (four per school), four among parents (males and females separately in each school) and two among teachers (one per school). Each group comprised 9 to10 participants and the discussions lasted for approximately one hour and thirty minutes. Table 2 provides the summary of the participants in the FGDs.

Data analysis

The audio-recordings and field notes were transcribed verbatim in English using Microsoft Word. The researchers read through transcripts and noted the emerging issues from the data. These were transformed into a codebook. The codebook contained various themes in the data, their definition and where such themes should be used in coding the data. The codebook was reviewed by the research team, imported into QSR NVivo 11 as nodes. The transcripts were also imported into QSR NVivo 11 for analysis. We first classified the data sources (FGDs, and IDIs) and assigned the classifications to the data sources. Various respondents were captured as cases and attributes such as designation, gender and age assigned to the respondents (cases). This allowed us

Table 2 Summary of Participants in FGDs

Participants	Number of FGD	Number of Participants
Female Students		
12–14 years	2	19
15–17 years	2	20
Male Students		
12–14 years	2	20
15–17 years	2	20
Parents		
Males	2	20
Females	2	19
Teachers		
Mixed male/female groups	2	18
Total	14	136

to run queries in NVivo to quantify the qualitative data sources and cases. Grounded theory was adopted for the analysis of the data. This approach involved three inter-related steps; open coding, axial coding and selective coding [46]. For the start, line-by-line coding of responses from various respondents was conducted based on the codebook. During the initial stages of the coding, items were coded unto the nodes as free nodes. However, as the coding proceeded, the relationship between nodes began to emerge, therefore these relationships were transformed into tree nodes. This continued until all the transcripts were coded. Afterwards, the nodes browser was reviewed to show the relationship between the various nodes. Queries were also run to obtain relations and main themes that emerged from the data in the form of axial relationship. Based on this relation, the data were reviewed and items coded selectively unto these nodes with the aim of developing a theory grounded on the dataset. At this stage hierarchical charts were drawn to explore the stakeholders' perspectives about the feasibility and acceptability of the use of psychologists and health workers to provide school-based ASRH. The results are complemented with quotes from the transcripts.

Results
Provision of sexual and reproductive health information and Services in Schools

There was unanimity among all respondents about the need for school-based provision of SRH information and services. This approach was viewed as the most appropriate way of addressing challenges that adolescent face in trying to access SRH information and services. Participants noted that there was an increase in enrollment in schools and that many adolescents were in school. Further, they noted that students spend majority of their weekly hours in school. They therefore noted that school-based channels would be the most appropriate platform to disseminate SRH information. The following quotes buttress these points by respondents:

"The most important place is school and at home. Because for especially these Christians you go to churches on Saturdays or Sundays. Isn't it? Once a week. But school, at least 5 days in a week, so it the best place for educating adolescents on sexual and reproductive health issues" (38-year married male parent, FGD).

"...first of all, the statistics show that most of our young people are in school, so if you want to meet adolescents with information then you might as well go to where they can be found where most of them are. And if most of them are found in schools as the statistics are telling us,

then it means that comprehensive sexuality education should start with the schools"(Health Manager 1, IDI).

"I also think that reproductive health services must be provided in schools. Children are exposed to a lot of information than we think. Many of them use the internet to seek information on certain things and the information they get may not be correct, so I think when the schools provide reproductive services, they will be informed on behavioral changes, positive behavioral changes that can help them to grow up as adults in future" (Education Manager-2, IDI).

Parents, education managers and health workers all agreed that there was a need to extend the SRH services in schools and there were little variations in views across the various respondents. Out of the 18 key informants interviewed, 15 supported school-based ASRH services. In FGDs among teachers, 14 of the 18 participants also supported this strategy of providing ASRH service. In FGDs with parents, 16 of 19 female parents and 14 of 20 male parent support this approach. Figure 1 shows a graph depicting the respondents' views on school-based ASRH services.

Some parents drew on their own experiences to highlight the negative effects of the lack of SRH information and services. One parent, for example, shared her experience with an unplanned pregnancy that led to her dropping out of school:

"For me with my child when I realized his behavior, - he likes being in obscure places with young girls, I cautioned him not to impregnate someone. He should bear in mind that I gave birth at 15 years and for that matter I couldn't continue with school, so the same thing

might happen to any lady so he should be very careful" (42-year female parent, FGD).

Views on range of services to be provided in schools

Participants mentioned health education, counseling services, and provision of sanitary pads as essential services for inclusion in any school-based adolescent health program. As shown in Fig. 2, there were mixed views on distributing condoms to students. Some respondents felt that it was appropriate to distribute condoms to students to enable them have protected sex should they wish to have sex. Those who held this view noted that some adolescents often engaged in unprotected sex and believed that the provision of condoms would prevent unplanned pregnancy and sexually transmitted infections. However, some respondents believed that distributing condoms would promote sexual activity as adolescents "experiment" with the condom. One respondent also noted that the current educational policy did not permit the distribution of condoms in school and suggested that condom distribution should be community-based. The following quotes from respondent illustrate these points:

"….But in our schools we provide the counselling services, we can have the health corner alright where counselling services are provided, where materials are provided for reading, where we could have the sanitary towels or pads and other things. But for now I won't subscribe to having condoms in school because of our socio-cultural background" (Education Manger 4, IDI).

"To me if they provide these services such as health education, distributing sanitary pad and condoms in school it is a good idea because nowadays if you advise

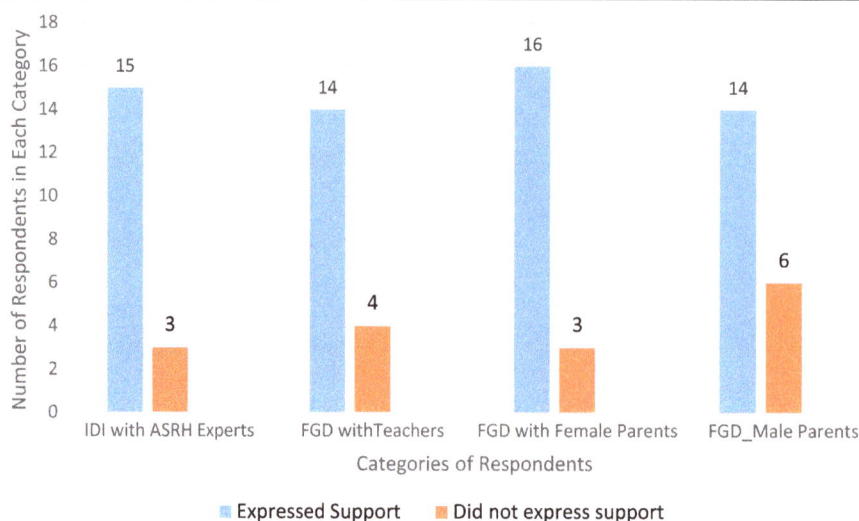

Fig. 1 Respondents' views on school-based sexual and reproductive health information and services

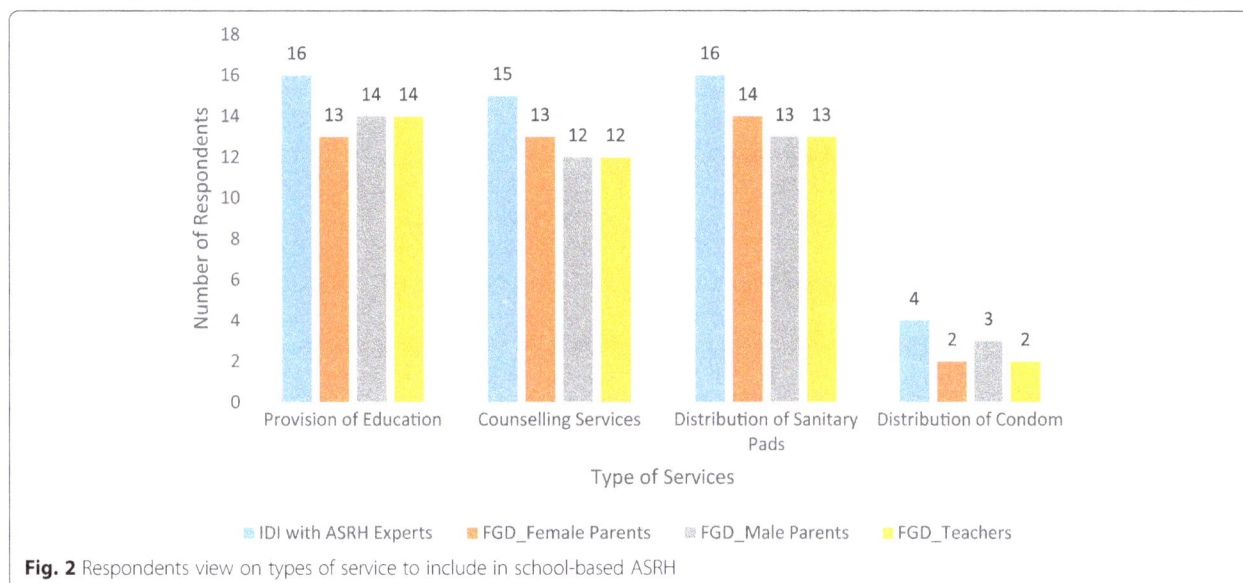

Fig. 2 Respondents view on types of service to include in school-based ASRH

the young ones not to have sex, they will have it. So it should be provided in schools for them to protect themselves" (Male Parent, FGD).

"My brother I told you from the very onset that for now Ghana Education Service doesn't permit the provision of condoms in our schools. Do you get the point? We have a few though of health corners in our schools... But because our schools we don't allow the provision of condoms, they don't give condoms to the children in the school but however just as I said and I reiterate, if you have any condoms to provide let it be community-based" (Education Manger 3, IDI).

Some respondents believed that it would be possible to revise the current prohibition of condom distribution within any school premise. Some education managers believed that if various stakeholders including parents were properly engaged it would be possible to obtain approval.

"Although the current system does not allow the provision of some reproductive health service within school compound, if good consultation among parents, teachers, education managers is done, it will be possible to revise the policy" (Education Manager 1, IDI).

Perceived benefits of providing school-based sexual and reproductive health services

Most participants believed that school-based provision of SRH information and services would help adolescents make good SRH choices and reduce the prevalence of unplanned pregnancies, abortions, and sexually transmitted infections. Participants also noted that access to SRH information and services could reduce school

dropout rate among females because those who become pregnant whilst in school are often compelled to drop out of school. The following quotes illustrate these points:

"With the services, it will go a long way in reducing the rate of abortion and teenage pregnancy" (Education Manager-1, IDI).

"My view is they should provide sexual health services in schools, it is a world known issue now that we are having girls getting pregnant in schools but if these services were provided to them, I don't think they will find themselves in this situations" (Education Manager 2, IDI).

"... it will help them delay becoming pregnancy, get pregnant when they want to, reduce the incidence of STIs and of course all these things will help them to improve their ability to stay in school and also improve their economic status in future" (Adolescent Reproductive Health Expert, IDI).

In FGDs with students, they acknowledged challenges in accessing reproductive health services at the community level. In their view, students who seek such services at the community are often perceived as bad boys/girls and service providers are unfriendly to them. They therefore believe the delivery of these services at the school can increase access and break social barriers inhibiting the uptake of such services at the community as illustrated:

"We cannot go to health facility to do family planning or go and buy condoms because the drugstore seller will

say you are a bad girl or boy and may tell your parents. So, those who cannot abstain from sex do it without any protection and some become pregnant in the process. One of our colleagues had to stop school because she became pregnant. So having access to this in the school will help address this" (17 years female student, FGD).

Potential challenges in introducing comprehensive school-based ASRH

Feedback from participants suggested that there might be some challenges in introducing school-based SRH programs. Respondents identified resistance from religious organizations, faith-based schools, teachers and parents as a key challenge. This notwithstanding, some respondents believed that with extensive consultation it would be possible to have wider acceptance. The following quotes illustrate these differing views:

"You see some churches will rise up against it. You know Catholics they are against the use of contraceptives, let alone providing the services at their school" (Education Manager 1, IDI).

"Yes, first is resistance from schools and from teachers but we need to do a lot of advocacy and some orientation for them to look at the benefits of such information before we rush into the school" (Education Manager 3, IDI).

"The only problem we'll have is our conservative nature as Ghanaians. That's the only challenge because, for instance, how will the parents feel if the child comes home to tell the mother that they shared condoms for us in school? Or they are doing family planning in schools. Every parent will be alarmed" (Health Manager 3, IDI).

Acceptability of the use of psychologists to provide ASRH services

While there were dissenting views on the use of psychologists to provide school-based SRH information and services (Fig. 3), majority of the participants believed that it was feasible and acceptable to use them for these services to adolescents.

Those who believed that it was appropriate to have trained psychologists noted that using psychologists would enable teachers to focus on their primary responsibility of teaching. To them, even though the current education system allows for the training of teachers to serve as guidance and counseling officers at school, these teachers are not effective because they are still expected to teach. Some participants also observed that some students may not feel comfortable discussing sexual and reproductive issues with their teachers and noted that a neutral person, such as a psychologist, would be more appropriate. Other participants felt that psychologists were better placed to identify students experiencing emotional challenges and to offer timely support and counseling. The following quotes illustrates these views from respondents:

"In our adolescent health program, we have a lot of psychology in it so they may not only provide the services and appropriate information but they are also able to provide the counselling that they need for children because they are many ramifications. A child may have some problem at home and that may manifest in inappropriate sexual behavior and we need such people to be able to delve into the details and be able to provide appropriate counselling for such kids" (Education Manager 3, IDI).

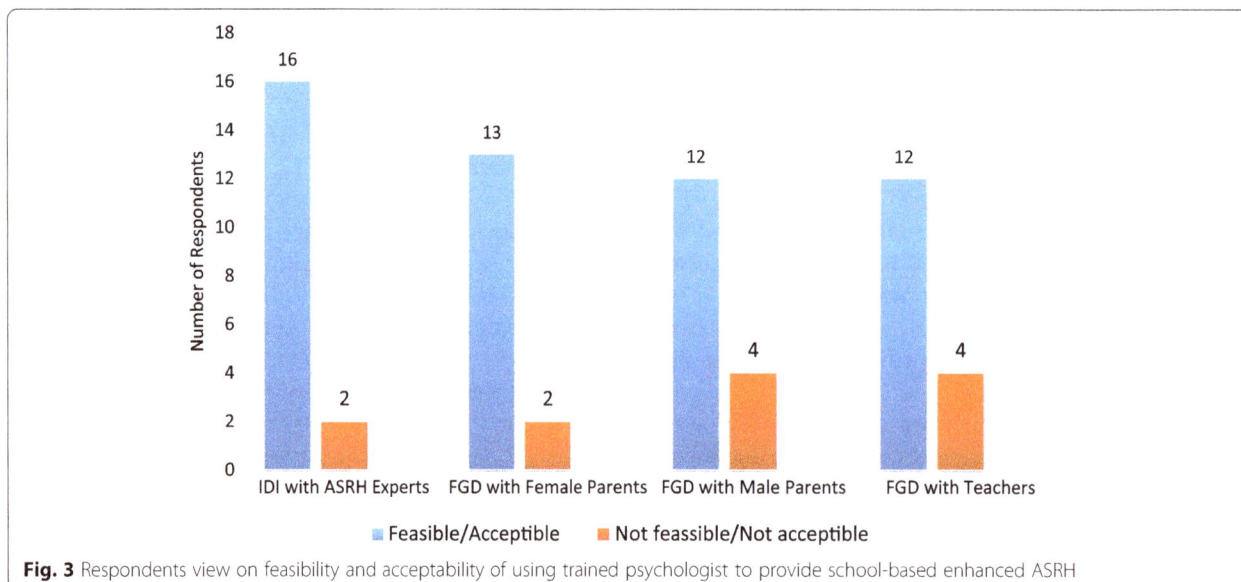

Fig. 3 Respondents view on feasibility and acceptability of using trained psychologist to provide school-based enhanced ASRH

"I think it will be a great advantage for them (psychologists) to come in because they will add to whatever teachers currently provide. Because these kids we have they are very complicated and sometimes when teachers are saying what they know, they will say oh you are supposed to come and teach me science, you are supposed to come and teach me maths, how do you think that you know about sex or you know about the changes that occur to me" (Male Teacher 2, IDI).

"Our parents don't have time or maybe they don't feel comfortable teaching us certain things and in the schools too, the teachers may not be able to teach us everything but if we have the psychologists or when we have these experts in the school based on the education and the counselling it can help reduce this teenage pregnancies" (Health Manager 2, IDI).

"Several, quite apart from providing the information, if it so happens that some children have some challenges, you know, there will be the opportunity to intervene with any of the psychotherapy... yes the psychologist can intervene with some form of help, and give some therapy when necessary" (Clinical Psychologist-1, IDI).

On the other hand, some respondents believed that using psychologists was not a feasible approach to addressing SRH challenges among adolescents largely because of the sustainability of such an approach. Specifically, respondents who were opposed to the use of psychologists generally raised concerns about the availability of trained psychologists and how to remunerate them for their services as illustrated:

"And also knowing the number of schools in Ghana and the number of psychologists that will be in the system, I think visiting a school or sometimes they might not be able to visit the school in that case it would not be effective" (Female Teacher, FGD).

"The idea [use of psychologist] is good but the problem will be placement and who to employ them and pay for their services. You know psychologist come with some level of higher education and the money to pay them will be the problem" (Male Teacher, FGD).

"Training psychologists to visit schools is not sustainable.... So just use available structures, we have guidance and counseling coordinators there and what GHS [Ghana Health Service] does is that we train the guidance and counseling coordinators in adolescent sexual and reproductive health so most at times they sometimes even do the referrals to the health facilities" (Health Manager 1, IDI).

"Ehhh, we have to strengthen our counselling department, we have, GES [Ghana Education Service] has counselling department and those department should be strengthened, more psychologist and counsellors would have to be trained, well equipped with an in-depth knowledge in adolescent reproductive health so that we could refer students to that department for a redress" (Headmaster, IDI).

Use of health workers to provide school-based SRH information and services

The results of the study also showed that stakeholders had a positive view on the use of health workers to deliver SRH services in school for adolescents (Fig. 4). According to respondents, using health workers would ensure that adolescents have access to accurate SRH information as well access to services. Using health workers was also perceived as a strategy that could be helpful in linking school-health services to the mainstream health care system for easy referral. These views are illustrated in the following quotes:

"Yes, I agree that health workers should visit schools to talk to the children about sexual and reproductive health. It will help them very well because the health workers can easily refer a student with a problem to hospital to get quick care" (Female Parent, FGD).

"You know that is the work of health workers. They have been trained and they have knowledge on sexual and reproductive health. So it would good to use them" (Male Parent, FGD).

"When we have this adolescent health centers with experts going there to work is very easy, for instance we have Nima, see Nima Cluster of schools for instance if we can establish one there, another cluster of school, Dansoman. You see, when we have these adolescent health centers it will rather help the nation, it will help Ghana, it will help Accra Metro" (Education Manager 1, IDI).

Views on operationalizing the use of psychologists and health providers to deliver school-based SRH services

Study findings underscored the need to address gender-related issues when operationalizing any school-based SRH programs. In FGDs with teachers, parents and students, it emerged that it would be preferable for male service providers to be assigned to male students and vice versa for females. According to respondents, matching the sex of service providers to the target students would increase students comfort in discussing sensitive SRH issues. Religious and cultural

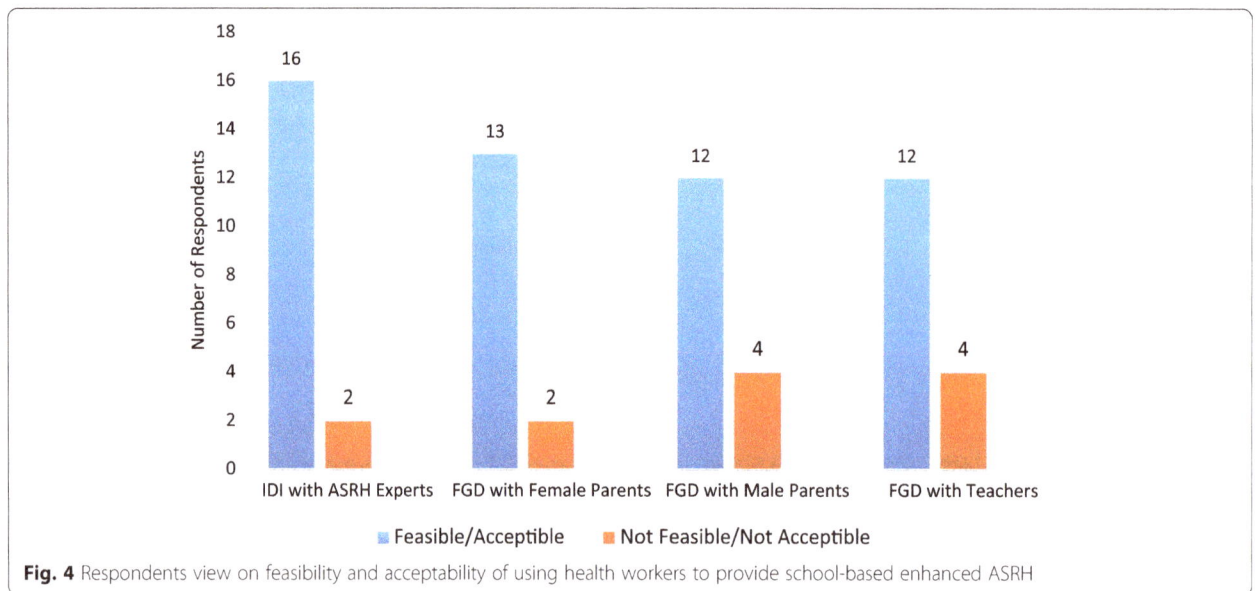

Fig. 4 Respondents view on feasibility and acceptability of using health workers to provide school-based enhanced ASRH

reasons for sex-separated programs were also highlighted. These views are illustrated in the following quotes:

"For our Islamic religion, what we are supposed to do is we have the females, we don't mix the females and the males. So we have to have a psychologist for the female and the psychologist for the male" (46-years Teacher, FGD).

"Madam like, they should separate the boys from the girls so that people can ask questions. When they are mixed, people feel shy to ask some questions which ermm is bothering them. So when they separate the boys from the girls' people will be able to ask questions and will be given a solution to all their problems" (15-years female student, FGD).

Female students were more concerned about separating male and female students. Female students reported that male students often make fun of them when female reproductive and sexual organs are mentioned. In addition, female students believed that female teachers and service providers have experienced what they may be going through and would therefore be in a better position to explain and provide support to them. The following quotes illustrates these points:

"A female teacher, because she is a woman and she has been what you are going through now. And she will more have knowledge of teaching" (17 years female student, FGD).

"…the boys they like when the teacher is teaching and will be saying, they will be saying vagina and those things about females. The boys will be happy and they will be laughing" (16 years female student, FGD).

The results of the study also showed that to be able to implement such a system will involve some work with the existing bureaucracies and good collaboration with various stakeholders including the Ministry of Education, Ghana Health Service and development partners who are currently engaged in SRH services and education in order not to run into challenges.

"As I said if you do not use the right channels the heads may not allow because they may think you are interrupting their contact hours and those would be the challenges. They will not be ready to give you access to the people so if you use the right channels I don't think you will have any problem" (Headmistress, IDI).

"This is [a] policy issue and will require bringing all stakeholders together to discuss. If Ghana Education Service make it a policy, than nobody can say no to it. We will implement it" (Teacher, IDI).

The study further found that one approach that could be used to implement school-based adolescent SRH is to organize schools into clusters and have one psychologist or health worker assigned to a specific cluster. This design was suggested to address the challenge of finding an adequate number of trained psychologists. The psychologist could provide age-specific education to a group of students and one-on-one counselling for those with specific psychological problems. These suggestion is illustrated in the following quote:

"What can be done is to group schools, a number of schools or students that can meet at a center, then a

trained psychologist can meet with about two hundred, three hundred, five hundred students in a big hall giving the same information at the same time so by that the target groups can be met, I mean the number of children that he can meet will expand and will be more" (Education Manager 2, IDI).

"Psychologist, how many are in the system? We may have to put schools together where you assign on psychologist in-charge" (Education Manager 4, IDI).

"The psychologist can educate a group of students on psychological changes and sexual and reproductive health and can provide counselling to individual students or do group counselling for people with similar problems" (Clinical Psychologist 2, IDI).

Further, stakeholders noted that the use of trained psychologists and health workers for the provision of adolescent and sexual health would require making some changes to the school timetables to cater for the time that would be used to provide such services. Further, some respondents highlighted the need to identify an appropriate service point or room where such services would be provided as privacy is required to assure adolescents that information provided would be treated as confidential. To implement this system of school-based provision of SRH would also require changes in existing policy and acquiring logistics that would be used in the delivery of the service.

"It will not be easy because sometimes the school will tell you they already have the time table for the term. So maybe giving you that enough time they [school] will not agree" (Health Manager 1, IDI).

"....You would have to start from the policy level come to the management and then it transcends to the school level. So the challenge is that you must have the materials that you would use for the education ready, err if you have any teaching and learning materials all these should be ready and it should be down to earth to reach the target group" (Education Manager 6, IDI).

"There should be a space or a room for them. So maybe there wouldn't be availability of a place for them to work. And then maybe we need to train more of the health personnel because this require extra training to deal with this thing. There should be [an] adolescent nurse, a nurse who... a guru, somebody who knows adolescent health, who has been trained, had extra training on adolescent health to tackle

them. So maybe shortage of staff will not allow us to err...reach our goal" (Health Manager 3, IDI).

The paradigm of school-based SRH programs using psychologists and health workers

Figure 5 is a framework developed from the data to explain the contextual issues in using health workers and psychologists to provide SRH services in schools. The study showed that existing sources of SRH information such as parents, teachers, peers, electronic media, community members, churches and mosques had practical challenges. Social norms especially made it difficult for parents and teachers to freely provide these services. The existing guidance and counseling services in school, which serve as channels for providing SRH education and support were being undermined by competing roles as the counselors still had to perform their primary role as teachers. The effect of the lack of access to SRH services is low knowledge among adolescents, high adolescent pregnancy and STIs. Adolescent generally need a positive SRH environment, high knowledge on sexuality, and access to SRH services to able to make informed decision which is not the case in Ghana. To that end, respondents generally believed existing systems were not achieving their objective and felt that it would be appropriate for both trained psychologists and health workers to provide school-based SRH to adolescents. In that opinion, using psychologists and health workers can create this positive environment and increase access to ASHR services. The use of health workers and trained psychologists was viewed to have additional benefits. Specifically, psychologists would be better able to identify and support adolescents with psychosocial problems, while health workers foster referrals to SRH services by creating a link between the school health service and formal health system delivery as diagrammatically presented in the figure. The types of services will include providing health education to various classes, individual counselling for those with psychological and physical problems. Group counselling sessions and family counselling could also be organized for students only and student who have family problems respectively (Fig. 5).

However, stakeholders perceived a number of practical challenges around how this could be implemented. Key among the challenges were how to pay for the services that health workers and trained psychologists would render, and availability of psychologists to cater for all schools. Another important challenge raised was around the acceptability of certain services such as distributing condoms and provision of contraceptives services especially in faith-based schools. Nonetheless, respondents believed that garnering enough support from parents and other stakeholders could help overcome this challenge. In designing school-based SRH programs that

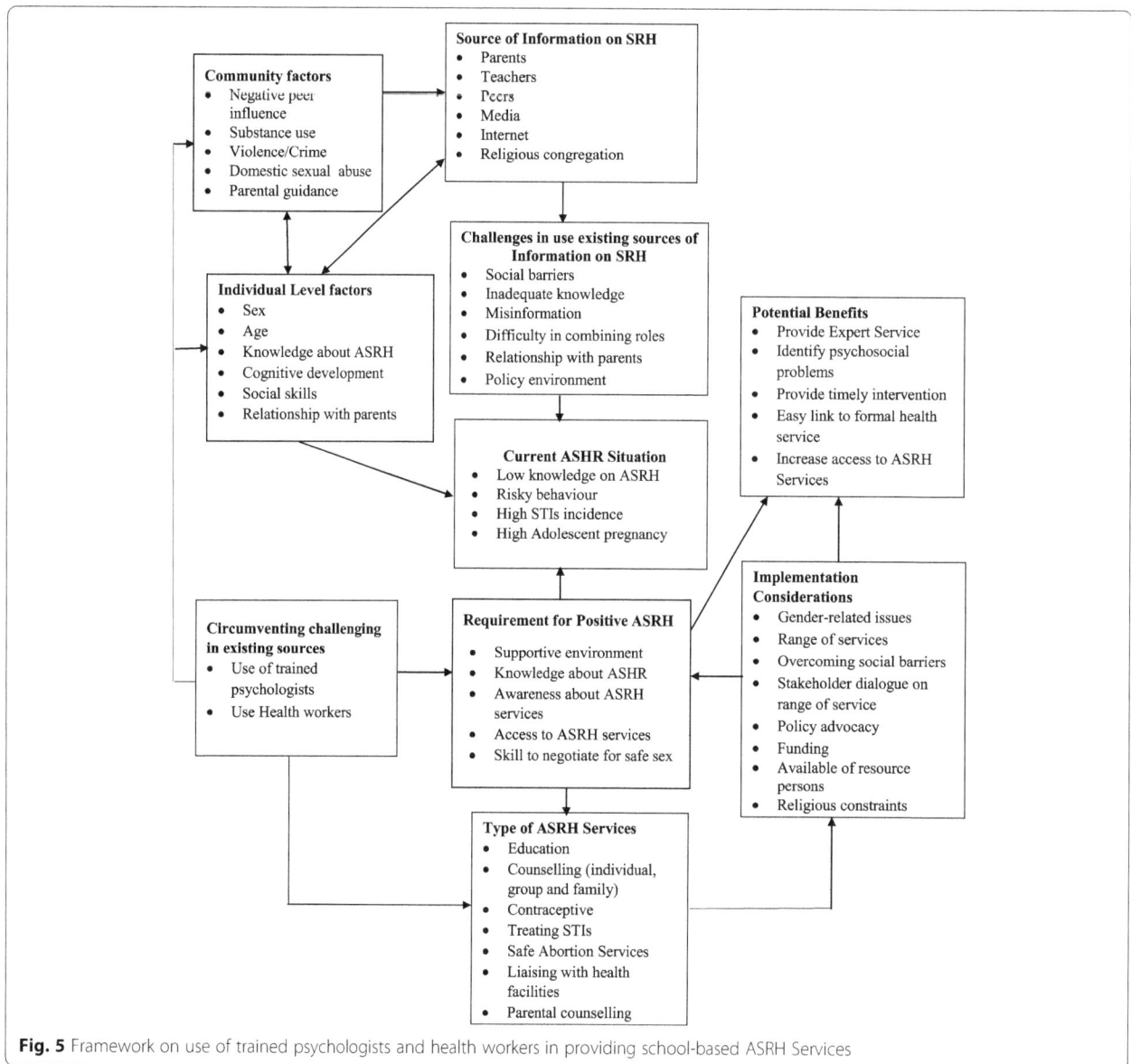

Fig. 5 Framework on use of trained psychologists and health workers in providing school-based ASRH Services

would rely on trained psychologists and health workers, our finding underscored the need for gender-sensitive programs that would enable both boys and girls to feel comfortable discussing sensitive issues. Once this is implemented, it is go to affect individual and community level factors that predispose adolescents to negative behavioral tendencies with its associated consequences.

Discussion

Acceptability of school-based SRH services

The study showed that stakeholders perceived the provision of SRH services in schools as laudable and an idea worth implementing. There was general consensus among all stakeholders, including parents, about the need to extend SRH services to school. Previous studies have demonstrated the importance of comprehensive

sexuality education. An earlier study in the United States found that adolescents who received comprehensive sex education in school were significantly less likely to report teen pregnancy than those who did not receive formal sex education [47]. In Indian, the introduction of sexual and reproductive intervention in school was also found to have resulted in a significant increase in the knowledge in both boys and girls. In that study, among girls, the percentage of poor knowledge reduced significantly from 64.1% (pre-intervention) to 8.3% (post-intervention) and among boys from 37.7% (pre-intervention) to 3.5% (post-intervention). Similarly, increase in knowledge level was also observed in various other aspects of reproductive and sexual health including, STI, HIV/AIDS and perceptions about premarital sex [48].

Although majority of respondents supported adolescents' access to comprehensive SRH information and services, they generally disapproved of providing contraceptive services in school because of concerns that contraceptive provision would promote sexual activity. Nonetheless comprehensive programs have been reported to be more beneficial. In a review of 56 adolescent SRH programs, it was found that abstinence programs did not delay initiation of sex but two third of comprehensive programs had positive impact on sexual behavior including delay in initiation, use of contraceptives and condoms [49]. Drawing from the findings of this study, it would be important for any discussions on designing a plan for school-based services to go beyond promoting abstinence only to making it possible for adolescent to access services that can ensure that adolescents who wish to engage in sex do that with protection against pregnancy and STIs.

Though distributing condoms and providing contraceptive services to adolescents was unacceptable to majority of respondents in this study, results suggested that it would be possible to garner more support for contraceptive service provision through extensive stakeholder engagement. Contraceptive service provision in schools may also require further studies to explore view of health workers on their attitude towards providing contraceptives services to adolescents as a study in Nigeria found that many healthcare providers have unfavorable attitudes towards the provision of contraceptives for unmarried adolescents [50].

Changes required to implement school-based SRH services

Though stakeholders in this study believed it was acceptable and feasibility to introduce school-based SRH programs delivered by psychologists and health workers, the implementation of such programs would require further consultation to inform the operationalization of the programs. Studies suggest that programs to promote access to and uptake of adolescent SRH services are reported to be most effective when adolescent-friendly facility-based approaches are combined with community acceptance and demand-generation activities [29]. In South Africa for example, a pilot study on school-based SRH services was found to be acceptable in the community and feasible with scale-up [51]. Ghana can draw on this experience to pilot this system in selected institutions where lessons learnt can then inform scale up. Locating health services in schools or providing outreach services has the potential to reduce transport costs, increase accessibility and provide links between schools and communities [52]. Moving forward, there is the need to organise stakeholders to deliberate on the findings of this study and fashion out an implementation plan. During the pilot phase there will be the need for an implementation research to inform scale up [53, 54].

Our findings also underscore the importance of allocating time for school-based ASRH services as there is need for enough time for interaction between the service provider and the students. In addition, schools must ensure that they identify a private space where the services can be provided. Importantly, school-based SRH service provisions requires a change in policy as the existing policy on school health does permit the inclusion of contraceptive services.

Views on the use of psychologists and health workers for delivery SRH services

The study showed that majority of the respondents perceived a system that will make it possible for sexual and reproductive services to be delivered in schools by trained psychologists as essential as the present system was not meeting the needs of adolescents. Teachers who are in-charge of guidance and counseling services were reported to perform those roles in addition to their primary role (teaching) and were less effective in guidance and counseling. Further, students were described as being unwilling to discuss sensitive issues with teachers. The study also showed that some adolescents might not be comfortable discussing sexual issues with their teachers, as they may be perceived to be immoral. When service providers are judgmental towards adolescents who seek services they may feel reluctant to go back due to shyness [55]. As such, 'neutral' service providers such as psychologists and health workers may increase young people's use of SRH services. Psychologists were also viewed to be better placed to detect emotional distress and offer timely counseling. For the purpose of social and cultural correctness, teachers were viewed as not been the right people to provide such information. The perception was that some teachers are likely to even take advantage of the adolescents and engage in sexual acts with them. Therefore, parents perceived finding a neutral person who will only visit to provide such information and services as a better option. In a systematic review of youth friendly programs, it was found that accessibility of health care; communication; staff attitude; medical competency; guideline-driven care; age appropriate environments; youth involvement in health care; and health outcomes were seen as core to the youth [56].

We found that stakeholders believed that using psychologists would also be beneficial in providing support to adolescents with diverse psychosocial needs. It is well documented that adolescents who exhibit delinquent behaviors are more likely to engage in risky sexual activities [56–59]. These behaviors often have psychological undertones that may be more accurately identified by psychologists who can then provide appropriate interventions.

Further, using health workers was believed to enhance linkages with the health system. A study in the United States showed that using a school nurse to deliver intervention aimed at encouraging adolescents to stop smoking was effective as intervention condition participants were almost twice as likely to be abstinent per self-report at three months compared with control participants [60]. In another study it was found that using school nurse to provide contraceptive service increased contraceptive use [61]. A study in Ethiopian also found that majority of the health workers had generally positive attitudes toward SRH to adolescents and this was reported to enhance the provision of services to adolescents [62]. Building from the evidence above, it is important to reflect carefully on using psychologists and health workers to deliver ASRH services in schools as it could contribute immensely to improving young people sexual and reproductive lifestyle. Opportunities therefore exist in the use of psychologists though now study has documented the use psychologist in providing adolescents SRH. The use of psychologists will be a novel intervention as using trained health workers have been widely reported in the studies referred to earlier.

Limitation of study

Although this study provides evidence on stakeholders' views about using health workers and psychologists to provide school-based adolescent SRH services, it is important to situate the conclusions in the context of one limitation. This study was conducted in one region in Ghana on a sample that is not representative, hence the findings cannot be generalized. This notwithstanding, in conducting the study, we followed the methodological requirements for a qualitative research such as the RATS checklist [63], Consolidated criteria for reporting qualitative research (COREQ), [64] and acceptable practice in fieldwork, analysis and interpretation [65].

Conclusions

Our study findings show that there is widespread acceptance of the need for enhanced school-based SRH programs as the present systems are not perceived to sufficiently meet adolescents' SRH needs. Results demonstrate that it is acceptable to use trained psychologists and health workers to deliver school-based SRH information and services in the Ghanaian school context. However, provisions must be made to cater for financial and other logistical considerations in the implementation of school-based SRH programs that rely on external human resources.

Abbreviations
AMA: Accra metropolitan assembly; ASRH: Adolescents sexual and reproductive health; CSE: Comprehensive sexual education; FGD: Focus group discussion; ICPD: International conference on population and development; IDI: In-depth interview; PTA: Parent teachers association; SRH: Sexual and reproductive health; STIs: Sexually transmitted infections

Acknowledgements
We wish to thank the research assistants for their role in conducting the FGDs and IDIs. The research assistants include; Justice Abuchow, Kofi Osei Appiah, and Addo Bright. We are also grateful to the headmasters of the schools that the study was conducted for their support in recruiting the study participants.

Funding
The study was funded by Population Council Ghana.

Authors' contributions
PT, TAB, HB, DKA and PBA conceived and designed the study, PT-NT PBA and ETM analyzed the data; PT-NT led the writing of the manuscript, all authors, critically reviewed the manuscript. All authors read and approved the final manuscript.

Competing interests
The authors declare that they have no competing interests.

Author details
[1]Department of Social and Behavioural Sciences, School of Public Health, University of Ghana, Accra, Ghana. [2]Department of Population, Family and Reproductive Health, School of Public Health, University of Ghana, Accra, Ghana. [3]Population Council, Accra, Ghana. [4]Population Council, City, Nairobi, Kenya.

References
1. UNFPA. International conference on population development: investing in people: National Progress in implementing the ICPD Programmme of action 1994-2004. A Summ. Rep. New York: UNFP; 2004.
2. World health organization. Making health services adolescent friendly -developing national quality standards for adolescent friendly health services. Geneva: World Health Organization; 2012.
3. Chandra-Mouli V, Svanemyr J, Amin A, Fogstad H, Say L, Girard F, et al. Twenty years after international conference on population and development: where are we with adolescent sexual and reproductive health and rights? J Adolesc Health. 2015;56:S1–6.
4. Gruskin S, Ravindran TKS. Realising the ICPD 20 years later: shifting the paradigms for research and education. Glob Public Health. 2014;1692:1–6.
5. Shaw D. Access to sexual and reproductive health for young people: bridging the disconnect between rights and reality. Int J Gynecol Obstet. 2009;106:132–6.
6. Bearinger LH, Sieving RE, Ferguson J, Sharma V. Global perspectives on the sexual and reproductive health of adolescents: patterns, prevention, and potential. Lancet. 2007;369:1220–31.
7. Okonta PI. Adolescent sexual and reproductive health in the Niger Delta region of Nigeria–issues and challenges. Afr J Reprod Health. 2007;11:113–24.

8. GSS/GHS/Macro International. Ghana demographic and health survey 2014. Accra: Ghana Statistical Service; 2015.

9. Nyarko SH. Prevalence and correlates of contraceptive use among female adolescents in Ghana. BMC Womens Health. 2015;15:60.

10. Kyilleh JM, Tabong PT-N, Konlaan BB. Adolescents' reproductive health knowledge, choices and factors affecting reproductive health choices: a qualitative study in the west Gonja District in northern region, Ghana. BMC Int. Health Hum. Rights. 2018;18:6.

11. UNESCO. Internatioanal Technical Guidance on sexuality education: an evidence-informed approach for schools, teachers and health educators. Paris: UNESCO; 2009.

12. Braeken D, Cardinal M. Comprehensive sexuality education as a means of promoting sexual health. Int J Sex Heal. 2008;20:50–62.

13. McCave EL. Comprehensive sexuality education vs. abstinence-only sexuality education: the need for evidence-based research and practice. Sch Soc Work J. 2007;32:14–28.

14. International Planned Parenthood Federation. From evidence to action: advocating for comprehensive sexuality education. Reprod Health. 2009;32:1-32.

15. Manu AA, Mba CJ, Asare GQ, Odoi-Agyarko K, Asante RKO. Parent-child communication about sexual and reproductive health: evidence from the Brong Ahafo region. Ghana Reprod Health. 2015;12:16.

16. Kyilleh JM, Tabong PT-N, Konlaan BB. Adolescents' reproductive health knowledge, choices and factors affecting reproductive health choices: a qualitative study in the west Gonja District in northern region, Ghana. BMC Int Health Hum Rights. 2018;18:6.

17. Awusabo-asare K, Bankole A, Kumi-kyereme A. Views of adults on adolescent sexual and reproductive Health : qualitative evidence from Ghana. Occas. Reeport no 34. New York: The Alan Guttmacher Institute; 2008. p. 1–48.

18. Essuman JK. The history of guidance and counselling in Ghana. IFE Psychol An Int J. 1999;7:22–43.

19. Esantsi SF, Onyango F, Quansah-Asare GJ, Kuffuor EOTP, Birungi H, Askew I. Understanding the reproductive health needs of adolescents in selected slums in Ghana: a public health assessment. Accra: Population Council Ghana; 2016.

20. Owusu SA, Blankson EJ, Abane AM. Sexual and reproductive health education among dressmakers and hairdressers in the Assin South District of Ghana. Afr J Reprod Health. 2011;15:109–19.

21. Coetzee J, Dietrich J, Otwombe K, Nkala B, Khunwane M, van der Watt M, et al. Predictors of parent-adolescent communication in post-apartheid South Africa: a protective factor in adolescent sexual and reproductive health. J Adolesc. 2014;37:313–24.

22. Fatusi A, Blum RW. Adolescent health in an international context. the challenge of sexual and reproductive health in sub-Saharan Africa. Adolesc Med State Art Rev. 2009;20:874–86.

23. Morris JL, Rushwan H. Adolescent sexual and reproductive health: the global challenges. Int J Gynecol Obstet. 2015;131:S40–52.

24. GSS. The 2010 Population and Housing Report Accra; 2011.

25. Abajobir AA, Seme A. Reproductive health knowledge and services utilization among rural adolescents in east Gojjam zone, Ethiopia: a community-based cross-sectional study. BMC Health Serv Res. 2014;14:1–11.

26. Rahman AA, Rahman RA, Ibrahim MI, Salleh H, Ismail SB, Ali SH, et al. Knowledge of sexual and reproductive health among adolescents attending school in Kelantan Malaysia. Southeast Asian J Trop Med Public Health. 2011;42:717–25.

27. Rajapaksa-Hewageegana N, Piercy H, Salway S, Samarage S. Sexual and reproductive knowledge, attitudes and behaviours in a school going population of Sri Lankan adolescents. Sex Reprod Healthc. 2015;6:3–8.

28. GSS/GHS/ICF Macro. Ghana demographic and health survey. Accra: Ghana Statistical Service; 2014.

29. Denno DM, Hoopes AJ, Chandra-Mouli V. Effective strategies to provide adolescent sexual and reproductive health services and to increase demand and community support. J Adolesc Health. 2015;56:S22–41.

30. Chilinda I, Hourahane G, Pindani M, Chitsulo C, Maluwa A. Attitude of health care providers towards adolescent sexual and reproductive health Services in Developing Countries: a systematic review. Health (Irvine Calif). 2014;6:1706–13.

31. Coley R, Votruba-Drzal E, Schindler H. Fathers' and mothers' parenting practices and responding to adolescent sexual risk behaviors. Child Dev. 2009;80:808–27.

32. Kincaida C, Jones DJ, Sterrettb E, McKeec L. A review of parenting and adolescent sexual behavior: the moderating role of gender. Clin Psychol Rev. 2012;32:177–88.

33. Kelley A, Schochet T, Landry CF. Risk taking and novelty seeking in adolescence: introduction to part I. Ann N Y Acad Sci Blackwell Publishing Ltd. 2004;1021:27–32.

34. Thomas R, Lorenzetti D, Spragins W. Cochrane Database Syst Rev. 2011;11: 1-18. CD007381.

35. Williams S, Dickinson A. The provision of nurse-led school based health services. Contemp Nurse. 2017;53:536–44.

36. Holmes BW, Sheetz A. Role of the school nurse in providing school health services. Pediatrics. 2016;137:e20160852.

37. Al-Dahnaim L, Said H, Salama R, Bella H, Malo D. Perceptions of school nurses and principals towards nurse role in providing school health services in Qatar. J Egypt Public Health Assoc. 2013;88:19–25.

38. Aniteye P, Mayhew SH. Shaping legal abortion provision in Ghana: using policy theory to understand provider-related obstacles to policy implementation. Heal Res Policy Syst. 2013;11:23.

39. GPC. List of Psychologists, Paraprofessional, and Lay Practitioners in Good Standing [Internet]. [cited 2018 Mar 15]. Available from 2018: http://www.ghanapsychologycouncil.org.gh/news/GPC Registered Members.pdf.

40. GPC. Benefits of Membership of Ghana Psychological Council [Internet]. [cited 2018 Apr 1]. Available from: 2018 http://www.ghanapsychologycouncil.org.gh/

41. Creswell JW. Qualitative inquiry and research design: choosing among five traditions. London: Sage Publications; 1998.

42. Green J, Thorogood N. Qualitative methods for Health Research. London: Sage Publications; 2004.

43. GSS. Ghana 2010 Population and housing census: national analytical report. Accra-Ghana: Ghana Statistical Service; p. 2013.

44. GSS. 2010 Population and housing census: district analytic report for Accra metropolitan area, vol. 2014. Accra: Ghana Statistical Service.

45. GES. Ghana education service report for Accra metropolitan assembly. Acrra: Ghana Statistical Service; 2013.

46. Creswell JW. Research design: qualitative, quantitative, and mixed methods approaches. Res Des Qual Quant Mix Methods Approaches. 2009;2;260. 3rd

47. Kohler PK, Manhart LE, Lafferty WE. Abstinence-only and comprehensive sex education and the initiation of sexual activity and teen pregnancy. J Adolesc Health. 2008;42:344–51.

48. Nair MKC, Paul MK, Leena ML, Thankachi Y, George B, Russell PS, et al. Effectiveness of a reproductive sexual health education package among school going adolescents. Indian J Pediatr. 2012;79(1):S64–8.

49. Kirby DB. The impact of abstinence and comprehensive sex and STD/HIV education programs on adolescent sexual behavior. Sex Res Soc Policy. 2008;5(3):18.

50. Ahanonu EL. Attitudes of healthcare providers towards providing contraceptives for unmarried adolescents in Ibadan. Nigeria J Fam Reprod Heal. 2014;8:33–40.

51. J a F, Mkhize N, Dellar RC, Mahlase G, Montague CT, Abdool Karim Q. Meeting the sexual and reproductive health needs of high-school students in South Africa: experiences from rural KwaZulu-Natal. S Afr Med J. 2014;104: 687–90.

52. Mason-Jones AJ, Crisp C, Momberg M, Koech J, De KP, Mathews C. A systematic review of the role of school-based healthcare in adolescent sexual, reproductive, and mental health. Syst Rev. 2012;1:49.

53. Proctor EK, Landsverk J, Aarons G, Chambers D, Glisson C, Mittman B. Implementation research in mental health services: an emerging science with conceptual, methodological, and training challenges. Admin Pol Ment Health. 2009;36:24–34.

54. Lobb R, Colditz GA. Implementation science and its application to population health. Annu Rev Public Health. 2013;34:235–51.

55. Malawi Goverment. Evaluation of youth-friendly health services in Malawi; June 2014. 2014.

56. Ambresin AE, Bennett K, Patton GC, Sanci LA, Sawyer SM. Assessment of youth-friendly health care: a systematic review of indicators drawn from young people's perspectives. J Adolesc Heal Elsevier Ltd. 2013;52:670–81.

57. Thompson RG, Auslander WF. Substance use and mental health problems as predictors of HIV sexual risk behaviors among adolescents in foster care. Health Soc Work. 2011;36:33–43.

58. Lohman BJ, Billings A. Protective and risk factors associated with adolescent boys' early sexual debut and risky sexual behaviors. J Youth Adolesc. 2008; 37:723–35.

59. Chen AC-C, Thompson EA, Morrison-Beedy D. Multi-system influences on adolescent risky sexual behavior. Res Nurs Health. 2010;33:512–27.

60. Pbert L, Druker S, DiFranza JR, Gorak D, Reed G, Magner R, et al.
    Effectiveness of a school nurse-delivered smoking-cessation intervention for
    adolescents. Pediatrics. 2011;128:926 36.

61. Gabzdyl EM. Contraceptive care of adolescents: overview, tips, strategies,
    and implications for school nurses. J Sch Nurs Off Publ Natl Assoc Sch
    Nurses. 2010;26:267–77.

62. Tilahun M, Mengistie B, Egata G, A a R. Health workers' attitudes toward
    sexual and reproductive health services for unmarried adolescents in
    Ethiopia. Reprod Health. 2012;9:19.

63. Clark JP. How to peer review a qualitative manuscript. In: Godlee F,
    Jefferson T, editors. Peer rev. heal Sci. London: BMJ books; 2003. p. 219–35.

64. Tong A, Sainsbury P, Craig J. Consolidated criterio for reporting qualitative
    research (COREQ): a 32- item checklist for interviews and focus group. Int J
    Qual Heal Care. 2007;19:349–57.

65. Barbour RS. The newfound credibility of qualitative research? Tales of
    technical essentialism and co-option. Qual Health Res. 2003;13:1010–27.

66. The Constitution of Ghana. The Constitution of the Republic of Ghana.
    Accra: Ghana Assembly Press; 1992.

11

Mapping the lack of public initiative against female genital mutilation in Denmark

Gro Møller Christoffersen[1], Peter James Bruhn[2*] (iD), Rosanna de Neergaard[3], Susanne Engel[4] and Vibeke Naeser[5]

Abstract

Background: Female genital mutilation (FGM) is a harmful practice prevalent in 35 countries, mainly in Africa, as well as in some Middle Eastern countries and a few Asian countries. FGM comprises all procedures that involve partial or complete resection of, or other injury to, external female genitalia for non-medical reasons. The practice of FGM has spread to Western countries due to migration. The European Institute for Gender Equality recommend that FGM be combatted by nationally coordinated efforts through implementation of national action plans, guidelines for professionals as well as comprehensive research in the field. FGM was outlawed in Denmark 2003, but no national actions plan has been implemented. Instead, the task of combatting FGM is currently under the responsibility of local governments in the form of the 98 municipalities. The aim of this study is to investigate the Danish municipalities' efforts to prevent FGM on the local level, and whether these initiatives are in accordance with international recommendations and standards.

Methods: All 98 Danish municipalities were invited to respond to a questionnaire regarding FGM in their respective municipalities. The inclusion process and questionnaire was designed after a pilot study, which included 29 municipalities. The questionnaire consisted of four overall areas of focus: "action plan", "registration", "information material" and "preventive initiatives". Demographic data were gathered from the 2017 census by Statistics Denmark. Risk countries were defined as countries with a tradition for FGM, identified from the 2016 UNICEF definition.

Results: A total of 67 municipalities participated in the study. At the time of census, 1.8% of the Danish population was immigrants with origins in risk countries. A total of 10.4% of the responding municipalities indicated to have implemented a specific action plan against FGM. A total of 7,5% had implemented specific preventive initiatives against FGM. Registration of reported FGM cases were indicated to be performed in 73.1% of the responding municipalities; however, only 17.9% stated to perform registration of FGM specifically as such, and not as general child abuse.

Conclusions: Our study shows that the current situation of FGM registration and prevention being under local administrative responsibility in the 98 Danish municipalities has led to a severe lack of coordinated public initiative against FGM.

Keywords: Female genital mutilation, Female genital cutting, Migrant health, Pricking

* Correspondence: peterjamesbruhn@gmail.com
[2]Department of Surgical Gastroenterology, Copenhagen University Hospital North Zealand, Dyrehavevej 29, 3400 Hillerød, Denmark
Full list of author information is available at the end of the article

Plain English summary

Female genital mutilation (FGM) is a harmful practice where female external genitalia are injured or partly or completely removed due to non-medical reasons. The practice of FGM has spread to European countries with immigration from countries with a tradition for FGM. The European Institute for Gender Equality recommends that FGM should be combatted by nationally coordinated preventive efforts in the form of, among other things, a national action plan. FGM was outlawed in Denmark in 2003, but no national action plan has been implemented. The task of combatting FGM is currently under the responsibility of local governments in the form of the 98 municipalities. We sought to investigate whether FGM is combatted in accordance with international standards on the local level. We invited the Danish municipalities to respond to a questionnaire regarding FGM prevention in their respective municipalities. We also analyzed demographic data regarding distribution of immigrants from countries that practice FGM, across the respective municipalities. We found that only very few Danish municipalities have implemented specific action plans against FGM, or have implemented specific preventive initiatives against FGM. Overall, only very few Danish municipalities live up to international recommendations and standards regarding FGM prevention. Thus, we conclude that the current situation of FGM registration and prevention being under local administrative responsibility in the 98 municipalities has led to a severe lack of coordinated public initiative against FGM in Denmark.

Background

Female genital mutilation (FGM) is a harmful practice prevalent in 35 countries, mainly in Africa, as well as in some Middle Eastern countries and a few Asian countries [1]. The practice is described by the World Health Organization (WHO) as follows: "Female genital mutilation (FGM) comprises all procedures that involve partial or total removal of the external female genitalia, or other injury to the female genital organs for non-medical reasons (...) FGM is recognized internationally as a human rights violation. It reflects deep-rooted inequality between the sexes, and constitutes an extreme form of discrimination against women" [2]. Due to migration over the past decades the practice of FGM has spread to European and other Western countries [3–10]. It has been estimated by the European Parliament that 500,000 women and girls have been subjected to FGM whereas 180,000 girls are in risk of being subjected to FGM [11]; though some argue that this is an under-estimation [4].

Female genital mutilation was outlawed in Denmark in 2003. In 2013, the European Institute for Gender Equality (EIGE) published an official recommendation for

Denmark to define and implement a national action plan such as "national guidelines for professionals across a variety of sectors as well as coordination of the effort to combat FGM. Comprehensive and in-depth research in the field is also needed as well as prevalence surveys of FGM in Denmark" [12]. However, several changing governments have not implemented a national action plan to prevent and combat FGM in Denmark. A proposal for a national action plan was drafted by Danish NGOs and a number of individual authors in 2007–2008 and was submitted to the Health Committee of the Parliament in 2009. This action plan was not implemented. Instead, the 98 Danish municipalities individually administrate the responsibility of combatting FGM on a local level.

The lack of political prioritization of the FGM issue in Denmark is unusual in a Nordic context. Finland, Sweden and Norway, along with several other European countries, have implemented comprehensive national and international guidelines to combat FGM [12–17].

In this study, our aim is to investigate the Danish municipalities' initiatives to prevent FGM on the local level, and whether these initiatives are in accordance with international recommendations and standards.

Methods
Questionnaire

In order to gain insight into if and how FGM is combated through public efforts on the local level in the 98 Danish municipalities, a questionnaire was developed. We designed the entirety of the questionnaire, since a validated questionnaire on the subject of FGM prevention on the local governmental level has not yet been published. During the questionnaire design process, we used a checklist proposed by Eysenbach et al. [18]. The questionnaire consisted of four main areas of focus, which we defined as "action plan", "registration of FGM", "information material" and preventive initiatives. These areas of focus were chosen in accordance with the concluding focus points described by EIGE in their 2013 report on the subject of FGM in Denmark, as well as efforts described in other Scandinavian action plans regarding FGM [12, 13, 16]. In those parts of the questionnaire where doubt about terminology could have an impact on answers, the question was supplemented with a definition, so as to ensure measurement validity. An action plan was defined as "A point to point guideline for professionals on how to act when being made aware of a case of FGM or of a girl in potential risk of FGM". Most questions were closed-ended with possible answers being yes/no/do not know. When questions were not close-ended, these could be answered with different given categories or free text (Additional file 1). The questionnaire was answered through a webpage and took few minutes to complete.

Pilot project

A total of 29 municipalities in the Capital Region in Denmark were invited to participate in a pilot project, which consisted of the questionnaire described earlier. The specific department in each of the municipalities with the main responsibility for children, reports of child abuse or likewise, were identified through the respective municipality's website or by telephone. By contacting the general manager with the overall responsibility for the department in question within each municipality, contact information for the individual employee appointed in charge of handling reports of cases of FGM, and with the most adequate knowledge about the particular area, was acquired. The questionnaire was then sent electronically to this person as the potential responder. If the initial contact did not result in a reply, the municipalities were then contacted by telephone or by email once more. The questionnaire was then revised, taking into account the feedback from the 29 municipalities in the pilot project. The revision simply consisted of the addition of a comment field to each question, enabling the respondents to elaborate their answers, if necessary. When revision of the questionnaire was complete, all 98 municipalities were invited to respond to the questionnaire through the process described above. Informed consent for study participation was obtained.

Demographics

Demographic data were gathered from the April 2017 census by Statistics Denmark, using the publicly available Statbank [19]. Data regarding the prevalence of citizens in each municipality originating in countries with tradition of FGM was gathered in order to compare the municipalities participating and not participating in the study, and to evaluate whether a high prevalence of citizens from risk countries was correlated with a higher possibility of having implemented a specific action plans against FGM.

First-generation immigrants are defined as individuals born in a different country than Denmark, and who have achieved status of permanent residents in Denmark at the time of the census. Second-generation immigrants are defined as individuals born in Denmark to two first-generation immigrant parents, and with a status of permanent residency in Denmark at the time of census. Risk countries were defined as countries with a tradition of FGM, and were identified in accordance with the UNICEF definition from 2016 [1], the Embará people of Colombia being excluded due to lack of data regarding the number of people from this ethnic group residing in Denmark. High-risk countries were defined as countries with FGM prevalence above 50%.

Statistics

Quantitative data are presented as frequencies and proportions. Statistical analysis was performed using IBM SPSS Statistics (version 19 for iOS, IBM Corporation, Armonk, NY). Figures were created using GraphPad Prism (version 6 for iOS, GraphPad Software, San Diego, CA).

Results

All 98 municipalities in Denmark were invited to participate in the study by responding to a questionnaire. A total of 67 municipalities participated in the study. The municipalities that did participate in the study had an average of 1.09% of the population with origins in countries with tradition of FGM and a median of 0.86%. The municipalities that did not participate in the study had an average of 1.21% and a median of 0.84%.

Demographics

As of the first of April 2017, a total of 91,121 first- and second-generation immigrants with origins in countries with a tradition of FGM resided in Denmark. This equals 1.8% of Danish population. A total of 41,896 of these were females. A total of 33,198 first- and second-generation immigrants originated from the 12 high-risk countries, comprising 0.7% of the total Danish population. A total of 14,929 of these were females.

The percentage of the population being first- or second-generation immigrants from countries with a tradition of FGM varied within the municipalities from 0% to 4.1% with a median of 0.8%. Only one municipality had 0% of the population originating in countries with a tradition of FGM. The ten municipalities with the highest prevalence of citizens with origins in risk countries were all situated within or in immediate proximity to the three most populated cities in Denmark (Fig. 1).

Questionnaire

Firstly, the municipalities were asked whether they regard FGM as a current problem in their municipality. One (1.5%) municipality regarded FGM as a current problem within its respective municipality, 59 (88%) answered "no" and seven (10.4%) answered "do not know". To the question of whether the municipality currently receives petitions concerning FGM from citizens and social workers, 47 (70.1%) municipalities answered "no", seven (10.4%) municipalities answered "yes" and 13 (19.4%) answered "do not know".

Action plans

A total of seven (10.4%) municipalities stated that they had implemented a specific action plan for cases regarding FGM. Of these seven, one municipality, Copenhagen, made their action plan available upon request, while the

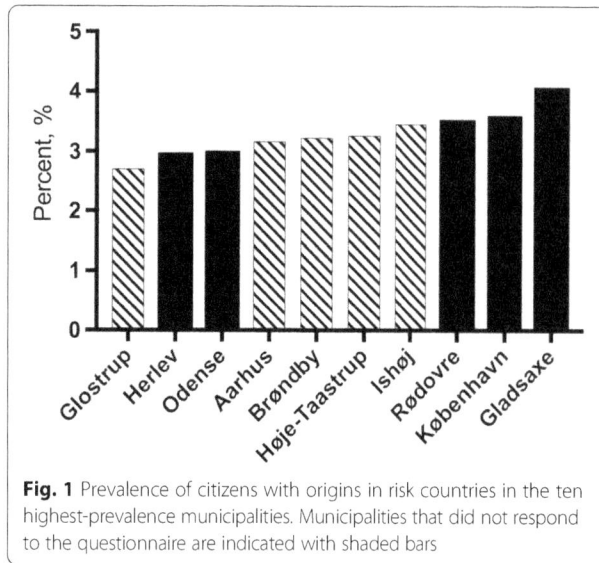

Fig. 1 Prevalence of citizens with origins in risk countries in the ten highest-prevalence municipalities. Municipalities that did not respond to the questionnaire are indicated with shaded bars

remaining six municipalities did not. A total of 57 (85%) municipalities stated that they do not have a specific action plan, while three (4.5%) replied, "do not know".

The municipality of Copenhagen was the only out of the aforementioned ten municipalities with the highest population share of citizens originating in a risk country, to state that they have implemented a specific action plan for combatting FGM.

Of the 57 municipalities where no specific action plan has been implemented, 13 (22.8%) municipalities indicated that FGM is included in other action plans within the given municipality. One municipality stated to be in the process of developing an action plan.

Thus, 46 municipalities (68.7%) indicated that they have not implemented a specific action plan regarding FGM, that FGM currently is not included in other action plans, that they are currently not in the process of developing a specific action plan towards cases of FGM or that they do not know whether an action plan has been implemented in their municipality.

Preventive initiatives

Five (7.5%) municipalities stated that they have developed and implemented preventive initiatives to combat FGM. These municipalities defined their initiatives in the comment field sections as follows: 1) outreach conversations with parents and families in relevant groups; 2) lectures about Danish legislation regarding FGM during Danish language courses for immigrants; 3) preschool interviews with the school nurse, and 4) outreach healthcare visits.

A total of 44 (65.7%) municipalities replied "no" to having implemented preventive initiatives against FGM. Of these, one (2.3%) municipality stated to be in the process of preparing implementation of specific initiatives and

preventive work against FGM, whereas 43 (97.7%) municipalities stated not to be. Eighteen (26.9%) municipalities answered "do not know", to whether they had implemented preventive initiatives against FGM.

Registration

A total of 49 (73.1%) municipalities indicated to have implemented routine registration of cases of FGM or suspicion hereof, whereas seven (10.5%) municipalities reported not to perform routine registration, and 11 (16.4%) were unaware if registration is performed. To the question of whether the municipalities register cases of FGM specifically and not under other categories of abuse or violence against children, 12 (17.9%) municipalities answered "yes". A total of 22 (32.8%) municipalities stated to register cases of FGM under other categories concerning abuse or violence towards children. To the question of whether data from these registrations were available upon request, two (3%) municipalities answered "yes". These two municipalities had unfortunately not made this data accessible to the public.

Information material

Five (7.5%) municipalities indicated that they offer booklets or other written information material to the citizens or relevant professionals regarding FGM, while 54 (80.6%) municipalities stated that no information material of any kind had been developed or were available. Eight (11.9%) municipalities responded "do not know" to this question. Of the 10 municipalities with the highest share of citizens from risk countries, one municipality stated to offer information material about FGM to citizens and/or relevant professionals.

Discussion

It was in the light of the fact that Denmark has not yet implemented a coordinated national action plan to combat FGM that we chose to undertake the present study to investigate whether the task of combating FGM was satisfactorily managed on the local level by the 98 Danish municipalities. Other Scandinavian countries have developed and implemented national action plans in order to create national as well as regional foundations for preventing FGM. In Sweden, FGM was prohibited in 1982, and several state prevention programmes was implemented from 1993. A national action plan was established in Sweden in 2003, as well as comprehensive guidelines from The Swedish Board of Health and Welfare to officials in the social sector. Johndottor et al. states that when dealing with cases of FGM, a crucial and facilitating factor is having guidelines so as to achieve knowledge of how to act practically when dealing with victims of FGM [13]. In Norway, a national action plan was developed and implemented in 2000 and a subsequent 3-year national project against FGM was launched in 2001 with continuous evaluations throughout the following years [16].

Our study showed that only 10.4% of the responding municipalities reported to have implemented a specific action plan to combat FGM. Our study also showed that only a small minority of Danish municipalities have implemented specific preventive efforts against FGM, have developed specific registration procedures for cases of FGM and/or have information material available for distribution. Furthermore, there seems to be no relation between the prevalence of immigrants with origins in risk countries and the probability of a certain municipality having implemented a specific action plan to combat FGM. Unfortunately, these facts are not in accordance with recommendations made by international actors in the field. It is recommended to implement a national action plan, and to combat and perform registration of FGM separately from other forms of abuse and violence towards children and adolescents [20–23]. A national action plan will furthermore ensure a consistent and uniform approach to the issue of FGM across municipality boundaries.

A total of seven municipalities reported to have received petitions regarding FGM cases; however, only one municipality stated that they view FGM as a current problem within the municipality. It can only be speculated whether the relatively rare occurrence of FGM petitions in Danish municipalities is a result of a general low incidence of FGM in Denmark, or is a result of a lack of coordinated registration and awareness among front workers.

In England, the introduction of coordinated registration systems in regards to cases of FGM revealed that over 1700 women and girls had undergone FGM and was treated by the NHS between in September 2014. This information was crucial so as to form a picture of the prevalence of FGM in the country and in order to support national prevention programmes [24]. There is currently no such national registration system in Denmark. Our study shows that registration of FGM specifically as such is performed in only 17.9% of Danish municipalities, and that 19.4% were unaware if there had been petitions received regarding FGM in their respective municipalities. These results suggest that Danish municipalities lack the necessary data to draw reliable conclusions as to whether or not FGM is a current problem.

A study by Van Baelen et al. based on demographic data from 2011 estimated that 7910 girls and women living in Denmark had been subjected to FGM before immigration [4]. The current prevalence of girls and women having been, or in risk of being, submitted to FGM in Denmark is unknown. A 2016 study by Ziyada

et al. on FGM prevalence in Norway, which has a comparable number to Denmark of immigrants with origins in risk countries, estimated a prevalence of 17,300 girls and women having been subjected to FGM, and a prevalence of 3000–7900 girls in risk of being subjected to FGM [7]. We strongly recommend further investigation into the current prevalence of FGM in Denmark using the definitions, models and methodological approaches as recommended by the 2013 and 2015 EIGE reports [25, 26].

It is a weakness of the study that it does not offer explanations as to the reasons why the respective municipalities have chosen not to implement specific preventive measures or action plans against FGM. It is also a weakness that we did not gather data describing the responders of the questionnaire with regard to their knowledge about FGM, laws and their respective amount of influence within the respective municipalities. Furthermore, it was not possible to externally validate our data collected from the questionnaire, given the fact that there is no existing studies or data sources containing information enabling us to corroborate our findings. It could also be considered a weakness of our study that only 67 of the 98 municipalities responded to the questionnaire. In particular, of the ten municipalities in Denmark with the highest prevalence of immigrants with origins in risk countries, five municipalities did not participate in the study. However, the response rate of 68% is in line with what is considered a successful response rate for an online survey [18, 27–29]. The questionnaire consisted of quite few categories, which limited the extent of the results, but it could also be argued that this was a strength considering the relatively high response rate for an online survey.

Conclusions

In conclusion, our study shows that the current situation of FGM registration and prevention being under local administrative responsibility, has led to a severe lack of coordinated public initiative against FGM in Denmark. Besides the lack of a coordinated, national action plan there seems to be a general lack of public awareness on the issue. In October 2017, the second conviction on FGM in Denmark was given to two parents for having their daughters subjected to FGM abroad. In the High Court of Western Denmark, the President of the court halved the sentence from the District Court from 18 to 9 months of prison, arguing "There has not been provided evidence of the procedure having consequences for the girls including consequences for their sexual health" [30]. This sentence was referred to in the national newspapers, but we have not been able to find any news articles questioning the sentence or the citation of the President of the High Court of Western

Denmark, despite the fact that the international research on FGM has shown all types of FGM to be harmful practices, severely jeopardizing the health of women and girls [1, 31–35].

As such, Denmark does not live up to international recommendations in the field and it should be considered to implement nationally coordinated efforts against FGM such as an elaborate action plan, coordinated data collection and research programs to ensure a consistent approach towards FGM throughout the nation.

Abbreviations
EIGE: European Institute for Gender Equality; FGM: Female genital mutilation; WHO: World Health Organization

Acknowledgements
We would like to acknowledge Lea Leas and Anne Christine Stender Heerdegen for their aid in data collection during the pilot project.

Funding
This study did not receive funding.

Authors' contributions
GC, PB, RN, SE, VN: Study conception and design. GC, PB, SE, VN: Data collection. GC, PB, VN: Data analysis and interpretation. GC, PB, VN: Manuscript preparation. PB, VN: Critical revision. All authors have read and approved the final manuscript.

Competing interests
The authors declare that they have no competing interests.

Author details
[1]University of Copenhagen, Faculty of Health and Medical Sciences, Blegdamsvej 3, 2200 Copenhagen N, Denmark. [2]Department of Surgical Gastroenterology, Copenhagen University Hospital North Zealand, Dyrehavevej 29, 3400 Hillerød, Denmark. [3]Department of Emergency Medicine, Zealand University Hospital Slagelse, Ingemannsvej 50, 4200 Slagelse, Denmark. [4]Department of Culture, Municipality of Sermersooq, Kuussuaq 2, 3900 Nuuk, Greenland. [5]Department of Obstetrics and Gynecology, Zealand University Hospital Næstved, Ringstedgade 61, 4700 Næstved, Denmark.

References
1. UNICEF. Female genital mutilation/cutting: a global concern. New York: United Nations Childrens Fund; 2016.
2. WHO: Female Genital Mutilation Fact Sheet, available at http://www.who.int/mediacentre/factsheets/fs241/en/. Accessed 11 Oct 2016.
3. Farina P, Ortensi LE, Menonna A. Estimating the number of foreign women with female genital mutilation/cutting in Italy. Eur J Pub Health. 2016;26(4):656–61.
4. Van Baelen L, Ortensi L, Leye E. Estimates of first-generation women and girls with female genital mutilation in the European Union, Norway and Switzerland. Eur J Contracept Reprod Health Care. 2016;21(6):474–82.
5. Teixeira AL, Lisboa M. Estimating the prevalence of female genital mutilation in Portugal. Public Health. 2016;139:53–60.
6. Goldberg H, Stupp P, Okoroh E, Besera G, Goodman D, Danel I. Female genital mutilation/cutting in the United States: updated estimates of women and girls at risk, 2012. Public Health Rep. 2016;131(2):340–7.
7. Ziyada MM, Norberg-Schulz M, Johansen REB. Estimating the magnitude of female genital mutilation/cutting in Norway: an extrapolation model. BMC Public Health. 2016;16:110.
8. Dubourg D, Richard F, Leye E, Ndame S, Rommens T, Maes S. Estimating the number of women with female genital mutilation in Belgium. Eur J Contracept Reprod Health Care. 2011;16(4):248–57.
9. Koukkula M, Keskimaki I, Koponen P, Molsa M, Klemetti R. Female genital mutilation/cutting among women of Somali and Kurdish origin in Finland. Birth. 2016;43(3):240–6.
10. Zurynski Y, Phu A, Sureshkumar P, Cherian S, Deverell M, Elliott EJ, for Australian Paediatric Surveillance Unit Female Genital Mutilation Study Steering C. Female genital mutilation in children presenting to Australian paediatricians. Arch Dis Child. 2017;102(6):509–15.
11. European Parliament resolution of 24 March 2009 on combating female genital mutilation in the EU. Available at http://www.europarl.europa.eu/sides/getDoc.do?pubRef=-//EP//NONSGML+TA+P6-TA-2009-0161+0+DOC+PDF+V0//EN. Accessed 2 Oct 2016.
12. EIGE. Study to map the current situation and trends of FGM - country reports. European Union, 2013. Available at http://eige.europa.eu/rdc/eige-publications/study-map-current-situation-and-trends-fgm-country-reports. Accessed 11 Oct 2016.
13. Johnsdotter, Carlbom. FGM in Sweden: Swedish legislation regarding "female genital mutilation" and implementation of the law. 2004 (Research Report in Sociology). Department of Sociology, Lund University.
14. van Kolfschooten F. Dutch government cracks down on female circumcision. Lancet. 2004;363(9420):1531.
15. PM outlines tough new measures to tackle FGM. J Fam Health Care. 2014;24(5):7.
16. The Norwegian Government's International Action Plan for Combating Female Genital Mutilation. 2014. Available at http://www.regjeringen.no/globalassets/upload/kilde/ud/bro/2003/0011/ddd/pdfv/197557-ud_kjonnslemlestelse_eng.pdf. Accessed 9 Oct 2016.
17. Ministry of Social Affairs and Health, Finland, Action Plan for the prevention of circumcision of girls and women 2012–2016. 2012. Available at https://julkaisut.valtioneuvosto.fi/bitstream/handle/10024/73924/URN%3ANBN%3Afi-fe201504226370.pdf?sequence=1%20. Accessed 9 Oct 2016.
18. Eysenbach G. Improving the quality of web surveys: the checklist for reporting results of internet E-surveys (CHERRIES). J Med Internet Res. 2004;6(3):e34.
19. Statistics Denmark census 2017, Statbank. available at http://www.statistikbanken.dk/statbank5a/default.asp?w=1280. Accessed 20 June 2017.
20. Berg K. Female genital mutilation: implications for social work. Soc Work. 1997;65(3):16–26.
21. Royal College of Midwives, Royal College of Nursing, Royal College of Obstetricians andGynaecologists, Equality Now and UNITE. Tackling FGM In The UK: Intercollegiate Recommendations for Identifying, Recording and Reporting. London: Royal College of Midwives, Royal College of Nursing, Royal College of Obstetricians and Gynaecologists, Equality Now and UNITE; 2013.
22. Morgan J. Working towards an end to FGM. Lancet. 2015;385(9971):843–4.
23. Creighton SM, Dear J, de Campos C, Williams L, Hodes D. Multidisciplinary approach to the management of children with female genital mutilation (FGM) or suspected FGM: service description and case series. BMJ Open. 2016;6(2):e010311.
24. Health and Social Care Information Center. Female Genital Mutilation (FGM), September 2014, experimental statistics, available at http://www.digital.nhs.uk/catalogue/PUB15711. Accessed 19 Oct 2016.
25. EIGE. Female genital mutilation in the European Union and Croatia. Lithuania: European Union; 2013.
26. EIGE. EIGE. Estimation of girls at risk of female genital mutilation in the European Union. Lithuania: European Union; 2015.
27. Cook JV, Dickinson HO, Eccles MP. Response rates in postal surveys of healthcare professionals between 1996 and 2005: an observational study. BMC Health Serv Res. 2009;9:160.

28. Fincham JE. Response rates and responsiveness for surveys, standards, and the journal. Am J Pharm Educ. 2008;72(2):43.

29. Asch DA, Jedrziewski MK, Christakis NA. Response rates to mail surveys published in medical journals. J Clin Epidemiol. 1997;50(10):1129–36.

30. Ritzau. Landsret halverer straf til forældre for omskæring af døtre. Berlingske Tidende. October 18th 2017. Available at http://www.b.dk/nationalt/landsret-halverer-straf-til-foraeldre-for-omskaering-af-doetre. Accessed 18 Oct 2017.

31. Ahmed MR, Shaaban MM, Meky HK, Amin Arafa ME, Mohamed TY, Gharib WF, Ahmed AB. Psychological impact of female genital mutilation among adolescent Egyptian girls: a cross-sectional study. Eur J Contracept Reprod Health Care. 2017;22(4):280–5.

32. Berg RC, Underland V. The obstetric consequences of female genital mutilation/cutting: a systematic review and meta-analysis. Obstet Gynecol Int. 2013;2013:496564.

33. Berg RC, Odgaard-Jensen J, Fretheim A, Underland V, Vist G. An updated systematic review and meta-analysis of the obstetric consequences of female genital mutilation/cutting. Obstet Gynecol Int. 2014;2014:542859.

34. Abdulcadir J, Tille JC, Petignat P. Management of painful clitoral neuroma after female genital mutilation/cutting. Reprod Health. 2017;14(1):22.

35. Yassin K, Idris HA, Ali AA. Characteristics of female sexual dysfunctions and obstetric complications related to female genital mutilation in Omdurman maternity hospital, Sudan. Reprod Health. 2018;15(1):7.

12

"My job is to get pregnant women to the hospital": a qualitative study of the role of traditional birth attendants in the distribution of misoprostol to prevent post-partum haemorrhage in two provinces in Mozambique

Karen Hobday[1*], Jennifer Hulme[2,3], Caroline Homer[4,5,6], Páscoa Zualo Wate[7], Suzanne Belton[1] and Ndola Prata[8]

Abstract

Background: Post-partum haemorrhage is the leading cause of maternal deaths in Mozambique. In 2015, the Mozambican Ministry of Health launched the National Strategy for the Prevention of Post-Partum Haemorrhage at the Community Level. The strategy included the distribution of misoprostol to women in advance at antenatal care and via Traditional Birth Attendants who directly administer the medication. The study explores the role of Traditional Birth Attendants in the misoprostol program and the views of women who used misoprostol to prevent post-partum haemorrhage.

Methods: This descriptive study collected data through in-depth interviews and focus group discussions. Traditional Birth Attendants between the ages of 30–70 and women of reproductive age participated in the study. Data was collected between June–October 2017 in Inhambane and Nampula Provinces. Line by line thematic analysis was used to interpret the data using Nvivo (v.11).

Results: The majority of TBAs in the study were satisfied with their role in the misoprostol program and were motivated to work with the formal health system to encourage women to access facility based births. Women who used misoprostol were also satisfied with the medication and encouraged family and friends to access it when needed. Women in the community and Traditional Birth Attendants requested assistance with transportation to reach the health facility to avoid home births.

Conclusions: This study contributes to the evidence base that Traditional Birth Attendants are an appropriate channel for the distribution of misoprostol for the prevention of post-partum haemorrhage at the community level. More support and resources are needed to ensure Traditional Birth Attendants can assist women to have safe births when they are unable to reach the health facility. A consistent supply of misoprostol is needed to ensure women at the community level receive this life saving medication.

Keywords: Maternal health, Traditional birth attendant, Mozambique, Post-partum Haemorrhage, Misoprostol, Community

* Correspondence: karen.hobday@menzies.edu.au
[1]Menzies School of Health Research, Charles Darwin University, Darwin, Australia
Full list of author information is available at the end of the article

Plain English summary

Bleeding after childbirth (post-partum haemorrhage) is the leading cause of maternal deaths in Mozambique. The majority of these deaths happen when women give birth at home, without a skilled or trained health worker. In 2011, the World Health Organization stated that they support the distribution of misoprostol (oral medicine tablets) to prevent bleeding after childbirth. These tablets are important for women who cannot get to a health clinic to give birth because they are easy to use, prevent bleeding and can save their lives. A woman simply swallows three tablets of misoprostol directly after the baby is born and before the afterbirth (placenta) is delivered.

In 2015, the Mozambique Ministry of Health launched a National Strategy to prevent bleeding after childbirth for women who give birth at home. The strategy included two ways for women to receive the misoprostol tablets. First, women can get misoprostol when they visit the health clinic for a maternal health check-up at 28 weeks in their pregnancy. Or second, they can receive it from a Traditional Birth Attendant, a community woman who helps other women give birth. Traditional Birth Attendants receive training about the medication and how to assist women in childbirth but is not a qualified health worker. The Traditional Birth Attendant gives the misoprostol to the woman directly after the baby is born. The study looks at the role of Traditional Birth Attendants in the misoprostol program and the views of women who used misoprostol to prevent bleeding after childbirth.

Background

The maternal mortality ratio in Mozambique is 489/ 100000 live births [1] and post partum haemorrhage (PPH) is a leading cause of maternal deaths [2, 3]. Mozambique experienced a 64.8% reduction in maternal mortality between 1990 and 2013 [1, 4] almost reaching the Millennium Development Goal target of a 75% reduction. Still, the lifetime risk of maternal death remains high; one in 40 Mozambican women will die during child birth [1]. The Mozambican Health Sector Strategy 2014–2019 prioritises the reduction of maternal mortality as a primary goal [2].

Results from a 2015 survey in Mozambique found that overall, 70% of births were assisted by Skilled Birth Attendants (SBA) [5]. The Ministry of Health marked significant improvement from the Demographic and Health Survey (DHS) in 2011 which found SBA coverage to be only 54% [1]. However, disparities exist; disaggregated results from urban and rural populations show heath facility births are much more prevalent in urban areas (91%) compared to rural areas (67%) [5]. Access to rural health services in Mozambique remains limited by geographic distance, lack of transport options, coverage and quality [6, 7].

In Sub-Saharan Africa, approximately 23% of all births are attended by a Traditional Birth Attendant (TBA, only half of which were formally trained in modern medical childbirth techniques with a focus on clean delivery [8]. A TBA is defined as, 'community-based providers of care during pregnancy, childbirth and the postnatal period' who are traditional, not-formally trained and work independent of the health system [9]. TBAs were largely ignored through the 1990s by governments and the global health community after multiple studies suggested that TBA training was cost ineffective and had minimal impact [10–12]. Notably, TBAs were not armed with birth kits or uterotonics alongside this training and thus some argue that new technology and evidence could improve outcomes [12, 13]. There is also growing evidence that TBA training may improve linkages with facilities and improve perinatal outcomes [10]. The aim of this paper is to analyse the role of TBAs in the provision of a maternal health innovation in Mozambique.

Context in Mozambique

Home births are a reality for women in rural and remote areas of Mozambique, despite the country's policy to achieve the highest possible coverage of facility births with SBAs. TBAs play an important role in promoting ANC, often accompany and attend facility births, and assist at home births when women cannot access the facility births. Women in rural Mozambique often give birth at home with a TBA who may have limited or no training and few resources to ensure a safe delivery.

Prior to 1985, the MoH largely discouraged the involvement of TBAs as they were seen to detract from facility based births [14]. Investment and training in TBAs commenced in the late 1980s in Mozambique as an acknowledgement of the shortage of SBAs and limited coverage of facility births amongst rural women. TBA training first took place between 1991 and 1998; 3734 TBAs were trained, one-third of which were located in Zambezia Province [14, 15]. In 1996, a study of TBA training in Manica Province found no significant difference in maternal, perinatal or infant mortality between trained and untrained TBAs [14]. This was published amongst mixed evidence on the utility of training TBAs for improving the quality of care and reducing the mortality of mothers/newborns [10–12]. The authors recommended that TBA training be balanced with improvements to health facility infrastructure and the provision of professional support to midwives working in remote locations. Since 2014, there has been a concerted effort in Mozambique to re-engage in promoting early antenatal care (ANC) and facility births [2]; they have also engaged TBAs in the use of both chlorohexidine for the prevention of neonatal sepsis and misoprostol for the prevention of PPH [16].

Misoprostol has proven to be a safe alternative utero-tonic where oxytocin is not available, such as at home births [17, 18]. Numerous countries have piloted the community-based distribution of misoprostol using either advanced distribution for self-administration during ANC visits or via Community Health Workers (CHW), or through distribution to TBAs who attend births [19–24]. Scale-up of community-based distribution of misoprostol remains limited; while there are early success stories emerging from Nepal and Bangladesh, many programs have been delayed or abandoned by donors or governments for political reasons and the lack of trust in community distribution [25].

The Mozambique MoH has committed to the expansion of misoprostol for the prevention of PPH alongside a network of CHWs known as Agentes Polivalentes Elementares (APEs) [15] and newly trained TBAs. A pilot distribution of misoprostol conducted in Nampula, Mozambique from November 2009–October 2010 found that distribution through both TBAs and Antenatal Care (ANC) achieved 99% misoprostol usage at home births [26]. In 2011, the Mozambican MoH formally approved the distribution of misoprostol at the community level for the prevention of PPH.

In 2014, the MoH launched the 'Strategy for the Prevention of PPH at the Community Level' (referred to as the National PPH Strategy), which included guidelines for the use of misoprostol for PPH where SBAs are not available [16]. The aim of the misoprostol program is to increase access to misoprostol for women who give birth in the community to reduce maternal mortality associated with PPH. The National PPH Strategy named 35 districts across the country to be included in the program for distribution. TBAs have a key role in the distribution and administration of misoprostol for the prevention of PPH. Pregnant woman at 28 or greater weeks of gestation may receive misoprostol in advance at ANC or they may receive it via a TBA in their neighbourhood. APEs act as the link between the health facility and the TBAs by providing misoprostol to the TBA in their zone. APEs are formally recognised by the health system, have a higher level of education than TBAs, often have a bicycle for transport, and receive a monthly subsidy [27]. Misoprostol for the prevention of PPH is branded as 'Misol' as a way to differentiate it between misoprostol used for inductions or abortion.

Implementation commenced in 2015 in six districts in Inhambane and Sofala provinces, and is ongoing in 35 districts across the country at the time this article was sent to publication. TBAs were recruited via recommendations by the health staff or APEs. Distance from the health facility was not considered in recruitment. Some TBAs prefer to remain autonomous and maintain their status outside of the formal health sector. Health staff,

TBAs and APEs all received training on the use and distribution of misoprostol in May 2015 in Inhambane Province and August 2016 in Nampula. TBAs received three- day training on safe birth practices and the use of misoprostol; 47 TBAs were initially trained in Inhambane and 80 in Nampula Province. Training was provided in a cascade 'Train the Trainers' approach and was supported by UNFPA and Jhpiego's Maternal and Child Survival Project. TBAs distribute misoprostol to women directly at the birth and are not permitted to provide the misoprostol in advance.

The aim of this study was to explore the role and perceptions of TBAs in the distribution of misoprostol for the prevention of PPH at the community level in two provinces in Mozambique. The facilitators and barriers that TBAs experienced working within the misoprostol program were also examined. We also sought to understand the views of women who had used misoprostol for the prevention of PPH.

Methods
Study design
This research was nested within a larger implementation study evaluating the distribution of misoprostol for the prevention of PPH in two provinces in Mozambique. A phenomenological qualitative approach was applied to understand the misoprostol program through the experience of TBAs and women who had used the medication. This approach is suited to understanding health care and health systems through the real world experiences of patients and health workers engaged in the system [28]. A combination of focus group and individual interviews allowed a broad range of themes, which were then further explored in focus group discussions. It also allowed inclusion of a more diverse group of participants whose availability and comfort with the two methods might differ.

This study was descriptive and used semi-structured qualitative interview guides for data collection. In-depth interviews and focus group discussions (FGD) were conducted by a trained research team who consisted of both local and international research assistants. Semi-structured interview guides ensured the main topics were covered including use and understanding of misoprostol, supply, safety, barriers and facilitators to participation in the program. A narrative review of the evidence base, challenges and scale-up of misoprostol was conducted by the authors [25]. This review in part informed the topics in the interview guide. The interview guides were pilot tested and then revised to ensure the questions were clear.

The majority of interviews and FGDs were conducted in local language or where appropriate, Portuguese. Interviews were held between 30 and 60 min and were recorded with permission from the participants. At the end of each day, individuals and/or the team debriefed their observations and provided further details about the interviews. Ethical clearance was granted by the Human Research Ethics Committee at Charles Darwin University, Australia (HREC 2015–2445) and the Mozambican National Bioethics Committee and Ministry of Health. Informed consent was sought and gained for all participants.

Setting

The study took place in three districts in Nampula Province and two districts in Inhambane Province in Mozambique. Inhambane and Nampula Provinces were chosen due to geographic region; one study site was located in the Southern region and one in the Northern Region of the country. Districts in each province were chosen based on inclusion in the national misoprostol for prevention of PPH program, geographical location and on discussions with Provincial and District Health Authorities.

Study participants

Female TBAs between the ages of 30–70 were the key participants in the study. Respondents were selected based on geographical location, involvement in the misoprostol program and selected with assistance from either the health facility staff and/or the CHW. Where possible, a research assistant would call the TBA directly to request the interview. In some cases, the District Maternal Health Director and/or Community Health Workers were asked to contact the TBAs in their designated district and invite them to the health facility to speak to the study team. Participants were given the option of withdrawing from the interview or the study at any point; no participants requested to withdraw. Additionally, interviews were conducted with women of reproductive health age in Inhambane and Nampula Provinces who had previously used misoprostol to prevent PPH during childbirth. These women were purposively selected on recommendation by the TBA, using snowball sampling to access this hard to reach population. Participant numbers were determined based on obtaining thematic saturation. Data were collected between June–October 2017.

Analysis

All interviews and debriefs were translated and transcribed in Portuguese, and then translated into English. Line by line thematic analysis was used to code and analyse the data using NVivo (v.11) [29]. KH and JH initially read all interviews twice to familiarise themselves with the data. Interviews were coded initially based on emerging themes, and then re-read and coded again resulting in additional themes. KH and JH coded the interviews and FGDs independently and reached consensus on key themes after several discussions; they discussed divergent cases as they arose and co-authors provided input when necessary [30]. Notes from debriefings and recordings

were reviewed and informed the analysis, particularly as a reminder of the context. KH is undertaking her PhD and JH is a medical doctor. They both have research and programming expertise in public health. Their views and life experiences may have influenced the data analysis.

Results

Qualitative semi-structured interviews were conducted with 16 purposefully selected Traditional Birth Attendants (TBA) (11 in Inhambane and 5 in Nampula Provinces). Four FGDs were undertaken with TBAs in Nampula Province with 3–5 women in each group. In total, we interviewed 11 women who had used misoprostol; 5 women were interviewed individually in Inhambane and Nampula Provinces and 6 women participated in a FGD in Nampula Province.

The findings were organized in the following themes: a)Understanding of misoprostol: correct use of misoprostol; misoprostol as risky b) TBA identity and role: satisfaction with misoprostol; encouraging facility births; trust between TBAs and health staff; sense of identity;, trauma and responsibility and c) Program operations: stock management;, resources limitations; and transport and distance. These themes were then organised in the context of facilitators (groups a and b) or barriers (group c and trauma and responsibility) to the misoprostol for prevention of PPH program. See Fig. 1.

Understanding of misoprostol
Correct use of misoprostol

The vast majority of TBAs correctly understood how to administer the misoprostol: three pills (600 micrograms) after the woman had given birth and prior to the removal of the placenta. For example, *"The mother, after giving birth, and before the placenta [is birthed], has to take three pills before the placenta leaves to reduce post-partum haemorrhage" (TBA1, FGD 2)*. Another TBA explained, *"In the training I was informed as soon as a mother finishes giving birth, I must immediately give three pills and she should swallow immediately to avoid bleeding" (TBA 4)*.

Three TBAs were unsure of how to administer the medication and they had not had the misoprostol provided to them since receiving the training. Because training took place in May 2015 in Inhambane Province and August 2016 in Nampula, there was often a time lag between training and the actual distribution of misoprostol. The majority of TBAs clearly described the administration of misoprostol prior to birth as 'dangerous' and knew the exact timing to give the medication. When asked if there were any other uses for misoprostol, none of them could name any, including when probed about use for abortion. However they were strictly told during their training to

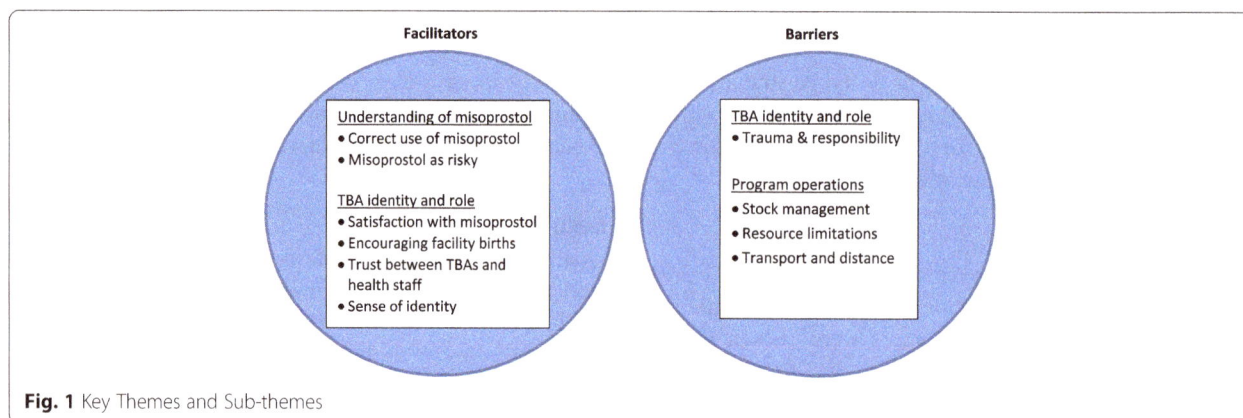

Fig. 1 Key Themes and Sub-themes

hide the medication from children and for others, saying for example:

Uhhhh, I personally have never heard of it [giving misoprostol before the birth], see even in the training about Misol we were not told that, we were told to give it after the birth, before the birth it should not be given. (TBA 9)

Misoprostol as risky

There was a strong focus on the risks and dangers (both real and fictional) associated with misoprostol as taught during the training and reinforced by the nurses. The TBAs receive three doses in a blister pack from the APE. If a zone or neighbourhood did not have an APE, the TBA received the doses directly from the Maternal Newborn and Child Health (MNCH) nurse at the health facility. Many TBAs were told that the medication, despite being in closed blister packs, attracted rodents and there would be a high risk of death if consumed by a child. One TBA explained,

They told us that we should be very careful with these tablets, keep them very well and safely, if they are opened even if it is a small opening, they become unusable, so we should not administer in this situation. (TBA 13)

One TBA mentioned that if the drug were to be sold, that the TBAs would experience severe consequences. "*...we were warned not to sell any pills, anyone found to do this could pay a fine of one million and go right to jail*" (TBA 14).

TBA identity and role
Satisfaction with distribution of misoprostol

Overall, the majority of TBAs stated that they had positive feelings about administering misoprostol and believed it

was useful for their work and the community. They made statements such as:

... the pills really help a lot, because there are times when the patient loses a lot of blood and if there are no pills it can be fatal, especially since everything here is distant, there is no transport and in the middle of the bush little can be done to save the patient. (TBA 15)

When we got the child out, I took out the Misol and gave it to the lady and removed the placenta. There was no bleeding problem. I am very pleased with this work. It is rewarding when everything goes well without bleeding, and even if the delivery goes well, I always advise her to go to a hospital for a brief check-up. (TBA3, FGD 3)

Women in the community who had taken misoprostol also spoke positively about the medication and felt that it made them strong and their 'body firm'. The majority of the women did not know the name of the medication; they referred to it as the pill that stopped the bleeding. All stated that they wanted the program to continue, for instance:

When I left the hospital I walked by myself until I got home. I did not need to stay in bed or be hospitalized, the pill had a good effect on my body. I was able to walk by myself. (Participant 3, FGD 6 Women who used misoprostol)

A few women spoke about some people who had not yet taken misoprostol that had worries about taking medication. They said that they encouraged other women in their community to use misoprostol as this woman explained.

People who have not yet taken it [misoprostol] say they are afraid to take it because they do not know what the reaction will be. Now we have tried to pass on to them the experience that it is a good medicine and that it does not harm the body and that it does not kill, we are here alive and healthy. (Participant 2, FGD 6 Women who used misoprostol).

The men when their wives have not taken it yet say that this pill is nothing, people are just excited, but for those of us who have already taken it our husbands have a contrary opinion because they have already seen the good effects of the Misol. (Participant 1, FGD 6 Women who used misoprostol).

Encouraging facility based births

All TBAs in both Inhambane and Nampula provinces emphasised that their primary responsibility was to bring women to the health facility to give birth. TBAs sometimes give talks to the community and women about seeking antenatal care, giving birth with an SBA and childhood vaccinations. APEs and community leaders also play a role to encourage health seeking behaviour and facility births. Women who used misoprostol also said that they encourage friends and relatives to seek care early and, if needed, use misoprostol in cases when they cannot get to the facility, for example:

...since the government has thought of putting a traditional midwife [TBA] in each neighbourhood or community, several advances have been recorded. In fact, it was a wise decision. And the mobilization or campaigns of sensitization is not only done here in the hospital, but also in the neighbourhoods. Local structures such as Ward Clerks, Community Leaders, are all aligned on spreading information about pregnancy and Misol. Even the structures of the district government have collaborated. When we met with a Director and asked for help to take a woman to the hospital, there was never anyone who refused. We all collaborate. (TBA 3, FGD 4)

It was commonly accepted that misoprostol was to be used only if a woman could not reach the health facility. Most of the informants, unprompted, described the importance of facility births as the safest option. TBAs described misoprostol as a medication only to be used in the event of a 'surprise' birth, or 'birthing along the way' to the facility. Any birth that they assisted with at home was either because the woman would give birth on the road, had progressed too quickly, could not walk, or a transfer could not be arranged despite her efforts. TBAs made comments explaining this including:

When I started this program, we were taught that we cannot perform births at home, but there may be some surprises and we have to deliver before we get to the hospital, so we should have these pills to give the woman after the baby is birthed. However, it is our duty to mobilize and sensitize pregnant women to the health unit. (TBA 6)

Some TBAs took a staunch approach to implementing the policy on health facility births and refused to assist home births. One TBA mentioned that 'their house was not a maternity' and they would outright refuse women to enter their house to give birth there, for example:

No, I do not usually take much time, when the place is far away I refuse (laughs), because I teach them to go to the hospital, going to the patient's house is also not accepted, only to call me, saying that she is on her way to the hospital. I do not accept to receive people in my house to give birth; they did not teach me to transform my house into maternity (laughs). (TBA 15)

Trust between TBA and health staff

Trust was identified as a major theme in the study and was a facilitator to the program being accessed in the community. Trust was central to allowing the health facility to move forward with community distribution. TBAs are well known in their community and respected which assisted in introducing misoprostol as a new intervention. Most TBAs enjoyed a positive relationship with those involved in the misoprostol program including the nurses, health staff and APEs.

TBAs often worked closely with the APE in their neighbourhood. They mostly described a good working relationship with the APE and were satisfied with the role the APEs played as the channel between themselves and the health facility for the distribution of misoprostol. For example,

"We take good care of them, along with our nurses, they do not abandon us nor despise us, in fact you just see between us and the nurses we have a good relationship...we understand each other" (TBA 7).

A strong, positive relationship with health staff also appeared to anchor the program and encourage facility births. Many TBAs spoke about attending the labour after assisting the woman to reach the health facility, some TBAs said they would observe or assist in the maternity ward. All TBAs appreciated and felt respected when the nurses included them in the maternity ward. Others mentioned that it was a good opportunity to learn from skilled birth attendants, as illustrated here:

We have good relations, we talk, we respect [each other], we help ourselves and we teach a little of everything, so that the service can go well, after all we all have the same objectives ...they always receive [us] with great professionalism, both the traditional midwives [TBAs] as well as the patients that we bring from our communities. Even when we arrive at midnight, the nurses get up and greet us. (TBA 1, FGD 4)

However, not all TBAs reported a positive relationship with the nurses and some were unhappy with the dynamic, for example:

That's why I said that when I arrive at the hospital with a patient, the nurses do not give me importance, until at some point they ask where you are going to sleep? They do not give me the opportunity to watch the work with the more informed colleagues, which is not good. (TBA 4)

Sense of identity

TBAs very strongly identified with their role, some stated that their skills to assist with births were a gift from God, or a skill passed on by their mother or family member. Often they were chosen by the community to work as a TBA.

I used to do many births, it was not by accident that I was taken to work in coordination with the hospital, although I could not read or write, but God gave me this gift to help women. Nowadays, since we started talking about the need for women to go to the hospital, these cases have greatly diminished. (TBA 8)

TBAs mentioned the importance of having t-shirts or capulanas (traditional material worn as a skirt, dress or to carry babies) with MoH logos to help with their identification in the community and to help them to gain acceptance and be respected in their work. The TBAs that had received a MoH printed TBA t-shirt wore it very proudly; it was clear this small incentive was a positive means to show they received support from the MoH. For example:

As we have this t-shirt, although it is the only one that was given to us in the hospital [a TBA printed MISAU shirt], it helps them to identify us and see that we work in coordination with the hospital and so they do not reject us. (TBA 7)

Trauma and responsibility

Very few TBAs experienced maternal mortality or newborn deaths, and several noted that they experienced

fewer cases of PPH after the introduction of misoprostol. Those that had experienced deaths described a deep sense of responsibility despite their limited skills and resources. This is highlighted in this quote:

There was this one time when I lost a girl here in the house, it was very difficult. Another time as well there was a woman whose family I counsel to go to the hospital but they took their time, and when they arrived at the maternity unfortunately it was too late, and she died. (TBA 10)

They also described significant fear and anxiety around attending homebirths without having the skills or the materials to respond adequately, for instance:

What usually is difficult for me is when you advise someone to go to the hospital and they resist until they give birth at home, it makes me very sad, because there may be a serious problem with the baby or the mother and I am held responsible for being the TBA of that person... Imagine that she gives birth and needs stitches, how will I do it? So I should be able to make the woman come to the hospital on time. (TBA 12)

Overall TBAs felt very accountable to their community and also worried about being blamed for any adverse outcomes. They had a clear sense of responsibility to respond to the needs of pregnant women and women in labour. This also manifested in fear and guilt, that they will not be able to provide for women when needed as explained here:

No, because as soon as you said that you are looking for the pills, for now there are none. This would be the only request because if you find someone in labour, outside the hospital, it is difficult without the pills, and we can only trust God, since we can not leave the person suffering. (TBA 16)

Program operations
Stock management

Stock outs were a source of stress and concern for both TBAs and women; there was concern for the women who would not benefit from the misoprostol. In the National PPH Strategy, the process for distribution of misoprostol is from the Health Facility to the APE to the TBA. TBAs receive the misoprostol in a blister pack from the APE. The APE acts as the link between the health facility and the TBA as they often have bicycles and a formal connection to the health system. APEs are responsible to submit monthly reports to the health facility and can then pick up more stock of misoprostol if needed. In practice, this system does not always function. In some instances, TBAs were not able to retrieve the misoprostol from their identified APE due to distance, unavailability or illness. In other cases, there may not have been an APE who lived in the same neighbourhood or community as the TBA. Some TBAs bypassed the APE "middle men" and picked up the misoprostol directly from the health facility. For example, *"They told us in the training that it should be the APE to give us but for my case it is difficult because my APE is far from me, so I come here to pick it up at the health unit with the nurse" (TBA 5).*

Other TBAs mentioned that the system whereby the TBA received the misoprostol from the APE was not always functioning due to the distances between the APE and TBA and the reliance on cell phones for communication. One TBA explained it as the following, *"We work well [together], but I'm very far from the APE, only my colleagues are close to them. I have more contact with the nurses" (TBA 13).*

In some districts, TBAs had been without stock for several months and in a few cases up to a year. Other TBAs said they had received training, but had not yet received any doses of misoprostol. This raised questions about the sustainability of the program; TBAs without regular access to misoprostol questioned whether the program would continue. In other cases TBAs reported that they had received stock but had to return it as the pills were expiring, for example:

When they do not have it we have a real despair. As it is a medicine that helps we run to the hospital to ask the nurse or the midwife. The sad thing is when they say they do not have it and are waiting for it. But when it's in the warehouse there's been no difficulty in giving us the pills. (Participant 2, FGD 6 Women who used misoprostol)

Surprisingly we did not speak to any TBAs that supervised the administration of misoprostol that mothers had previously received at ANC. TBAs who lived further away from the facilities were often those who directly administered misoprostol, probably to women who were less likely to have had received ANC after 28 weeks. A reliable supply of misoprostol which is easy to access, either via the APE or directly from the health facility was seen to be an essential component of the functioning of the program.

Resource limitations

Lack of financial and material resources were prominent underlying barriers to the TBAs involvement in the misoprostol program. TBAs do not receive any salary, incentives or resources for their participation in the program. While this did not seem to have negative implications on the relationships between the TBA and APEs or health staff, all of the TBAs mentioned that they would appreciate support from the government to perform their jobs safely. TBAs that we spoke with did not have any other employment or additional income and were very poor, for example:

Unfortunately I am not lucky enough to earn money for the work I do, I have already brought many people into the world by my hands. If it were a case of working for a boss, I think I would be in retirement now and earning money for the time spent in this activity. (TBA 15)

Many TBAs spoke about their lack of soap and gloves, and resulting fear of infection. They explained that they did not receive gloves or soap to assist with their work as their role, as per MoH policy, was solely to accompany woman to give birth at the health facility, as explained here:

Well, they tell me that my job is to get pregnant women to the hospital, but if it happened before I was there, I should get some plastic [from a 1kg sugar bag], and put it on my hands, that's how I do it, they did not give me gloves, they said they wear the gloves in the hospital. (TBA 10)

Just a few things saddens me in this work, we do not want much, just soap, imagine you my daughter, we are dirty and we have to go home to wash us with the little that our husband tries to arrange, with many difficulties, he even gets annoyed because he says that this work does not help me at all and he threatens to forbid me. Still, I keep doing it because I like to help. Therefore, we do not need much, just soap because it is inevitable that the blood will make us dirty and it is not easy without cleaning ourselves. (TBA 7)

Poverty and shame was also an underlying theme in discussions with women who had used misoprostol. Women spoke of poverty in terms of the lack of resources to deliver comfortably; being transported to the health facility, with a new capulana (traditional cloth) for the baby, and having food to eat after the birth of the baby, for example:

For example when a child is born they do not let it be covered with this capulana that I used, in the hospital they say it must be a new capulana ... where will I get money for a new capulana if my only capulana is this one? So we do not know ... this price we are paying for our misfortune is very high. The nurses only know to say that we should produce vegetables to be able to sell to get money ... but here who will buy what we produce if we are all farmers and poor people? (Participant 3, FGD 6 Women who used misoprostol)

Transportation and distance

In addition to a lack of resources, the majority of TBAs spoke about the challenges they faced reaching the health facility. One of the key roles of TBAs is to accompany women to the health facility to give birth; however transportation was never provided, and many TBAs reported they had to walk or pay for transport out of pocket as highlighted here:

Another problem is transportation, I live far from the health unit, I must pick up two cars and pay 40 meticais just to come, so, round trip is 80 meticais and no one gives me that money, its personal effort. We are told that this is voluntary work and that we should do it of our own free will, so I do it without gaining anything. (TBA 13)

A few TBAs refused to assist in home births, even when transport or walking was impossible, and seemed concerned about being blamed or punished by heath staff if and when they did. 'Birthing along the way' or on the side of the road in transit to the health facility was a challenge for both TBAs and women. TBAs described the challenges of walking and assisting women to give birth in the dark without gloves, soap or water. TBAs and women explained that often they only had an unwashed capulana (traditional cloth) with them to wrap the baby.

Women in the community vividly described the hardship of walking 3 hours or more to the health facility in late pregnancy or in labour. The imperative for safe reliable transport to the health facility was a key request by women in the community:

We want to continue to receive your medicines the Misol tablet. Of the many difficulties that women here face the greatest of all is transportation. We need a car to help us. Our bodies are already getting tired, we have to raise children, take care of the house and still go to the fields. We are asking for a lot [a car]... with this, expensive Misol would reach the most distant people... (Participant 5, FGD 6 Women who used misoprostol)

Discussion

This study aimed to understand the role and perceptions of TBAs in the distribution of misoprostol for the prevention of PPH at the community level in two provinces in Mozambique. The facilitators and barriers that TBAs experienced working within the misoprostol program were also examined.

We encountered tremendous support for the misoprostol program from TBAs and women themselves. Women who had used misoprostol appreciated the medication and encouraged community members, relatives and friends to use it. TBAs highly valued the program, and spoke confidently about distributing misoprostol and understood its role in preventing PPH. Similar to other studies in Nigeria [31] and Nepal [32], most TBAs correctly explained how and when to administer misoprostol.

TBAs expressed a strong sense of identify and pride in their work, and described their role as a respected member in their community. Many TBAs spoke of the calling they had either from God or a family member to assist women to give birth. T-shirts and capulanas with the MoH logo provided them with a uniform and a means of identification in the community. TBAs felt a heavy responsibility to the women they assist which at times caused them to feel stress. Few TBAs were present when a woman passed away in labour or shortly after giving birth; however many discussed the risk of death and their fear of being able to assist with complications.

TBAs described strong, positive relationships with the APEs and MNCH nurses which often bolstered their sense of identity as a link between the informal and formal heath system; other studies have also seen an increase in referrals and awareness of medical care with the engagement of TBAs [33, 34]. TBAs were satisfied that their work was recognized by the formal health sector, and interestingly some appreciated the opportunity to observe the facility delivery as a learning tool. These findings are in keeping with a systematic review which found that including TBAs within health facilities increases skilled birth attendance and the more involved the TBA was with the health facility, the greater the impact [35]. Facility births can be improved with the creation of a supportive environment that links TBAs and SBAs and also removes barriers to women's access to health facilities and SBAs [32].

TBAs consistently described accompanying pregnant and labouring women to the health facility, a finding in keeping with the strong commitment by informal and formal health care workers and community members in southern Mozambique to promote ANC and births at the health facility [7]. TBAs were aware of the national policy to encourage health facility births, and understood that misoprostol should be used only in the event of emergencies or unexpected births. Findings from a recent systematic review of task shifting in Active Management of the Third Stage of Labour support this approach; first promoting facility birth and then including additional interventions, such as community distribution of misoprostol, in place as a safeguard [36]. While it is encouraging that misoprostol is being used only as a last resort, it is important also that health providers and TBAs receive the message that it is a life saving medication and therefore they should not be overly cautious and avoid using it for fear of repercussions.

This study unveiled several unintended consequences of promoting facility deliveries without major investments in transport or communication systems. While some communities did have access to a maternal waiting home, often women were not able to leave their children at home without care and/or husbands did not see it as appropriate for their wife to be away from the home. Giving birth "on the way" to the facility, with no protection from the elements has also been described in Malawi, where women had to give birth on the roadside often due to a delay to seek assistance from a TBA or SBA at the health facility [37].

Some informants attributed their lack of resources for safe and clean birth as a way the health facility emphasised their role to promote facility births. Almost all TBAs discussed the lack of soap and gloves as having a negative impact to their work and motivation. Some TBAs spoke about using alternatives like used sugar bags or plastic sheets as makeshift gloves or none at all. They were fearful of contracting blood-borne illnesses themselves. Clean birth kits are not available to the TBAs; this includes soap, gloves, plastic sheets, razor blade and a cord clamp or string [38]. Clean birth kits are an affordable intervention and relatively easy to implement; they are used in at least 51 low-income countries with high prevalence of home births [38]. Lack of gloves and soap was seen to be a greater barrier to the work of TBAs than any other, including transportation and lack of financial incentives.

Poverty was the root of discussions around TBA and women's lack resources, and transportation. TBAs do not receive payment for services besides what the community or households may offer informally – food, material or other small gifts. APEs are supported by the national program and receive a monthly subsidy of approximately 20 USD. Despite not receiving a stipend or incentives, the majority of TBAs said that they did not feel resentment towards the APEs for their earnings or expect a salary. However, many were impoverished by the out of pocket transportation costs associated with accompanying women to the health facility. All TBAs in the study said they would appreciate basic resources to assist with their work. Many described the hardship of encouraging facility based births coupled with the reality of the great distances, lack of transportation, lack of money and poor access. These barriers to healthcare are widespread across Mozambique as cited in other studies [6, 7, 39].

This study supports the notion that TBAs can be effective partners in delivering maternal and child health interventions to improve safe delivery until health facility birth is accessible to all women [10, 13]. The results of this study provide insight into the role and daily work of TBAs in Mozambique, with implications for minor modifications to the operations of the national misoprostol program, and implications for maternal health policy more broadly. Recommendations in Table 1 reflect a combination of global best practices and conclusions from this study.

Limitations

Participant recruitment was established through purposive sampling. A mapping of all TBAs in the country has not been conducted and very little reporting takes place due to a number of factors, including illiteracy and the fact that TBAs are not officially part of the formal health sector. Therefore it is very difficult to know details about the number of TBAs and their catchment areas.

The majority of TBAs that participated in the study and were involved in the misoprostol program live relatively near to the health facility. Therefore there is a risk of potential selection bias as TBAs were referred by the health facility or CHWs. Due to time limitations and participant availability we were only able to reach a small sample of women who had previously used misoprostol. The perspectives from TBAs who live further from the health facility are different than those who live relatively closer, especially in terms of access to the health facility and participation in the misoprostol program.

Table 1 Recommendations

Operational recommendations for the misoprostol program:

- Allow TBAs to pick up the medication from the health facility where necessary and appropriate to ensure a stable supply of misoprostol.

- Heighten communication of the Strategy for the Prevention of PPH at the Community Level to TBAs. TBAs and MNCH nurses should feel confident distributing and administering misoprostol to women who will have a home birth as part of the National Strategy.

- Provide clear information to the community via heath facility staff, CHWs and TBAs about misoprostol and how to use it correctly, alongside messages encouraging facility-based birth to dispel fears and myths in the community.

- Consider clean birth kits distributed through ANC, APEs, and/or directly to TBAs. This would alleviate the concerns TBAs have about infections to themselves, women and newborns while reducing neonatal mortality. This study found no concerns that this might undermine facility deliveries.

Recommendations to increase coverage of births attended by SBAs:

- Transportation, while costly, is a necessary investment to ensure women have access to health facilities. Women and TBAs both strongly support facility deliveries, but requested assistance with transport and communication.

As with many qualitative studies, it is difficult to generalise the findings of this study due to the small sample size and varied context.

Conclusion

This paper contributes to the growing body of research supporting the community distribution of misoprostol for PPH prevention in settings where births that take place outside of health facility are still a significant proportion of all deliveries, and provides particular contextual findings for the role of TBAs in two provinces of Mozambique. TBAs play an important role in the distribution of misoprostol, encouraging facility based birth and advocating key messages for safe motherhood. This study adds to the evidence that TBAs are appropriate channels for the distribution of misoprostol for prevention of PPH; they are willing, capable and understand how and when to safely distribute the medication. Many TBAs highly valued their inclusion in the health system, receiving training and being provided with misoprostol.

A consistent supply chain of misoprostol is necessary to ensure the sustainability of the program. TBAs request resources such as birth kits, communication and transport options to heighten their efforts to ensure women can access to the safest birth possible. The MoH should expand their support to TBAs as allies with the health system to improve maternal and child health outcomes.

Abbreviations

ANC: Antenatal care; APE: Agentes polivalentes elementares; CHW: Community health worker; FGD: Focus group discussion; MNCH: Maternal newborn and child health; MoH: Ministry of Health; PPH: Post-partum haemorrhage; SBA: Skilled birth attendant; TBA: Traditional birth attendant

Acknowledgements

The authors would like to sincerely thank all of the Traditional Birth Attendants and women who participated in the study. We would also like to extend our gratitude to the research assistants who worked tirelessly to collect the data. We acknowledge the support of the Ministry of Health and Department of Women and Child Health, especially Dra Elsa Jacinto. Thank you also to the Provincial and District Health Authorities of Nampula and Inhambane Provinces. Finally, a sincere thank you to everyone who helped with the logistics of making this study possible and Jennifer Barrett for her support in Maputo.

Funding

KH is undertaking her PhD at Menzies School of Health Research at Charles Darwin University. This study was part of her PhD thesis. KH was a recipient of a Research Training Program Scholarship from the Australian Government. Funding from this scholarship was used to undertake this research.

Authors' contributions

KH designed the study, coordinated and oversaw data collection, conducted data analysis, and wrote the manuscript. JH contributed to the design of the study, coordinated and oversaw data collection, performed data analysis and provided critical manuscript revision. PW adapted the study design to the local context and contributed to the manuscript. CH, SB and NP provided input into the conception and design of the study and contributed to the manuscript. All authors read and approved the final manuscript.

Competing interests

The authors declare that they have no competing interests.

Author details

[1]Menzies School of Health Research, Charles Darwin University, Darwin, Australia. [2]Department of Emergency Medicine, University Health Network, University of Toronto, Toronto, Canada. [3]Department of Family and Community Medicine, University of Toronto, Toronto, Canada. [4]Centre for Midwifery, Child and Family Health, Faculty of Health, University of Technology Sydney, Sydney, Australia. [5]Honorary Fellow, Menzies School of Health Research, Charles Darwin University, Darwin, Australia. [6]Maternal and Child Health Program, Burnet Institute, Melbourne, Australia. [7]Centre for Midwifery, Child and Family Health, Faculty of Health, University of Technology Sydney, Sydney, Australia. [8]Bixby Center for Population, Health and Sustainability, School of Public Health, University of California, Berkeley, USA.

References

1. WHO, UNICEF, UNFPA, World Bank Group and the United Nations Population Division. Trends in maternal mortality: 1990 to 2015: estimates by WHO, UNICEF, UNFPA, World Bank Group and the United Nations population division. Geneva: WHO; 2015.
2. Ministério da Saúde (MISAU). Health Sector Strategic Plan PESS 2014-2019. Maputo: MISAU; 2014.
3. David E, Machungo F, Zanconato G, Cavaliere E, Fiosse S, Sululu C, Chiluvane B, Bergström S. Maternal near miss and maternal deaths in Mozambique: a cross-sectional, region-wide study of 635 consecutive cases assisted in health facilities of Maputo province. BMC Pregnancy and Childbirth. 2014;14:401.
4. Alkema L, Chou D, Gemmill A, Hogan D, Mathers C, Mills S, Moller AB, Say L, Suzuki E. Trends in maternal mortality: 1990 to 2013. Estimates by WHO, UNICEF, UNFPA, the World Bank and the United Nations population division. Geneva: WHO; 2014.
5. Ministerio da Saude Moçambique (MISAU), Instituto Nacional de Estatística Moçambique (INE) and ICF International. Inquérito de Indicadores de Imunização, Malária e HIV/SIDA em Moçambique 2015. Maputo and Rockville: INS, INE and ICF International; 2016.
6. Schwitters A, Lederer P, Zilversmit L, Gudo PS, Ramiro I, Cumba L, Mahagaja E, Jobarteh K. Barriers to health care in rural Mozambique: a rapid ethnographic assessment of planned Mobile health clinics for ART. Glob Health Sci Pract. 2015;3(1):109–16.
7. Munguambe K, Boene H, Vidler M, Bique C, Sawchuck D, Firoz T, Makanga PT, Qureshi R, Macete E, Menendez C, et al. Barriers and facilitators to health care seeking behaviours in pregnancy in rural communities of southern Mozambique. Reprod Health. 2016;13(Suppl 1):31.
8. UNICEF. The state of the world's children 2009: maternal and newborn health. New York: UNICEF; 2009.
9. World Health Organization. Making pregnancy safer: the critical role of the skilled attendant a joint statement by WHO, ICM and FIGO. Geneva: WHO; 2004.
10. Darmstadt GL, Lee ACC, Cousens S, Sibley L, Bhutta ZA, Donnay F, Osrin D, Bang A, Kumar V, Wall SN, et al. 60 million non-facility births: who can deliver in community settings to reduce intrapartum-related deaths. Int J Gynaecol Obstet. 2009;107(Suppl 1):S89–112.

11. Sibley LM, Sipe TA, Koblinsky M. Does traditional birth attendant training increase use of antenatal care? a review of the evidence. J Midwifery Womens Health. 2004;49(4):298–305.

12. Bergström S, Goodburn E. The role of traditional birth attendants in the reduction of maternal mortality. In: De Brouwere V, Lerberghe V, editors. Safe motherhood strategies: a review of the evidence, studies in health services organization and policy. Volume 17. Antwerp: ITG Press; 2001.

13. Prata N, Passano P, Rowen T, Bell S, Walsh J, Potts M. Where there are (few) skilled birth attendants. J Health Popul Nutr. 2011;29(2):81–91.

14. Gloyd S, Floriano F, Seunda M, Chadreque MA, Nyangezi JM, Platas A. Impact of traditional birth attendant training in Mozambique: a controlled study. J Midwifery Womens Health. 2001;46(4):210–6.

15. Ministerio da Saude Moçambique (MISAU). National Plan for Health Human Resources Development (NPHHRD) 2008-2015. Edited by Institute of Hygiene and Tropical Medicine L, Portugal, The National Health Institute, Human Resource Directorate, School of Medicine in Maputo. Maputo: Ministry of Health National Directorate of Human Resources; 2008.

16. Libombo A, Bique C, da Luz VM, Jamisse L, Reis V, David E, Chavane L, Carbonell A, Modan A, Amade N. Strategy for the prevention of postpartum hemorrhage at the community level. Maputo: Republic of Mozambique Ministry of Health; 2013.

17. Derman RJ, Kodkany BS, Goudar SS, Geller SE, Naik VA, Bellad MB, Patted SS, Patel A, Edlavitch SA, Hartwell T, et al. Oral misoprostol in preventing postpartum haemorrhage in resource-poor communities: a randomised controlled trial. Lancet. 2006;368(9543):1248–53.

18. Walraven G, Blum J, Dampha Y, Sowe M, Morison L, Winikoff B, Sloan N. Misoprostol in the management of the third stage of labour in the home delivery setting in rural Gambia: a randomised controlled trial. Int J Obstet Gynaecol. 2005;112(9):1277–83.

19. Mobeen N, Durocher J, Zuberi N, Jahan N, Blum J, Wasim S, Walraven G, Hatcher J. Administration of misoprostol by trained traditional birth attendants to prevent postpartum haemorrhage in homebirths in Pakistan: a randomised placebo-controlled trial. Int J Obstet Gynaecol. 2011;118(3):353–61.

20. Prata N, Ejembi C, Fraser A, Shittu O, Minkler M. Community mobilization to reduce postpartum hemorrhage in home births in northern Nigeria. Soc Sci Med. 2012;74(8):1288–96.

21. Diadhiou M, Dieng T, Ortiz C, Mall I, Dione D, Sloan NL. Introduction of misoprostol for prevention of postpartum hemorrhage at the community level in Senegal. Int J Obstet Gynaecol. 2011;115(3):251–5.

22. Dao B, Ngabo F, Zoungrana J, Rawlins B, Mukarugwiro B, Musoni P. Increasing access to prevention of postpartum hemorrhage interventions for births in health facilities and at home in four districts of Rwanda. Afr J Reprod Health. 2015;15(4):58–67.

23. Bell S, Passano P, Bohl DD, Islam A, Prata N. Training traditional birth attendants on the use of misoprostol and a blood measurement tool to prevent postpartum haemorrhage: lessons learnt from Bangladesh. J Health Popul Nutr. 2014;32(1):118–29.

24. Vallely L, Homiehombo P, Walep E, Moses M, Tom M, Kelly-Hanku A, Andrew V, Nataraye E, Ninnes C, Mola GD, et al. Feasibility and acceptability of clean birth kits containing misoprostol for self-administration to prevent postpartum hemorrhage in rural Papua New Guinea. Int J Gynaecol Obstet. 2016;133(3):301-6. doi.org/10.1016/j.ijgo.2015.10.018.

25. Hobday K, Hulme J, Belton S, Homer CSE, Prata N. Community-based misoprostol fo the prevention of post-partum haemorrhage: a narrative review of the evidence base, challenges and scale-up. Glob Public Health. 2018;13(8):1081-97. https://doi.org/10.1080/17441692.2017.1303743.

26. Bique C, Prata N, Holston M, Moran M, Weinrib R. Community-based prevention of postpartum hemorrhage with misoprostol in Mozambique: final report. Maputo: Venture Strategies Innovations; 2011.

27. Chilundo B, Cliff J, Mariano A, Rodriguez D, George A. Relaunch of the official community health worker programme in Mozambique: is there a sustainable basis for iCCM policy. Health Policy Plan. 2015;30:ii54–64.

28. Mc William CL. Phenomonology. In: Bourgeault I, Dingwall R, de Vries R, editors. The SAGE handbook of qualitative methods in health research edn. London: SAGE; 2010. p. 229–48.

29. Ezzy D. Qualitative analysis: practice and innovation. London: Routledge; 2002.

30. Pope C, Ziebland S, Mays N. Qualitative research in health care: analysing qualitative data. Br Med J. 2000;320(7227):114–6.

31. Orobaton N, Abdulazeez J, Abegunde D, Shoretire K, Maishanu A, Ikoro N, Fapohunda B, Balami W, Beal K, Ganiyu A, et al. Implementing at-scale, community-based distribution of misoprostol tablets to mothers in the third stage of labor for the prevention of postpartum haemorrhage in Sokoto state, Nigeria: early results and lessons learned. PLoS One. 2017; 12(2):e0170739.

32. Ejembi CL, Norick P, Starrs A, Thapa K. New global guidance supports community and lay health workers in postpartum hemorrhage prevention. Int J Gynaecol Obstet. 2013;122(3):187–9.

33. Mir AM, Wajid A, Gull S. Helping rural women in Pakistan to prevent postpartum hemorrhage: a quasi experimental study. BMC Pregnancy Childbirth. 2012;12:120.

34. Geller SE, Adams MG, Kelly PJ, Kodkany BS, Derman RJ. Postpartum hemorrhage in resource-poor settings. Int J Gynaecol Obstet. 2006;92(3):202–11.

35. Byrne A, Morgan A. How the integration of traditional birth attendants with formal health systems can increase skilled birth attendance. Int J Gynecol Obstet. 2011;115(2):127–34.

36. Raams TM, Browne JL, Festen-Schrier VJMM, Klipstein-Grobusch K, Rijken MJ. Task shifting in active management of the third stage of labor: a systematic review. BMC Pregnancy Childbirth. 2018;18(1):47.

37. Kumbani L, Bjune G, Chirwa E, Malata A, Odland JØ. Why some women fail to give birth at health facilities: a qualitative study of women's perceptions of perinatal care from rural southern Malawi. Reprod Health. 2013;10:9–9.

38. Healthy Newborn Network. Clean birth kits - potential to deliver? Evidence, experience, estimated lives saved and cost. 2010. Available from: https://www.healthynewbornnetwork.org/resource/clean-birth-kits-potential-to-deliver-evidence-experience-estimated-lives-saved-and-cost/.

39. Firoz T, Vidler M, Makanga PT, Boene H, Chiaú R, Sevene E, Magee LA, von Dadelszen P, Munguambe K, the CLIP Working Group. Community perspectives on the determinants of maternal health in rural southern Mozambique: a qualitative study. Reprod Health. 2016;13(Suppl 2):112.

13

Healthcare provider-patient communication: a qualitative study of women's perceptions during childbirth

Precious Madula[1,2]* (iD), Fatch Welcome Kalembo[2], Hong Yu[1] and Atipatsa Chiwanda Kaminga[2]

Abstract

Background: There is limited information on the impact of effective healthcare provider-patient communication on facility-based delivery in Malawi. The purpose of this study was to examine the nature of communication in the maternity ward, identify facilitators and barriers to healthcare provider-patient communication, and understand how they affect maternal healthcare.

Methods: This was a descriptive study that used qualitative data collection and analysis methods. Data were collected through face-to-face in-depth interviews using a semi-structured interview guide to collect information about women's perceptions of their communication with healthcare providers. A total of 30 in-depth interviews were conducted with women admitted for delivery in six health facilities drawn from three administrative regions in Malawi. The information collected focused on the communication that pregnant women had with healthcare providers, their perception of that communication, and the barriers to effective communication. A thematic approach was used for data analysis.

Results: The main themes that emerged regarding the nature of communication between healthcare providers and patients were: 1) good healthcare provider-patient interaction; 2) verbal abuse and lack of respect; 3) failure by healthcare providers to answer or entertain questions; 4) linguistic barriers to communication and lack of competency in non-verbal communication; and 5) discrimination due to one's status.

Conclusion: This study has revealed the existence of some communication barriers such as disrespecting and verbally abusing pregnant women, language limitations by some healthcare providers and discrimination due to one's status which are affecting maternal service delivery in some health facilities in Malawi. The study has also shown that pregnant women who are happy with the way healthcare providers communicate with them have the motivation to deliver at a health facility. There is a need, therefore, to develop an intervention that could help healthcare providers to communicate better with their patients.

Keywords: Maternal mortality, Communication, Pregnant women, Traditional birth attendants, Skilled birth attendant, Health facility

* Correspondence: preciousmadula@yahoo.co.uk
[1]School of Journalism and Information Communication, Huazhong University of Science and Technology, 1037 Luoyu, Road, Wuhan 430074, People's Republic of China
[2]Mzuzu University, Private Bag 201, Luwinga, Mzuzu 2, Malawi

Plain English summary

Effective healthcare provider-patient communication is a key element in optimal maternal service delivery. In order to build a good relationship, there is a need for healthcare providers and patients to communicate effectively. When there is positive communication between healthcare providers and women in the maternity ward, women are encouraged to utilise maternal services at a health facility. On the other hand, poor patient-healthcare provider communication results in some pregnant women deciding not to deliver at a health facility with skilled attendance in favour of delivery with a traditional birth attendant (TBA) or delivery at home, which might lead to pregnancy complications and maternal mortality. It has been reported that some healthcare providers in Malawi communicate poorly with their patients. We, therefore, conducted this study in order to examine the nature of communication in the maternity ward between healthcare providers and their patients. The study has revealed that some healthcare providers communicate poorly with pregnant women in the maternity ward. There is, therefore, a need to develop an intervention which could help healthcare providers to improve their communication to better serve women in the maternity ward.

Background

In order to build a positive relationship between healthcare providers and patients, there is a need for the existence of effective healthcare provider-patient communication. This will help to ensure that all parties involved are able to listen to each other and fully understand what is being said [1]. Effective healthcare provider-patient communication can be facilitated by healthcare provider behaviours such as establishing a positive rapport by avoiding shouting and rudeness, encouraging two-way dialogue, bridging any social gaps between healthcare providers and patients, effectively using both verbal and non-verbal communication, allowing patients ample time to tell their sickness story and exhibiting positive attitudes when talking to patients [2]. Lack of effective communication between healthcare providers and patients can result in negative health outcomes. For instance, a study in rural Zimbabwe showed that rudeness, unfriendly and abusive behaviour by nurses discouraged pregnant women from accessing maternal services at a healthy facility, a major contributor to maternal mortality and pregnancy complications [3].

Healthcare provider-patient communication is a fundamental component in effective maternal service delivery [4]. Alongside expertise, effective healthcare provider-patient communication is a prerequisite to building a therapeutic healthcare provider-patient relationship [5, 6]. Thus, a good relationship between health workers and pregnant women remains an important precursor in encouraging pregnant women to utilise maternal services at

a health facility [7]. Furthermore, "where effective communication prevails between patients and healthcare providers, immediate outcomes include patient satisfaction and information recall; intermediate variables include adherence to recommendations; and long-term outcomes include changes in health status or lifestyle" [8].

Empirical data indicate that in health care settings, effective interactions between healthcare providers and patients are essential for a shared understanding of the feelings and symptoms experienced by patients as well as the goals of the provider [9]. Effective communication is particularly important in the provision of maternal services because labour and birth are vulnerable and stressful times where lapses in communication can result in health complications, failure to access health facilities for maternal services and, in worst case scenarios, maternal mortality [10, 11].

In Malawi, a number of studies have reported about poor communication between some healthcare providers and pregnant women [4, 7, 12]. Poor communication may be one of the contributing factors to maternal deaths and complications that are experienced in Malawi. According to a World Health Organisation (WHO) (2016) report, approximately 830 women die every day from preventable causes related to pregnancy and childbirth around the world [10]. Ninety-nine per cent of all maternal deaths occur in low and middle-income countries, and maternal mortality is higher (546 deaths per 100,000 livebirths) in women living in rural areas and among the poor - 511 deaths per 100,000 livebirths in urban areas and 652 deaths per 100,000 livebirths in rural areas [10]. Malawi is a low-income country where the maternal mortality rate is estimated at 439 deaths per 100, 000 births [13] and the neonatal mortality rate is 31 per 1000 live births with skilled attendance [4].The current maternal mortality rate is very high compared to the target of Sustainable Development Goal number 3 which aims to reduce the global maternal mortality ratio to less than 70 per 100,000 live births by 2030 [http://www.who.int/en/news-room/fact-sheets/detail/maternal-mortality].

WHO [http://www.who.int/en/news-room/fact-sheets/detail/maternal-mortality], asserts that in Sub-Saharan Africa and South Asia, women in rural areas do not receive adequate health care due to the low number of skilled health workers and that lack of information is one of the factors that prevent women from receiving or seeking care during pregnancy and childbirth. Better healthcare provider-patient communication could mitigate some pregnancy-related problems and complications.

Reduction of maternal mortality is a global health priority, and one way to combat maternal and pregnancy complications is by encouraging pregnant women to use maternal health services. Research that was conducted in Chikhwawa and Mangochi in southern Malawi, indicates that women are dissuaded from utilising maternal services offered by skilled healthcare providers because of rudeness, insults and disrespect by some health personnel [14, 15]. This clearly demonstrates that despite the existing policy of the Malawi Government encouraging all women to deliver in health facilities where they can be cared for by skilled attendants, not all pregnant women do. Poor attitudes and behaviours by health workers are one of the documented reasons why some women may not choose to deliver at a health facility [4]. There is a need for healthcare providers to ensure that they conduct themselves in a manner that will motivate women to utilise professional maternal health services [16]. Good communication with pregnant women could be one of the ways of persuading them to deliver at a health facility in line with the government policy. The objective of this study was therefore, to explore the nature of communication between healthcare providers and pregnant women in some hospitals in Malawi with the view to establishing whether communication is one of the reasons behind women's choice to deliver at a health facility or not.

Methods

Setting

Malawi is an African country located in Southern Africa. It is a member state of Southern African Development Community (SADC). It is bordered by Tanzania on the northern and eastern sides, Mozambique on the eastern, southern and south-western sides and Zambia on the western side. The World Bank estimated that the population of Malawi in 2016 was 18.2 million [17]. The country is divided into three administrative regions, namely Northern, Central, and Southern Regions. These regions exhibit great diversity in socio-economic, cultural, and geographical features. Each region has a city; Lilongwe in the Central Region, Blantyre in the Southern Region, and Mzuzu in the Northern Region. The population of Lilongwe is estimated at 1.2 million people. Blantyre has about 1 million people whereas Mzuzu is estimated to have a population of approximately about 300, 000 people [18, 19].

Healthcare in Malawi is primarily delivered by two sectors; the government run public sector, and the private sector, which includes the Christian Health Association of Malawi (CHAM) and other private providers [20]. The Government provides 60%, the CHAM 37%, and the other private providers the remaining 3% [20] http://www.cham.org.mw. Healthcare facilities in the country are organised into three tiers: primary, secondary, and tertiary [21]. The levels are linked through a referral system [21]. At the primary level, healthcare is provided through community-based outreach programmes, dispensaries, health posts, healthcare centres and community hospitals. The primary level facilities refer obstetric emergencies and patients requiring in-patient medical, surgical or paediatric care to secondary level facilities. Secondary level care is provided through district hospitals (for the public sector) and CHAM hospitals (for the private sector). Patients who require special care from the secondary level facilities are referred to tertiary level facilities [21]. The tertiary healthcare service is provided by four central hospitals with two in the Southern Region (Queen Elizabeth and Zomba Central Hospitals), one in the Centre (Kamuzu Central Hospital) and another in the Northern Region (Mzuzu Central Hospital) [20]. The tertiary hospital in each region caters for all primary and secondary level facilities for that particular region. Each of the three tertiary public hospitals included in this study, provides specialist referral services including obstetrics and gynaecology for their respective regions.

Data were collected from three tertiary hospitals and three private hospitals located in the three administrative regions of the country. One tertiary hospital and one private hospital were identified as research sites in each region. Although the three private hospitals are not as big as the government tertiary hospitals, they provide specialised obstetric and gynaecological care but for a fee.

Study design, and study participants

The study was a descriptive qualitative study that used a semi-structured interview guide. The qualitative research design was chosen because it was important to hear the views and experiences of pregnant women and those who had just given birth in their own words on what they feel about patient-healthcare provider communication that they had experienced in the maternity ward. We collected data through interviews with women admitted to six tertiary hospitals (three government and three CHAM hospitals also referred to as public and private health facilities respectively) drawn from three administrative regions of Malawi (Northern, Central and Southern). We conducted 30 interviews across the three regions of Malawi, with five interviews conducted per hospital. Data collection started in the Southern Region, then Central Region before winding up in the Northern Region. Saturation was reached within the first 19 interviews, but we still completed the remaining 11 interviews in order to obtain sample heterogeneity [22]. Participants were heterogenous because they were recruited from hospitals and regions that exhibit great diversity in cultural, geographical, historical, political, and religious background. Saturation level of data was considered to have been reached if there was no new information arising from the interviews [16].

The six hospitals were selected as research sites for the following reasons: 1) to obtain a deep understanding of women's perception of their communication with healthcare providers in the maternity ward given the fact that women who are admitted to these hospitals tend to have complications with their pregnancies and are likely to be engaged in deep and long conversation with healthcare providers; 2) to achieve a good representation of participants from all the three administrative regions of the country that could help to provide a deep understanding of women's perception of healthcare provider-patient communication in the maternity wards in Malawi; and 3) to compare the perception of women regarding their communication with healthcare providers between public and private healthcare systems in Malawi. Participants were recruited in the study if they were 18 years or older (the legal age to provide consent to participate in a study in Malawi); were admitted to maternity ward at the participating hospital; had given birth at the participating hospital within 5 days of the interview, regardless of their mode of delivery; and if they were able to give consent.

Data collection procedure

Following approval from the management of the hospitals, the principal researcher approached midwives working in the maternity ward to start the recruitment process. We anticipated that many women would be willing to participate in the study. However, we only needed a limited number of participants per hospital. As such, we used systematic random sampling using admission numbers to recruit study participants. Normally women admitted to the maternity ward in Malawi are given admission numbers. The first person to be admitted is assigned one, and the last person is assigned the last number according to the number of people admitted to the ward on that particular day. We recruited five women with the first five odd admission numbers per hospital. The principal researcher conducted all the interviews while the women were still admitted to the health facility. The interviews were conducted in a separate room where nobody could hear the conversation between the researcher and the participant. In addition, all interviews were conducted after working hours (after 4.30 p.m) when the women were not being seen by doctors or midwives. On average, each interview took 30–50 min to be completed. The interviews were conducted in the Malawian local language (Chichewa). During the interviews, follow-up questions using probes were asked in order to acquire deeper understanding when an explanation provided by the interviewee was unclear or ambiguous. Data were collected between February and March, 2017.

Study instrument

An interview guide was developed in Chichewa through review of literature. The guide was piloted with five maternity patients at a hospital which did not participate in the main study. The interview guide had questions that focussed on: (a) patients' communication with healthcare providers; (b) the perception of patients on their communication with their healthcare providers; and (c) barriers to effective communication between patients and healthcare providers. The principal researcher (a doctoral student) interviewed all the participants and where necessary, he asked further probing questions in line with the participants' answers in order to gain more clarity on the issue and obtain as much information as possible. All interviews were digitally recorded and transcribed verbatim.

Data analysis

A thematic analysis of the interviews was conducted to generate an understanding of how women in the maternity ward perceived their communication with healthcare providers. This was done in accordance with Braun and Clarke's [23] six steps of thematic analysis. The six steps include: 1) familiarisation with data; 2) initial coding; 3) searching for themes; 4) reviewing themes; 5) defining and naming themes; and 6) writing up the research report. Prior to data analysis, the recorded interviews were transcribed by the research team in Chichewa before being translated into English. The principal researcher verified the transcriptions by reading them while listening to the recordings and any identified errors were corrected. To ensure that no original meaning was lost in the translation process, an expert translator was involved in order to check both the recordings and transcripts. Inductive thematic analysis was employed in this study since the analysis was based on what the participants reported during the interviews. The principal researcher developed a list of codes from the transcript which were discussed with members of the research team. The research team had several meetings during which they discussed and verified if the codes were coming from the transcription. Thereafter, the research team identified extracts and themes captured by the codes.

Ethical consideration

Ethical approval for the study was granted by the National Commission for Science and Technology (Protocol PO1/17/153). A written permission to conduct the study at each of the six health facilities was also obtained from the Hospital Directors and officers responsible for research activities at each institution. All participants were informed about the purpose of the study and only participated after providing informed consent. Literate participants signed consent forms while a thumbprint was used for those who were illiterate. Since participation was voluntary, participants were free to withdraw from the study at any time without facing any penalties. All participants were assured that anonymity would be observed at all times.

Results

Demographic characteristics

Thirty in-depth interviews were conducted. The majority of participants were married ($n = 25$) and over half ($n = 16$) of participants had received secondary education or higher. There were five participants from each health facility. Table 1 provides the demographic characteristics of the participants.

Identified themes

The following themes were identified through thematic analysis: good healthcare provider-patient interaction, verbal abuse and lack of respect by healthcare providers, failure by healthcare providers to answer questions or entertain questions from clients, linguistic barriers to communication and lack of competency in non-verbal communication, attitudes of some healthcare providers, and discrimination due to one's status. The results of the study indicate that generally some women admitted to the maternity wards in both public and private hospitals had good communication with healthcare workers. The study also shows that verbal abuse and lack of respect by

Table 1 Demographic characteristics of the participants ($N = 30$)

Variable Name	Total number of participants	Percentage of participants
Name of health facility		
Public hospital in Central Region	5	16.7
Public hospital in Southern Region	5	16.7
Public hospital in Northern Region	5	16.7
Private hospital in Southern Region	5	16.7
Private hospital in Central Region	5	16.7
Private hospital in Northern Region	5	16.7
Age range		
18–25	14	47
26–40	16	53
Marital Status		
Single	4	13.3
Married	25	83.3
Widowed	1	3.3
Educational Qualification		
No formal education	8	26.7
Primary education	6	20
Secondary education	12	40
Tertiary education	4	13.3

healthcare providers were frequently reported by the participants recruited from both types of health facilities.

Good healthcare provider-patient interaction

Half of the participants, from both public and private health facilities, indicated that healthcare providers were very good and treated them with warmth, sympathy and respect. They even indicated that they were very happy and impressed with the way healthcare providers were communicating with them. One participant in a post-natal ward had this to say:

"I have been at this hospital for two weeks now. I came here well in advance to wait for my labour. I delivered three days ago. My child has a minor complication, and that's why I am still here. Honestly, the nurses and midwives I have been dealing with here are very friendly, loving and talk to me in a good manner. Before coming here, I was told that some nurses are rude and that they shout at patients but for me all has been well, and I have been well taken care of. I am very satisfied with the relationship I am having with the nurses here. This is my first pregnancy, but next time I fall pregnant again, I will certainly come back and deliver here" (A woman who recently delivered at a public hospital)

From the above discourse, it can clearly be seen that the participant was absolutely happy with her experience at the health facility not just because of the medical care she was given, but also because of the way the nurses and midwives interacted with and treated her. Surprisingly, some participants from private health facilities complained that their communication with healthcare providers was not good. From the outset, the lead researcher's experience was that participants in private health facilities, where fees are paid for treatment, would have mostly positive perceptions of their communication with healthcare providers. However, this was not the case. Some participants in both public and private health facilities indicated that their communication with healthcare providers was poor.

Verbal abuse and lack of respect

About half of the participants from both government and private health facilities said that some midwives and nurses abused them verbally. They indicated that this abuse was generally in the form of scolding and shouting at them. None of the participants however, did not explain why they were abused. The majority of the participants who complained about verbal abuse and lack of respect were from public health facilities. Only a few participants from private health facilities described the abuse, but their complaints showed a serious degree of verbal abuse and lack of respect. One participant in a labour ward at a private health facility had this to say:

"Midwives and nurses shout at us and talk to us in a rude manner. At times they talk to us in a mocking manner and use words as if we are children. And when we fail to follow instructions, they shout at us instead of just talking to us in a normal way or correcting the mistake that we have made. I really don't like such nurses, and it makes me wonder whether I do come at this hospital just to be ridiculed. One day I experienced a nasty thing. There was a pregnant woman who was in labour. She called the midwife on duty for help. Sadly, instead of the midwife coming to help she just yelled at her. My friend and I had to go and help her deliver. By the grace of God, she managed to deliver a bouncing baby boy. But I don't feel happy here. What is happening here is not good. Being a private hospital, we pay a lot of money and expect good services. Sadly we are being given a raw deal. Next time I will never come here again" (A woman waiting to deliver at a private hospital)

It is apparent that the patient was very frustrated with the services offered, no wonder she expressed the above sentiments.

More than half of the participants from both the public and private health facilities indicated that some healthcare providers were rude, disrespectful and acted towards them and indeed talked to them as if they were children. One participant in a labour ward said this:

"Sometimes when they are talking to us, some nurses talk as if they are talking to kids. Whenever they give us some instruction, and we fail to act accordingly, they talk to us in a rude manner, using demeaning and derogatory words. They also look at us as if we are stupid and don't deserve their time. Their tone of talking does not even show respect, and it clearly shows that they don't care about us nor do they have respect for us. This is bad because we expect them to show a caring heart and correct us in a good manner when we make mistakes". (A woman waiting to deliver at a private hospital)

Failure by midwives and nurses to answer some questions or entertain more questions from pregnant women

The majority of the participants in both public and private health facilities indicated that generally the nurses and midwives did not give them a chance or enough time to ask some questions about subjects or issues they do not understand concerning their pregnancy. When asked why they thought healthcare providers behaved in this way, the majority of the respondents said they suspected the healthcare providers feared the workload of being bombarded by inquisitive patients if they were generous in entertaining questions. One respondent at a public health facility said the following:

"Nurses do not help us when we want extra information on what they normally give us. Whenever we try to ask questions, the nurse just looks away and does not even attend to us. Sometimes the nurse pretends as if she or he did not hear our questions. So yea, it's pretty frustrating to fail to get crucial information from the experts who are supposed to attend to us and meet all our needs" (A woman waiting to deliver at a public hospital).

Linguistic barriers to communication and lack of competency in non-verbal communication

Our analysis also revealed that language is another barrier to effective communication between some healthcare providers and pregnant women in Malawi. This is particularly true in multilingual health facilities where healthcare providers and patients speak different languages. For instance, some participants at a public health facility in Mzuzu in the Northern Region of Malawi, indicated that they would have been more comfortable if most of the healthcare providers were proficient in the region's lingua franca (Chitumbuka) even though they accepted that most of the healthcare providers communicated with them in a positive and polite manner. One participant in a post-natal ward made the following statement:

"The nurses at this hospital are good and talk to us in a polite manner. I only have problems with nurses who do not speak Chitumbuka because we can't communicate effectively since my Chichewa is very bad, and I can't speak English either" (A woman who recently delivered at a public hospital).

Furthermore, the study has also revealed the problems that healthcare providers face when dealing with pregnant women who can only communicate using sign language. In this study, one of the respondents in a post-natal ward at a public health facility had speech-impairment but could hear and write. She noted that most of the healthcare providers treated her in a polite, friendly and caring manner. She also indicated that sometimes she uses her relative to translate sign language if she cannot write her responses for the healthcare providers. However, she bemoaned lack of sign language expertise by healthcare providers. She described the following:

"Generally, I can't say that healthcare providers mistreat me nor talk to me in an impolite or unfriendly manner. They have all been good. But my biggest concern is that all the nurses I have been interacting with do not possess any knowledge of the sign language which I use, so if I can't have a chance to write down what I want to say I don't think I can manage to communicate with them. How I wish hospitals had experts in sign language who could attend to us!" (A woman who recently delivered at a public hospital)

Discrimination due to one's status

A few participants from the public health facilities said that some healthcare providers discriminate against patients who are poor or come from rural areas. Participants from the private health facilities did not indicate that healthcare providers were discriminatory. That was not surprising because there were fewer poor patients in facilities where patients pay in order to access health services. Those participants who talked about discrimination indicated that some healthcare providers changed the way they communicated depending on the person they were talking to. They said that healthcare providers sometimes shouted and used demeaning words when addressing poor patients and chose a more respectful way of communicating when talking to patients from urban areas. A participant who came from a rural area shared the following:

"The nurses here discriminate against us and have a negative attitude towards us poor people. Every time they want to talk to us, they shout and use threats like... "If you continue behaving the way you are I will not help you. You are not the only one, I deal with many people here. Do you think I have time to waste with you?" On the contrary, they do not do the same when they are talking to pregnant women from urban areas" (A woman waiting to deliver at a government hospital).

The theme of discrimination due to one's status also dominated the interviews with illiterate women in the public hospitals. There were no illiterate participants from the private health facilities, so the theme did not emerge there. Some participants in the public health facilities felt that they were failing to understand simple instructions or very basic information because of their illiteracy and that the healthcare providers were discriminating against them by not recognising the need to help them understand. This could explain why some healthcare providers were not willing to entertain questions from some patients if they were not recognising whether

patients had not understood instructions or information. One participant had this to say:

"I did not go to school, so sometimes I don't understand what the nurses are saying. It is even worse when the nurse mixes English and Chichewa in her discourse. Now the frustrating thing is that when I want to ask for clarification, I am shouted at and at times stopped or denied any opportunity to ask questions. This is why in my first pregnancy I decided to deliver at a TBA because there she never shouted at me. She was more caring than the nurses here who take advantage of our illiteracy" (A woman who recently delivered at a public hospital).

Discussion

This study has explored factors that can both facilitate and inhibit effective communication between healthcare providers and women in the maternity ward. The factor that is facilitating communication between healthcare providers and patients is good interaction which entails providers treating patients with warmth, sympathy and respect. On the other hand, factors that inhibit healthcare provider-patient communication include healthcare provider's verbal abuse of women, failure by healthcare providers to take questions from maternity patients, linguistic barriers and poor quality of non-verbal communication, and discrimination due to one's status. Furthermore, the study has also revealed that both private and public hospitals in Malawi have some healthcare providers who communicate poorly with their patients.

The study identified healthcare providers' good attitude and behaviour by some healthcare providers in both private and public health facilities as one of the effective facilitators in the provider-patient communication. This study has shown that women who experienced good communication at a health facility appreciated the maternal services and were satisfied. They were even committed to returning to the same hospital facility for their next delivery. Interestingly, some respondents at a private health facility indicated that some healthcare providers had a bad attitude and communicated to them poorly. This was a surprising finding because one might expect a better quality of service in private hospitals where patients pay a fee to access healthcare services. Those participants described their lack of desire to utilise that health facility again in future. This finding is similar to previous research that indicates that good provider-patient communication is the bedrock for patient satisfaction [24–26]. The more a patient is satisfied, the more likely she will utilise maternal services, follow instructions and adhere to all treatment regimens [27].

Another finding in this study is that many healthcare providers in public health facilities and some in private health facilities disrespect patients by talking to them rudely and shouting at them. This finding is consistent with other studies in Malawi which found that some health workers are impolite, rude, and shout at patients, which consequently dissuades pregnant women from delivering at health facilities where they can be helped by a skilled birth attendant [4, 7, 14, 28–30].

In addition, this study also supports the finding of Mtotha [12] which showed that some healthcare providers are negligent in their duty of care and instead of providing support they shout at women in labour. In the current study, no participant from public health facilities complained about being neglected by healthcare providers. On the contrary, it was reported that at one private hospital a skilled health worker did not assist and shouted at a patient who was about to give birth. Such behaviour is unacceptable, could have resulted in serious complications and will likely discourage women from seeking maternal services at health facilities [7, 28–30]. Previous research has shown that delivery with the assistance of professional health providers can shorten the length of labour, lower rates of intervention such as caesarean section and instrumental deliveries, lower levels of reported pain and increase maternal satisfaction [31–34].

This study also established that some healthcare providers discriminate against patients due to social status and place of residence. Discrimination was only mentioned by pregnant women in public health facilities. This discrimination is counterproductive and is likely to discourage patients from rural areas from accessing maternal service at a health facility. Even though all participants in this study appreciated the need for a pregnant woman to access maternal service at a health facility, some participants said that they would consider seeking help from a TBA if they knew that a healthcare provider would not treat them with respect and dignity. This finding is consistent with the findings from a study that was conducted in Nigeria that indicated that discrimination due to one's ethnicity, literacy level and place of residence was contributing to the low proportion of births supervised by skilled birth attendants [35–37]. To change the current status, there is an urgent need to remove any form of discrimination by healthcare providers so that they are able to effectively communicate with their patients. Frequent supportive supervision of healthcare providers and provision of refresher courses on communication skills can also greatly help to improve healthcare provider-patient communication.

Discrimination due to one's status was also observed in the way healthcare providers communicate with illiterate patients in public health facilities. No participant from the private health facilities was illiterate in our sample. Some participants reported that they sometimes fail to grasp information from the healthcare providers due to illiteracy. Unfortunately, they said that when they tried to ask questions to better understand what was being communicated to them, some healthcare providers did not give them the opportunity to ask questions or seek clarification. This widens the information gap. It is important for healthcare providers to exercise empathy and provide information to all patients regardless of their education levels. This finding is in agreement with another study that was conducted in Mangochi, Malawi which revealed that the education gap between healthcare providers and patients was one of the barriers in accessing maternal services [7]. To address this, healthcare providers should strive to increase patients' understanding of their own health needs because there is a direct correlation between understanding and compliance. Training on how providers ought to communicate with patients could help to address this problem [38, 39]. In addition, it is the responsibility of the healthcare providers to offer patients clear and concise means to understand health information regardless of patients' education levels. Thus, communication by healthcare providers has to be designed for the average or illiterate person to understand and must be put in simple language [38].

Finally, this study has revealed that language is another barrier that is inhibiting patient- provider communication. This resonates with the findings of a study that was conducted in Canada which showed that a failure to address language barriers can result in misunderstandings, problems with informed consent, inadequate comprehension of diagnoses and treatment, dissatisfaction with care, preventable morbidity and mortality, disparities in prescriptions, test ordering and diagnostic evaluations [9]. Language barriers can inhibit a healthcare provider's ability to elicit patient symptoms, often resulting in increased use of diagnostic resources or invasive procedures, inappropriate treatment and diagnostic errors. Other studies [40–43] have also found that linguistic barriers were one of the problems affecting provider-patient communication. This barrier may be challenging to overcome due to current policies in Malawi where civil servants and other personnel are posted to any part of the country without consideration of their ability to speak the dominant languages of those areas. Kamwendo [40] has argued that posting staff according to the languages that they speak would in some cases mean that civil servants work in their home district or region, which could exacerbate regionalism and ethnic loyalties at the expense of national cohesion. Where a healthcare provider does not speak the same language as a patient, an interpreter should be employed to bridge the communication gap [40, 42, 43, 44].

The findings of this study should be interpreted with some limitations in mind. Since the interviews were conducted in Chichewa and then translated into English, the translations might have lost the original meaning in the translated language. To minimize this problem, an expert translator was involved to check both the recordings and transcripts to ensure that no original meaning was lost. Another potential limitation is the small sample of participants only attending urban hospitals which means the study is unlikely to be representative of all health facilities in Malawi. Another limitation is that there was no triangulation in this study. This study only focused on patients. Comparing information from patients and healthcare providers in order to fully understand all facets of this complex situation would have strengthened the findings. There is, therefore, a need to conduct another study that will include data from both patients and healthcare providers.

Conclusions

This study has identified some of the challenges affecting interpersonal communication between healthcare providers and pregnant women in the maternity ward in both public and private health facilities in Malawi. The study has underscored the importance of effective patient-provider communication in the provision of maternal healthcare. It is, therefore, important for the healthcare providers to ensure that they are effectively communicating with pregnant women. In all the health facilities, both public and private, healthcare providers need to have good communication skills in order to encourage as many pregnant women as possible to seek maternal services at a health facility with a skilled attendant. This is particularly critical in line with Sustainable Development Goals and WHO efforts to reduce mortality rate in low and middle-income countries. In view of the study findings, it is necessary to develop an intervention to help healthcare providers to improve their communication with patients. This intervention could entail provision of in-service training or refresher courses on communication skills to healthcare providers in order to change their behaviour towards patients. Finally, since this study only focused on urban areas and patients, there is need to conduct a large scale research study involving health facilities based in rural areas that includes healthcare providers' perceptions in order to comprehensively explore the nature of healthcare provider-patient communication in Malawi.

Abbreviations

CHAM: Christian Health Association of Malawi; NSO: National Statistical Office; TBA: Traditional birth attendant; UNSG: United Nations Sustainable Goals; WHO: World Health Organisation

Acknowledgements

The authors are greatly grateful and indebted to all participants in the study for giving their time and information during the interviews. The authors also give special thanks to all Hospital Directors and staff from the research sites for their support during data collection.

Authors' contributions

PM conceptualized the study, collected, analysed data and drafted the manuscript. HY is the Principal supervisor of the study who together with FWK and ACK critically reviewed drafts, edited and provided important intellectual content. All authors read and approved the final manuscript.

Competing interests

The authors declare that they have no competing interests.

References

1. Improving Interpersonal communication between healthcare providers and patients. Bethseda, MD: Quality Assurance Project. 1997.
2. The Joint Commission. Advancing communication, cultural competence, and patient-and family-centred care: A roadmap for hospitals. 2010. Retrieved from: http://www.jointcommission.org/assets/1/6/ARoadmapforHospitalsfinal version727.pdf. Accessed 15 Oct 2016.
3. Mathole T, Lindmark G, Majoko F, Ahlberg BM. A qualitative study of women's perspectives of antenatal care in rural area of Zimbabwe. Midwifery. 2004;20:122–32.
4. Kumbani L, Bjune G, Chirwa E, Malata A, Odland J. Why some women fail to give birth at health facilities: a qualitative study of women's perceptions of perinatal care from rural southern Malawi. Reprod Health. 2013;10:9.
5. Stewart MA. Effective physician-patient communication and health outcomes: a review. Canad Med Assoc J. 1995;152(9):1423–33.
6. Ruben BD. Communication theory and health communication practice: the more things change, the more they stay the same. Health Comm. 2016;31:1–11.
7. Seljeskog L, Sundby J, Chimango J. Factors influencing women's choice of place of delivery in rural Malawi: an explorative study. Afr J Reprod Health. 2006;10(3):66–75.
8. Harrington J, Noble LM, Newman SP. Improving patients' communication with doctors: a systematic review of intervention studies. Pat Edu Counsel. 2004;52:7–16.
9. Higginbottom GMA, Hadziabdic E, Yohani S, Paton P. Immigrant women's experiences of maternity services in Canada: a meta-ethnography midwifery. Midwifery. 2014;30(5):544–59.
10. Binder P, Borne Y, Johnsdotter S, Essen B. Shared language is essential: communication in a multi-ethnic obstetric care setting. J Health Commun. 2012;17:1171–86.
11. Degni F, Suominen S, Essen B, El Ansar W, Vehvilainen-Julkunen K. Communication and cultural issues in providing reproductive healthcare to immigrant women: healthcare providers' experiences in meeting the needs of [corrected] Somali women living in Finland. J Mino Health. 2012;14:330–43.
12. Mtotha DM. An exploratory study of government health policy with special reference to maternal mortality in Malawi. PhD Thesis, University of AZTECA (2013).
13. National Statistical Office Malawi and ICF. Malawi Demographic and Health Survey 2015-2016. Zomba, Malawi, and Rockville, Maryland, USA National Statistical Office and ICF 2017.
14. Kambala C, Morse T, Masangwi S, Mitunda P. Barriers to maternal health service use in Chikhwawa. Southern Malawi Mal Med J. 2011;23(1):1–5.
15. O'Donnell E, Utz B, Khonje D, van den Broek N. 'At the right time, in the right way, with the right resources': Perceptions of the quality of care provided during childbirth in Malawi. BMC Preg Childbir. 2014;14:248.

16. Tuckett A. Qualitative research sampling-the very real complexities. Nurse Res. 2004;12(1):47–61.

17. The World Bank. (2016). Malawi. Retrieved from https://www.google.com.au/search?q=the+world+bank_population+of+Malawi&oq=the+world+bank_population+of+Malawi&aqs=chrome..69i57j0.10460j1j8&sourceid=chrome&ie=UTF-8. Accessed 13 Mar 2017.

18. Population Reference Bureau and Malawi Government. Malawi Population Data Sheet 2012. 2012 Retrieved from https://www.prb.org/malawi-population-2012/. Accessed 4 Aug 2018.

19. National Statistical Office (NSO) of Malawi, UNICEF. Malawi, multiple indicator cluster survey (2006). Final Report. NSO and UNICEF, Lilongwe Malawi 2008.

20. World Health Organisation. Human resources for health country profile, Malawi. 2010. Retrieved from Lilongwe: http://www.who.int/workforcealliance/knowledge/resources/hrh_profile_malawi/en/. Accessed 13 Jan 2017.

21. Chirwa M. Knowledge synthesis on Malawi health system: literature review. 2013. Retrieved from Malawi: http://41.87.6.35:8080/xmlui/bitstream/handle/123456789/904/Knowledge%20synthesis%20on%20Malawi%20health%20system%20literature%20review.pdf?sequence=1. Accessed 7 Aug 2014.

22. Guest G, Bunce A, Johnson L. How many interviews are enough?: an experiment with data saturation and variability. Field Meth. 2006;18(1):59–82. https://doi.org/10.1177/1525822X05279903.

23. Braun V, Clarke V. Using thematic analysis in psychology. Qual Research Psycho. 2006;3:77–101.

24. Mrisho M, Schellenberg JA, Mushi AK, Obrist B, Mshinda H, Tanner M. Factors affecting home delivery in rural Tanzania. Trop Med Int Health. 2007;12:862–72.

25. D'Ambruoso L, Abbey M, Hussein J. Please understand when I cry out in pain: women's accounts of maternity services during labour and delivery in Ghana. BMC Public Health. 2005;5:140.

26. Bazant ES, Koenig MA. Women's satisfaction with delivery care in Nairobi's informal settlements. Intern J Quality Health Care. 2009;21:79–86.

27. Hall JA, Roter DL, Katz BA. Meta-analysis of correlates of provider behaviour in medical encounters. Med Care. 1988;26:657–75.

28. Chadwick RJ, Cooper D, Harries J. Narratives of distress in south African public maternity settings: a qualitative study. Midwifery. 2014;30:862–8.

29. McMahon SA, George AS, Chebet JJ, Mosha IH, Mpembeni RNM, Winch PJ. Experiences of and response to disrespectful maternity care and abuse during childbirth; a qualitative study with women and men in Morogoro region. Tanzania BMC Pregnancy Childbirth. 2014;14:268.

30. Austad K, Chary A, Martinez B, Juarez M, Juarez MY, Ixen C, Rohloff P. Obstetric care navigation: a new approach to promote respectful maternity care and overcome barriers to safe motherhood. Reprod Health. 2017;14:148.

31. Scott K, Klaus P, Klaus M. The obstetrical and post-partum benefits of continuous support during childbirth. J Women's Health Gender-Based Medicine. 1999;8:1257–64.

32. Sauls D. Effects of labour support on mothers, babies, and birth outcomes. J Obstetrics, Gynecol Neonatal Nurs. 2002;31:733–41.

33. Rosen P. Supporting women in labour: analysis of different types of caregivers. J Midwifery Women's Health. 2004;49:24–31.

34. Brown H, Hofmeyr J, Nikodem C, Smith H, Garner P. Promoting childbirth companions in South Africa: a randomised pilot study. BMC Med. 2007;5:7.

35. Kifle D, Azale T, Gelaw YA, Melsew YA. Maternal health care service seeking behaviours and associated factors among women in rural Haramaya District, Eastern Ethiopia: a triangulated community-based cross-sectional study. Reprod Health. 2017;14:16.

36. Okafor II, Ogwu EO, Obi SN. Disrespect and abuse during a facility-based childbirth in a low-income country. Int J Gynecol Obstet. 2015;128:110–3.

37. Bolde MD, Bangoura A, Diallo BA, Sall O, Bolde H, Niakate AS, Vogel JP, Bohren MA. A qualitative study of women's and health providers' attitudes and acceptability of mistreatment during childbirth in health facilities in Guinea. Reprod Health. 2017;14:4.

38. Bohren M, Hunter EC, Munthe-Kaas HM, Souza JP, Vogel JP, Gulmezoglu AM. Facilitators and barriers to facility-based delivery in low- and mid-income countries: a qualitative evidence synthesis. Reprod Health. 2014;11:71.

39. Weinstock D. Deer in the headlights: improving patient literacy. J Medical Practice Manag. 2015;30(4):273–5.

40. Okonofua F, Ogu R, Agholor K, Okike O, Abdus-salam R, Gana M, Randawa A, Abe E, Durodola A, Galadanci H, The WHARC, WHO, FMOH, MNCH Implementation Study Team. Qualitative assessment of women's satisfaction with maternal health care referral hospitals in Nigeria. Reprod Health. 2017;14:44.

41. Kamwendo G. Language policy in health services: a sociolinguistics study of Malawian referral hospital: Helsinki University Printing House; 2004. Retrived on: https://helda.helsinki.fi/bitstream/handle/10138/19198/language.pdf?sequence=1/.

42. Divi C, Koss RG, Schmaltz SP, Loeb JM. Language proficiency and adverse events in U.S. hospitals: a pilot study. Intern J Quality Health Care. 2007;19(60):60–7.

43. Arungwa OT. Effect of communication on nurse-patient relationship in National Orthopaedic Hospital, Igbobi, Lagos. WA J of Nurs. 2014;25(2):37–46.

44. Ong LML, De Haes JCJM, Hoos AM, Lammes FB. Doctor-patient communication: a review of the literature. Soc Science Med. 1995;40(7):903–18.

14

Adolescents' perceptions and experiences of pregnancy in refugee and migrant communities on the Thailand-Myanmar border

Carine Asnong[1][*] ⓘ, Gracia Fellmeth[2], Emma Plugge[1], Nan San Wai[3], Mupawjay Pimanpanarak[3], Moo Kho Paw[3], Prakaykaew Charunwatthana[4], François Nosten[1,3] and Rose McGready[1,3]

Abstract

Background: Adolescent pregnancy remains a global health concern, contributing to 11% of all births worldwide and 23% of the overall burden of disease in girls aged 15–19 years. Premature motherhood can create a negative cycle of adverse health, economic and social outcomes for young women, their babies and families. Refugee and migrant adolescent girls might be particularly at risk due to poverty, poor education and health infrastructure, early marriage, limited access to contraception and traditional beliefs. This study aims to explore adolescents' perceptions and experiences of pregnancy in refugee and migrant communities on the Thailand-Myanmar border.

Methods: In June 2016 qualitative data were collected in one refugee camp and one migrant clinic along the Thailand-Myanmar border by conducting 20 individual interviews with pregnant refugee and migrant adolescents and 4 focus group discussions with husbands, adolescent boys and non-pregnant girls and antenatal clinic staff. Inductive thematic analysis was used to identify codes and themes emerging from the data.

Results: Study participants perceived adolescent pregnancy as a premature life event that could jeopardise their future. Important themes were premarital sex, forced marriage, lack of contraception, school dropout, fear of childbirth, financial insecurity, support structures and domestic violence. Supportive relationships with mothers, husbands and friends could turn this largely negative experience into a more positive one. The main underlying reasons for adolescent pregnancy were associated with traditional views and stigma on sexual and reproductive health issues, resulting in a knowledge gap on contraception and life skills necessary to negotiate sexual and reproductive choices, in particular for unmarried adolescents.

Conclusions: Adolescents perceive pregnancy as a challenging life event that can be addressed by developing comprehensive adolescent-friendly sexual and reproductive health services and education in refugee and migrant communities on the Thailand-Myanmar border. Creating a more tolerant and less stigmatising environment in these communities and their governing bodies will help to achieve this goal.

Keywords: Adolescent pregnancy, Refugee, Migrant, Myanmar, Qualitative, Sexual and reproductive health, Contraception, Stigma, Forced marriage, Domestic violence

* Correspondence: carina.asnong@ndm.ox.ac.uk
[1]Centre for Tropical Medicine and Global Health, Nuffield Department of Medicine, University of Oxford, Oxford OX3 7FZ, UK
Full list of author information is available at the end of the article

Plain English summary

Globally 17 million girls under the age of 19 give birth every year, among them one million under the age of 15. Early pregnancy and motherhood put these adolescents at a higher risk of death, health problems, social stigma, school dropout, unemployment, poverty and domestic violence. Their babies are more likely to die and to have long-term health problems.

This study was set up to get a better understanding of the views and experiences of adolescent pregnancy in refugee and migrant communities on the Thailand-Myanmar border, where poverty, poor education and health facilities, early marriage, difficult access to contraception and traditional beliefs may cause particular difficulties.

The investigators conducted 20 interviews with pregnant refugee and migrant adolescents, as well as four focus group discussions with husbands, adolescent boys and non-pregnant girls and antenatal clinic staff.

Most of the adolescents agreed that unplanned teenage pregnancy is a negative life event during a time that needs to be spent in school. Important themes were premarital sex, forced marriage, lack of contraception, school dropout, fear of childbirth, financial insecurity, insufficient support and domestic violence. Supportive relationships with mothers, husbands and friends were considered to be helpful.

Among the reasons for adolescent pregnancy were traditional views and stigma on sexual and reproductive health issues, resulting in a knowledge gap on contraception and life skills necessary to negotiate sexual and reproductive choices, in particular for unmarried adolescents. Better adolescent-friendly sexual and reproductive health services and education can address this gap in refugee and migrant communities on the Thailand-Myanmar border. In addition a more tolerant and less stigmatising environment could encourage open communication between adolescents and their families and within sexual relationships.

Background

Adolescent pregnancy is an important global health issue and is linked to seven of the Sustainable Development Goals (SDG 1–5, 8, 10) [1]. Every year an estimated 16 million girls aged 15–19 years and another one million girls under the age of 15 give birth; 95% of these births occur in low- and middle-income countries, with the highest rates in sub-Saharan Africa and south Asia. Births to adolescents under 20 years represent 11% of all births worldwide but 23% of the overall burden of disease in this age group [2].

Complications of pregnancy and childbirth, including unsafe abortions, make pregnancy one of the leading causes of death in adolescent girls. Health problems such as anaemia, malaria, sexually transmitted infections, in particular HIV, postpartum haemorrhage and mental disorders are strongly associated with negative outcomes of adolescent pregnancy. About 65% of all obstetric fistulae develop during adolescence, generating significant physical, social and psychological consequences. In addition infants of adolescent mothers are more likely to die, have low birth weight and experience long-term adverse health effects in comparison with infants of adult mothers [2–4]. Premature motherhood significantly reduces the chances of continuing education, developing skills and finding paid work, thus creating a negative cycle of adverse health, economic and social outcomes [5]. A large body of evidence has highlighted the damaging consequences for adolescent mothers and their babies [6–9].

Although some adolescents want and plan their pregnancy, for most of them pregnancy is unplanned and associated with poverty, living in rural areas, difficult access to health care and family planning, early marriage and lack of (sexual and reproductive health) education [3]. Migrant and refugee adolescent girls may be even more at risk [10, 11]. Numerous married adolescent girls cannot access existing family planning services because their husbands or family do not approve due to traditional beliefs. Unmarried adolescents may have particular difficulties accessing contraception because premarital sex is judged as inappropriate and unacceptable [12–14].

The Thailand-Myanmar border (Fig. 1) is home to large populations of refugees who initially fled civil war in Myanmar [15]. Currently an estimated 100,000 refugees live in ten camps on the Thai side of the border. For the past 10 years camp life has been relatively safe and stable, but education, employment and access to the outside world are restricted [16]. Despite poverty and confinement, people feel safe and are reluctant to leave, now that voluntary return and relocation programmes have been negotiated between the Thai and Myanmar governments, envisioning closure of all refugee camps within a not yet defined time period [17].

This region also has an estimated 200,000 migrant workers from Myanmar who have come to Thailand for employment in agriculture or construction, earning higher salaries than in Myanmar [18, 19]. Migrants remain at risk of arrest, extortion and deportation unless they or their employer can afford official registration. The migrant and refugee populations in this region include many ethnic groups such as Karen, Burman and Burman Muslim, each with their own culture, language and religious backgrounds. In this area a number of non-governmental organisations (NGOs) provide basic humanitarian, education and health services, including prenatal care [16].

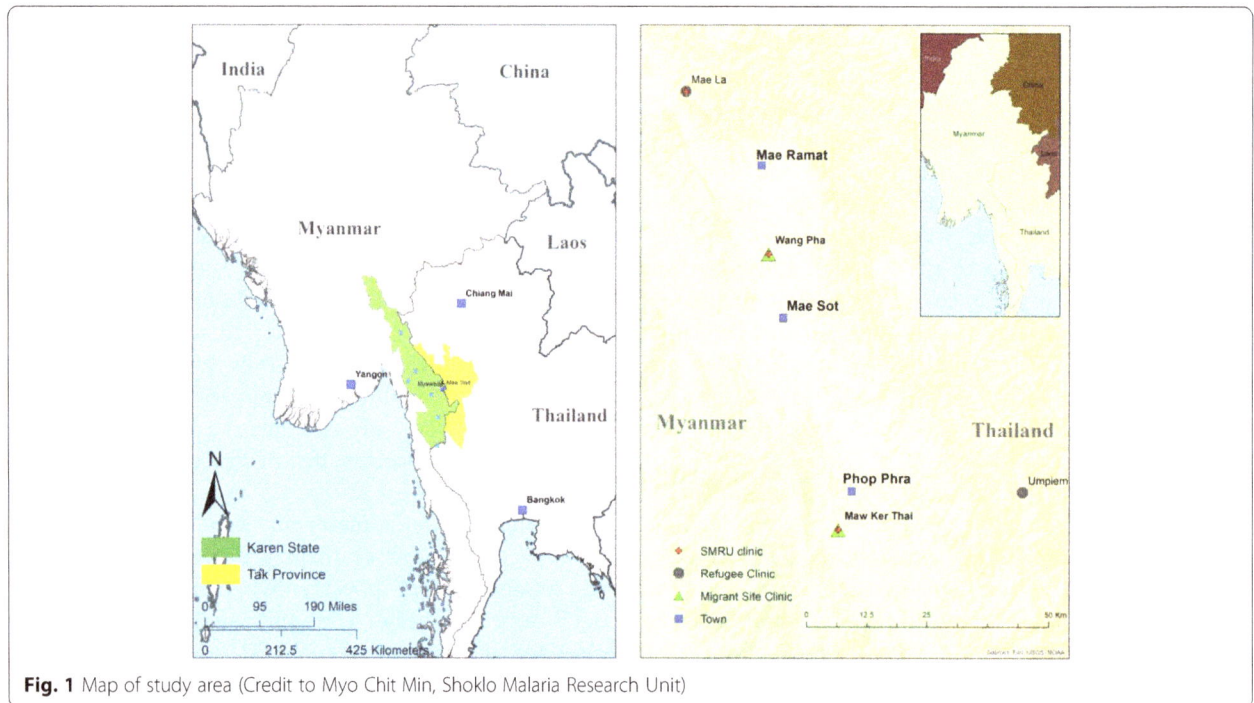

Fig. 1 Map of study area (Credit to Myo Chit Min, Shoklo Malaria Research Unit)

Little is known about adolescent pregnancy and motherhood in this setting. Previous research has focused on pregnant adolescents with refugee backgrounds after resettlement in developed countries [20, 21]. A 2010 study in two refugee camps on the Thailand-Myanmar border assessed young refugees' reproductive health knowledge, attitudes and sources of information and identified early marriage as a major problem [22]. The aim of the current study was to develop a better understanding of adolescent pregnancy, including sexual and reproductive health knowledge and family and community support structures on the Thailand-Myanmar border. In this paper we report on the findings relating to the adolescents' perceptions and beliefs of early motherhood.

Methods

Setting

Since 1986 the Shoklo Malaria Research Unit (SMRU) has provided free antenatal care to displaced populations on the Thailand-Myanmar border and has extensive experience of working with local refugee and migrant communities. The antenatal clinic (ANC) in Mae La refugee camp (MLA) serves the refugee community in the largest camp on the Thai side of the border, while the Maw Ker Thai (MKT) ANC serves rural migrant communities on both sides of the border, south of Mae Sot, Thailand. ANC staff consist mainly of locally trained medics, midwives, nurses and counsellors, supported by a minimal international team of clinicians and researchers [23]. Based on clinic data an estimated 16–18% of all pregnant women seen at SMRU ANC are adolescents under the age of 18.

Study design [24]

Pregnant adolescents younger than 18 years were recruited for in-depth interviews. Eligible participants were pregnant adolescents who registered for a first antenatal visit between 1 September 2015 and 15 June 2016 in the MLA or MKT ANC. A total of 76 adolescents were identified in the clinic database, 40 in the MLA ANC and 36 in the MKT ANC, using convenience sampling, i.e. we selected participants who were coming to the clinic for antenatal visits during the data collection period. A senior midwife approached them individually in the ANC waiting area to explain the purpose of the study and explore their interest in participating.

Additional focus group discussions (FGDs) were held in MLA with husbands of pregnant adolescents, adolescent boys and non-pregnant girls younger than 18 years, and locally trained ANC staff members. Participants for the FGDs were recruited by various methods. Husbands of pregnant adolescents were recruited through snowballing, by asking pregnant adolescents to invite their husbands to attend the clinic on a Saturday morning. Adolescent boys were recruited in a MLA boarding school, where students from villages outside the camp on both sides of the border receive free education, while non-pregnant adolescent girls were recruited by asking locally trained ANC staff members to invite their adolescent daughters and friends. ANC staff members rostered onto the daytime shift were recruited on a voluntary basis after a professional skills training for ANC staff of different camps.

All sessions were conducted in private meeting rooms in proximity to the ANC waiting area and planned to last between 45 and 60 min. Since four different languages are spoken in this setting (Sgaw Karen, Poe Karen, Burmese and English), all interviews and FGDs were co-facilitated by the principal investigator (CA) and a senior midwife (NSW in MLA, MP and MKP in MKT). Topic guides were discussed with facilitators beforehand to check cultural appropriateness and familiarise them with the content. Similar topic guides were used for the interviews and FGDs with husbands and adolescent boys and non-pregnant girls. For the FGD with ANC staff some extra questions were added to explore their willingness to discuss contraception with (unmarried) adolescents (Table 1). The facilitators translated the questions into Karen or Burmese and the participants' responses into English, while the principal investigator took notes to enhance

later data analysis and interpretation. All interviews and FGDs were audio recorded for future reference. Participants received a towel and a bar of soap at the end of the interview or FGD as a token of thanks.

Notes from the interviews and FGDs were reviewed and discussed with the facilitators at the end of each day of data collection. Due to time limitations data saturation was not formally aimed for and assessed.

A Karen refugee student (DK) transcribed all voice recordings and translated them into English. Complete transcripts of the interviews and FGDs were only available at the end of the data collection period. A senior administrative SMRU staff member performed accuracy checks and back-translations of a random 10% of transcripts. NVivo for Mac v11.3.1 was used to organise the data set and prepare it for thematic analysis. Inductive thematic analysis was conducted in six consecutive steps, as outlined by Braun and Clarke [25, 26]. Two authors (CA and EP) separately coded the transcripts and agreed on key emerging themes.

Table 1 Interview/FGD topic guide

1. At what age most women become pregnant?
   Do you think this is young/old to have a baby?
   What is a young age to have a baby?
   What advice do you give to your best friend on the best age for pregnancy?
2. Why do women become pregnant at a young age?
   Are the fathers also young/older?
   Who decides to have a baby? Father? Mother? Together?
3. Which things can make pregnancy and motherhood difficult?
   Which things can make pregnancy and motherhood easier?
   Can you give examples?
   Can you explain more?
4. Is pregnancy/motherhood at a young age different from pregnancy/motherhood at an older age?
   How is it different?
   Can you give examples?
5. Do you know pregnant adolescents or young mothers who are not happy and lonely?
   Why do you think they are not happy and lonely?
   How do you know they are not happy and lonely?
6. Who can help these young pregnant women/mothers when it gets difficult?
   Could you explain how that will help young pregnant women/mothers?
   What can happen if they have nobody to help them?
7. Have you heard of ways to prevent or stop pregnancy? Can you give examples?
   If adolescents can get contraception, will they use it?
   Can you explain why they will use it/ not use it?
8. What do schools teach young girls about pregnancy, contraception?
   Do you want schools to teach young girls about pregnancy, contraception?
   Where can they find this information?
   Can you explain that more? Can you give examples?
9. What do young men know about pregnancy/contraception?
   Do they need more information/education on pregnancy/contraception?
   Why do you think that is important?
   Where can they find this information?
10. FGD ANC staff only:
    Can you describe ways to improve the knowledge of adolescents about sexual health, pregnancy and contraception?
    Are you comfortable discussing this with adolescents?
    Would you like to learn more about this?

Ethics

Participant information and informed consent/assent were administered verbally to all participants. Adolescents under the age of 18, the legal age of consent in Thailand, were invited to provide written assent, co-signed by a parent, husband, sister or guardian prior to participation in the study. Low-literacy participants provided a thumbprint instead of a signature. A copy of the consent/assent form was given to each participant. Ethical approval for this study was obtained from the University of Oxford's Tropical Research Ethics Committee (OxTREC Ref [13–16]), the Mahidol University Faculty of Tropical Medicine Ethics Committee (TMEC16–025) and the Tak Border Community Advisory Board (T-CAB-04/01/2016).

Results

We conducted a total of 20 individual interviews with adolescents who were pregnant at the time of recruitment: ten in the MLA and ten in the MKT ANC. In addition four FGDs were conducted in MLA only: FGD1 with three husbands of pregnant adolescents, FGD2 with six adolescent boys, FGD3 with six non-pregnant adolescent girls and FGD4 with five locally-trained ANC staff members. All eligible adolescents and staff members who were approached for an interview or FGD agreed to participate and signed a consent form. No participants left during any of the interviews, but one participant of FGD1 left after 5 minutes without providing a reason. The duration of the interviews varied between 14 and 45 min. The FGDs were longer and lasted between 62 and 115 min. Tables 2 and 3 give an overview of the socio-demographic characteristics of the study participants.

A preliminary analysis of the data transcripts showed that similar themes were emerging from the

Table 2 Socio-demographic characteristics of interview participants

Reference number[a]	Age of participant	Age of husband	EGA (weeks)[b]	Language	Years in school	Prior employment
MLA01	16	18	8	Burmese	4	No
MLA02	15	15	38	Burmese	2	Shop auntie
MLA03	16	25	19	Karen	11	Agricultural work
MLA04	15	20	12	Burmese	4	Home shop
MLA05	16	25	Post-partum	Karen	5	Household
MLA06	15	18	Miscarriage	Karen	3	Agricultural work
MLA07	15	19	27	Karen	4	Care siblings
MLA08	17	18	31	Karen	9	Agricultural work
MLA09	17	25	34	Burmese	3	Agricultural work
MLA10	14	15	–	Karen	8	No
MKT01	16	18	8	Burmese	4	Agricultural work
MKT02	15	25	26	Burmese	0	Agricultural work
MKT03	17	20	36	Burmese	2	Agricultural work
MKT04	16	23	18	Karen	3	Agricultural work
MKT05	13	20	36	Karen	0	Agricultural work
MKT06	17	22	17	Burmese	4	Agricultural work
MKT07	16	20	22	Burmese	9	Agricultural work
MKT08	16	19	16	Karen	4	Agricultural work
MKT09	15	18	25	Karen	6	Agricultural work
MKT10	17	24	20	Karen	7	Household

[a]MLA: participants attending antenatal clinic in Mae La refugee camp; MKT: participants attending antenatal clinic in Maw Ker Thai migrant clinic
[b]EGA estimated gestational age at time of interview

individual interviews and FGDs, as were refugee and migrant participants' views, and therefore all results were analysed together.

Two overarching themes emerged, "getting pregnant" and "becoming a mother", each including different levels of closely interrelated sub-themes.

Getting pregnant
Too young

All adolescents agreed that they were too young for pregnancy and motherhood and that a minimum age of 20 was more appropriate. While adolescent girls worried mostly about physical difficulties in childbirth and financial hardship, adolescent boys thought that missed educational opportunities and social consequences could make the future difficult. One participant in the husbands' focus group noted that it was problematic for young fathers under the age of 20 because 'their education is still too low and they are not ready to take responsibility for everything.'

"If girls get pregnant and become mothers at such young age, it is difficult for them, like ... not having enough money... If a husband cannot earn some money, it will be a problem." (MLA10 pregnant refugee)

Marriage

In this context premarital sex and pregnancy outside of marriage are disapproved and not tolerated by general society and culture. As is common in many rural and traditional societies, interaction between unmarried boys and girls can only take place in public or in the presence of a family member or friend, in particular in the evening hours, when adolescents are expected to experiment with sexuality. Consequently a rendezvous between two young people without a chaperone can result in a forced cover-up marriage, sometimes even within the next 24 h. ANC staff members clearly described the stigma that is associated with premarital sex in their community.

"So how does the community react when they catch young couples sleeping together, they force them to get married, even if they don't agree. Once they're married, then the issue is over... the people don't talk about it anymore. You will be dead if you don't get married after you've slept together!" (FGD4 ANC staff)

Talking about premarital sex was an extremely sensitive topic for most adolescents. They avoided the words, indicated that they did not wish to discuss it, replied by 'I don't know' or referred to it in different

Table 3 Socio-demographic characteristics of FGD participants

Reference number	Age of participant	Years in school	Employment	Language
Husbands of pregnant adolescents				
1FGD1	16	3	Agricultural work	Karen
2FGD1	15	7	No	Karen
3FGD1	18	11	Teacher	Karen
Adolescent boys				
1FGD2	14	7	Student	Karen
2FGD2	19	10	Student	Karen
3FGD2	17	3	Student	Karen
4FGD2	16	9	Student	Karen
5FGD2	16	8	Student	Karen
6FGD2	18	5	Student	Karen
Adolescent non-pregnant girls				
1FGD3	14	7	Student	Karen
2FGD3	17	10	Student	Karen
3FGD3	16	9	Student	Karen
4FGD3	13	6	Student	Karen
5FGD3	16	9	Student	Karen
6FGD3	16	9	Student	Burmese
Antenatal staff (all locally trained)				
1FGD4	–	–	Ultrasound technician	Karen
2FGD4	–	–	Midwife	Karen
3FGD4	–	–	Nutrition counsellor	Karen
4FGD4	–	–	Midwife	Karen
5FGD4	–	–	Midwife	Karen

ways. Out of the 20 interviewed pregnant adolescents, four refugees and three migrants indicated that they were forced to marry after they got pregnant. As one pregnant refugee noted, 'Some end up getting pregnant because they indulge themselves in the wrong track in their lives.'

However some pregnant refugees and migrants explained that they themselves decided to marry and that free-choice adolescent marriages out of love were more common than arranged and cover-up marriages. A 15-year old pregnant refugee, who lived most of her life in Myanmar before moving to Mae La camp, defended a rather liberal viewpoint, similar to that of most western countries and very unusual in this conservative setting, stating that 'couples just decide to live together and get married when the girls become pregnant.'

For one refugee girl marriage was a coping strategy to escape a poor and abusive home environment. She ran away in search for a better life in the Bangkok area, where she married a co-worker. The unplanned pregnancy however forced her to return to Mae La and live with her parents again.

"After my father left, my mother married another man. He does not like me and he always yelled at me. I had to do all the hard work in the house, so I ran away."

"I didn't plan for this, my pregnancy, but it just happened. And my husband told me that we would not get pregnant until we were financially doing well. If we have the baby now, both for us and for the baby, we'll be in trouble. My mother has to live with her husband and if she wants to help me or give me money she needs to get permission from my stepfather. When I feel sad, I have to make myself feel better, because I cannot talk to my mother anymore." (MLA09 pregnant refugee)

Marriage at a young age, arranged by parents or other family members, is less common in this setting and occurs mostly in Muslim families. One interviewee explained that her widowed mother had married her off at 13 years of age to secure support for her family.

Planned or unplanned pregnancy?

Of all interviewees only two migrant girls (16 and 17 years old) confirmed that they made a positive choice to marry and have a baby after prior use of contraceptives. More than half of all pregnancies took the young couples by surprise. It 'just happened', mostly because they were not using contraception or their contraception failed due to irregular use.

"My husband's aunt saw me and asked me how long I had missed my period? I told her about two months. So she asked me if I were pregnant and I told her that I didn't know." (MLA09 pregnant refugee)

In only one case, an arranged Muslim marriage, a religious explanation was given for the unplanned pregnancy.

"It is just the way it is because God gives blessings to them for their pregnancies." (MLA01 pregnant Muslim refugee)

Some adolescent girls had to give in to the strong wish of their husband or parents to have a (grand) child.

"After the marriage I took some pills. But my husband told me to stop ... his mother wanted him to have a baby. Then the whole family discussed together and made the final decision." (MKT08 pregnant migrant)

"However now I have to follow the decisions by my husband because I'm very young. You can't say 'no.' ... It's just ..." (MKT09 pregnant 15 year-old migrant)

There was however a fine line between forced sex and a husband's wish to have a baby. Some girls indicated that they were not assertive enough to negotiate reproductive choices with their husbands. This was too sensitive an issue to explore further in the individual interviews, but it was discussed in the adolescent boys' FGD2.

Q: "For example, a boy asks his girlfriend to sleep with him but the girl refuses, what do you think of this situation?"

A: "It would be forced sex and the boy should respect the girl's decision. A boy shouldn't force her to sleep with him because it would be a kind of rape, although they are boyfriend and girlfriend. It's so wrong!" (FGD2 adolescent boys)

Contraception

The knowledge and beliefs about contraception play a crucial role in adolescent pregnancy in this setting and are tightly interwoven with the taboo around sexual and reproductive health (SRH) education for unmarried adolescents.

"So it is difficult to talk to unmarried boys and unmarried girls about family planning and safe sex. People do not accept it because they think that such education can corrupt their children's minds, like they think it teaches them to be more sexually active. We used to provide family planning education to the community. When we showed for example, how to use condoms, some girls felt embarrassed about it, even the married people ... they never looked at that demonstration! If even the married people felt very embarrassed, you can imagine the unmarried people." (FGD4 ANC staff)

SRH education in camp and village schools is limited to biological facts on puberty and pregnancy and does not include any information on contraception, sexual relationships and life skills.

"Sometimes teachers teach us about reproductive stages, a female's thing and a male's thing. We don't get to learn about sex and pregnancy or family planning. We only know that from neighbours." (FGD3 adolescent girls)

"In school I only learned about menstruation and the boys laughed about this when the girls were explained ..." (MLA02 pregnant refugee)

"We don't know how to make the right decisions and we do not talk about it with our wife. But school is not a good place to teach about contraception. I think it can give the students bad habits, if they know about prevention." (FGD1 husbands)

Most adolescents received information on contraception elsewhere, from mothers, sisters, aunties, neighbours and friends. Some adolescents preferred to talk to friends only, because they dreaded their parents' judgement when showing an interest in contraception. One participant in the adolescent girls' focus group was clear that 'we don't feel comfortable to talk about this with our mothers: without getting married, talking and discussing with our mothers about this is a bit ... our mothers may think that their daughters are pregnant ... we will end up being scolded.' Only a few participants mentioned health professionals as the best resource.

Many adolescents had heard about contraceptives, but did not know how to use them correctly. A common misconception was the idea that the use of contraception before a first pregnancy causes the uterus to shrink.

"Umm... I have heard that taking contraception pills can sometimes lead to uterus contraction, and a girl can no longer conceive a baby after that." (MLA04 pregnant refugee)

Most antenatal and family planning clinics offer information on contraception and provide condoms, contraceptive pills and injectable hormones free of charge. However sometimes staff members refuse to provide contraception to unmarried adolescents.

"They seem to only give medications and condoms to the married couples. If some of them are still in school, they wouldn't be given anything to prevent pregnancy." (MLA08 pregnant refugee)

Adolescents are hesitant to use the clinic services because of the associated stigma and social control vis-à-vis premarital sex: a clinic visit in itself could show the community that the adolescent is sexually active or interested in premarital sex. A participant in the adolescent boys' group stated that, 'I feel shy for getting a condom, we feel a bit uncomfortable to get condoms from the health-workers working in our villages.'

Often adolescents ask a relative or friend to get contraceptive pills or condoms on their behalf in pharmacies and regular shops because they do not want to be caught in the act of buying contraceptives.

"For contraception it is better to live in a big city. Nobody will know you there when you want to buy contraceptives or condoms. In the village everybody will know and they will talk." (FGD2 adolescent boys)

School dropout
Across all interviews and FGDs adolescent pregnancy was believed to cause major disruptions in the lives of unmarried adolescents. Some schools expelled students if they knew about premarital sex while other schools allowed students to stay if they got married. However the pregnant adolescents and their partner always chose to leave school, some because they felt embarrassed and teased by their classmates, others because the new responsibilities as parents caused pressure to find work and support the young family.

"I didn't want to go to school anymore because I feel embarrassed about me getting married earlier. Some

of my friends seem a bit different, looking down at me like 'oh, you're a married man now...' They tease me like that. And it is the same for the girls." (FGD1 husband)

" In my point of view, once you get married, you have a different life. So for me, I have to work for my life and family now when my friends are going into different directions of life. Now, I have to take responsibility for my family." (FGD1 husband)

While the boys voiced more feelings of regret about missed educational opportunities, the pregnant girls seemed to have less of a problem with this school dropout and some really cherished the thoughts of motherhood,.

"Since I'm married, I'll need to take care of the baby soon and I don't want to be in school anymore." (MLA08 pregnant refugee)

Becoming a mother
Most interviews and FGDs were saturated with negative experiences, stories and examples. Few participants raised positive experiences spontaneously and most of them only talked about them when asked for explicitly.

Wellbeing of mother and baby
For most pregnant adolescents feeling healthy and physically comfortable seemed to give them more confidence and resilience towards the future. Knowing that the baby was healthy and growing well made them happy, especially when sharing and comparing their bellies with some of the other pregnant women in the ANC waiting room.

"I have two new friends in my neighbourhood and they are also pregnant. We come to the clinic together; there is one in the waiting room over there. We often talk about our babies and how they get bigger." (MLA08 pregnant migrant)

Besides nausea and minor pregnancy-related ailments there were few examples of physical difficulties during adolescent pregnancy. The only important topic that emerged from the interviews and discussions was physical labour. Most pregnant migrants had been working in the fields and indicated that they had already stopped or were planning to stop their work soon. One pregnant refugee however complained that she had to work hard in the third trimester of her pregnancy to 'pay' for support from her relatives. To protect her in the last weeks before childbirth she was admitted to the antenatal ward by the local midwives.

"Some women can live comfortably during their pregnancy whereas I have to work without any rest at my aunts' house, including cooking, going out to sell stuff... the whole day. My aunts... they usually come back around 11 o'clock then go out elsewhere ... I am left behind to do chores if I want to live in their house." (MLA02 pregnant refugee)

Necessary support

Perceptions of health and physical comfort were closely linked to the daily living conditions of the young mother-to-be. Having financial support and family around made the pregnancy a lot easier, as one pregnant refugee noted, 'it is all easy for me, because my uncles and aunts from abroad support me. And I also have my mother and a younger sister in the house.'

Supportive and caring relationships were seen as indispensable assets. Most pregnant adolescents declared that having family around, especially their mother, was the best support they could wish for. They preferred their mother or female relatives over their husband for emotional and practical support and advice during and after the pregnancy. For more 'planned' adolescent pregnancies, based on mature relationships, the support preferences were similar. Mothers were not only perceived as experts in pregnancy and childcare, both 'women's businesses', but even more as unconditional supporters, in spite of social pressure and community disapproval. When mothers were unavailable older sisters and aunties tended to take over this role. On the other hand a good and caring relationship with their husband was perceived as a condition for a stable and financially sound future life. Sometimes the embarrassment of adolescents towards their family was just too overpowering and friends were the first resource for emotional support.

"Talking to mother is still the best thing to do because yes, she may scold you, but she will finally take care of you." (FGD3 adolescent girls)

The young fathers perceived it as a duty to work and protect their young wives. They acknowledged the importance of family support for the young mothers, but some also emphasised the adolescent father's need for knowledge and involvement in baby care.

"But young fathers should also receive support about caring for their baby if they want to be involved. But in my opinion, the young father needs to support his wife in physical things... She always needs company

with her when going somewhere at night too, for safety, I mean." (FGD1 husbands)

Perceived challenges

Nearly every pregnant adolescent expressed fear of physical difficulties and pain during childbirth. They had all heard that having a baby at a young age can be difficult and that a Caesarean section is sometimes necessary. The financial burden of an operation in the Mae Sot hospital represented an additional concern for these young women and their families.

One migrant's story was very emotional because she was only 13 years old.

"When I first got pregnant, I thought of myself that I was going to die because I'm young. I was worried and cried. Then I talked to my mother. My mother just told me 'it's nothing'. And my husband said that it is a girl's thing and that I have to be ready for the pain." (MKT05 pregnant migrant)

Many of the pregnant adolescents worried about financial hardship in the immediate and far future. Most pregnant refugees had been in school until they got pregnant. Without financial support from their parents, relatives or their husbands, they would have to find work to support their family, a difficult task for a woman living in Mae La refugee camp.

"I didn't have any money for today to cook, I didn't have rice. Then I had to go ask some from others and if they didn't give me some rice, I had to go to some other places to find food." (MLA09 pregnant refugee)

Apart from two pregnant migrants who planned their pregnancies, feelings of unpreparedness, struggle and unhappiness emanated from many stories. Instead of completing their education in school and spending time with friends, they had to dedicate their life to a baby, organise their household or earn a living. In some stories young mothers refused to accept this new role, disliked and even neglected their baby.

"I have seen a very young pregnant girl, about 14 years old, around my house. She gave birth to a big and healthy baby at the hospital. However, about two weeks after she was discharged from the hospital, she went out to join her friends and play. When she came back her baby was already dead. Some of her neighbours felt sorry for what just happened, but she kind of felt nothing." (MLA08 pregnant refugee)

Some pregnant adolescents admitted that they had considered abortion as a solution to their unplanned pregnancy, but fear and traditional beliefs prevented them from carrying it out.

"In my village, we believe that when a person tries to make an abortion and has succeeded, afterwards in her next life, she has to eat back the things she aborted in a previous life. Also you cannot get pregnant anymore! That's why it scared me!" (MKT09 pregnant migrant)

Domestic violence and suicide

Unplanned adolescent pregnancy and the subsequent cover-up marriage were generally perceived as major risk factors for troubled relationships both within families and within marriages. Social pressure and traditional culture kept some parents from supporting their pregnant daughter and made them use violence instead to solve the problem. One adolescent boy related a sad story about one of his friends who 'was beaten by her mother because she didn't like her daughter getting pregnant early, so she lost the baby.'

Numerous were the stories about husbands not supporting their young pregnant wife or family, often resorting to alcohol and drug abuse, gambling, domestic violence and divorce.

"She loves her husband, but her husband doesn't love her. She lives with her mother-in-law, but that mother in law treats her badly. Her mother-in-law and her husband always beat her up. Her husband drinks alcohol, uses drugs... umm... he treats his wife badly." (MKT03 pregnant migrant)

In more extreme situations suicide was perceived as the only way out.

"For other people, their husbands are not good to them. Sometimes they commit suicide as they feel young and are in such a complicated situation. Their husbands drink alcohol a lot and there is domestic violence, so that the wives do something when becoming depressed ... like committing suicide by drinking poison." (MLA02 pregnant refugee)

Discussion

In the refugee and migrant communities on the Thailand-Myanmar border adolescents perceive pregnancy as a premature and usually unplanned life event that can jeopardise their future chances in life. Pregnant adolescents are fearful of childbirth and premature motherhood, but most of all the uncertainty to secure a well supported and financially sound future. These findings endorse the large body of evidence that highlights the disadvantages and risks of teenage pregnancy and keeps it high on the global health agenda [6–9].

Despite their initial negative reactions, mothers or other women in the family are perceived as a major asset to encourage adolescents during pregnancy and teach them how to be a good mother after childbirth. In this setting many husbands work outside the refugee camp or in the Bangkok area to earn higher wages, and they are physically not present to support their pregnant wives. This may have played an important role in the experiences of marital support that is mostly perceived as a means of financial security. A qualitative study exploring the experiences of teen pregnancy of African Australian refugee women after resettlement in Australia by Ngum Chi Watts et al. [21] describes similar findings. The importance of support structures in teenage pregnancy and parenthood are also highlighted by Letourneau et al. [27] on family and partner support, and Bunting et al. on the role of young fathers [28].

On the other hand, many participants' stories demonstrate how the lack of support and troubled relationships, including social stigma, domestic violence and alcohol abuse, can drive young families into dire living conditions and young mothers into despair and even suicide. This reflects the findings reported by Fellmeth et al. [29] in the same setting, that economic and family-related causes are the most commonly raised issues among the causes of mental illness. A study by Falb et al. [30] documenting violence against Karen refugee women along the Thailand-Myanmar border, reports that 7.9% of all surveyed women, irrespective of age, were recent victims of intimate partner violence often linked to alcohol abuse. Fear of women to speak out could have caused underreporting and the real numbers were likely to be higher [30]. In our study both refugee and migrant participants reported domestic violence and hence this phenomenon does not seem to be limited to the refugee camp context only.

The main underlying causes for adolescent pregnancies in refugee and migrant communities on the Thailand-Myanmar border can be linked to traditional and stigmatising views on premarital sex. Communication about sexual and reproductive health between parents and unmarried adolescents is mostly perceived as non-existent because it is deemed inappropriate and corrupting young people's minds, as previously described by Srikanthan et al. [31] in an overview of religious and cultural influences on contraception. Even health workers are reported to refuse contraceptive information and services to unmarried adolescents, similar to the results of Brand et al. [32]. Likewise schools offer a very limited sexual and reproductive health programme, avoiding the topics of contraception, sexual behaviour and life skills necessary to negotiate informed and healthy reproductive choices.

The subsequent adolescent SRH knowledge gap contributes to a highly unmet need for contraceptive services by unmarried adolescents, enhanced by perceptions of social control by the community, in particular in the more isolated refugee camp setting. This corresponds with the findings of Benner et al. [22], demonstrating how youth in refugee camps on the Thailand-Myanmar border are not supposed to have premarital sex or to need reproductive health services, and with a review of contraception barriers for adolescents in low- and middle-income countries by Chandra-Mouli et al. [13]. Once married, adolescents can get information about contraception from their mothers, older siblings or friends, but open communication between husband and wife on reproductive choices is often experienced as uncomfortable and not done. Family planning counsellors and midwives in the antenatal clinics confirm these experiences. In addition they explain how they have to counter deeply ingrained misconceptions and fears for compromised future fertility when they try to recommend contraception for adolescent girls.

Strengths and limitations

This study is based on limited numbers of individual interviews and focus group discussions, both qualitative research methods that are well suited to explore sensitive and complex social issues. Its findings are not representative of all pregnant refugee and migrant adolescents in this or other settings. Due to time and budget restrictions the study design and recruitment strategy were determined by pragmatic considerations rather than by achieving data saturation.

There was a striking difference in depth, richness and length between the individual interviews and the FGDs, suggesting that the FGD group dynamics were more effective in eliciting stories, perceptions and explicit views on the sensitive topic of teenage pregnancy than individual in-depth interviews. This may be because of the sense of community so that it was more 'natural' to speak in groups than to spend a long period of time talking to one person individually. Previous studies confirm that the FGD format works well in the SMRU setting [29] and that Karen refugees in the USA have been notably shy in individual in-depth interviews [33].

All adolescent FGD participants, boys and girls, were secondary school students, who were highly talented and used to voicing their opinion. The unheard voices in this study were the low-literacy, less educated migrant adolescents living in villages and shelters along the border and working in the fields for a living. Future research on this topic should target these groups specifically.

Conducting qualitative research in a setting with different languages may have influenced participants' responses. The indirectness of communication between an English-speaking researcher and study participants leaves, to a large extent, the contents and flow of conversations into the hands of the facilitators and out of control of the researcher. Three different senior midwives facilitated the interviews and FGDs, each approaching and encouraging the participants in their own style. Notes from the interviews and FGDs were reviewed and discussed with the facilitators at the end of each day of data collection, but we did not perform any cross-checking for accuracy of interpretation of results among the facilitators involved in data collection. A young refugee student translated all participant documents and transcribed all voice recordings with only partial accuracy checks. Due to budget restrictions the transcription of all Karen and Burmese interview and FGD recordings was done directly in English instead of by a two-step process.

Finally, despite rigorous informed consent procedures, adolescent participants may have felt intimidated or afraid to decline participation, particularly in the presence of a non-local researcher.

As far as we can ascertain this appears to be the first publication where the views of pregnant adolescents in Asian refugee camps and amongst Myanmar migrants in Thailand have been directly obtained. The findings of this study can help to identify and support initiatives in the refugee and migrant communities, schools and local health centres to improve adolescent health and empower adolescents towards a healthier life-course, in preparation for the uncertainties of a future return and resettlement to Myanmar or third countries [17].

They are particularly important for the refugee camp community and their governing body and they will be used to inform policy. When presenting preliminary findings of this project to local stakeholders, they expressed their concerns and acknowledged the urgency of comprehensive SRH education in the camps to better prepare their youth. Follow-up meetings were planned to address these issues. Further research needs to be done on the strategy, cultural and religious barriers, timing, and contents of comprehensive SRH education initiatives in the communities on the Thailand-Myanmar border. Informal discussions with the midwives and counsellors of the MLA refugee and MKT migrant antenatal clinic also highlighted their interest in new adolescent-friendly SRH initiatives and additional training to deliver them [33–36].

Conclusion

Adolescent pregnancy remains a major global health issue that contributes significantly to the morbidity and mortality in this age group and can create a negative cycle of adverse health, economic and social outcomes. In this study most refugee and migrant adolescents perceive their unplanned pregnancy as a challenging life event, not only for themselves, but also for their babies and families. They describe how traditional views and stigma on sexual and reproductive health issues have contributed to an important knowledge gap on contraception and life skills necessary to negotiate sexual and reproductive choices, especially for unmarried adolescents. The perceptions and views on adolescent pregnancy presented in this study can help to identify and develop effective strategies to provide comprehensive adolescent-friendly sexual and reproductive health services and education in refugee and migrant communities on the Thailand-Myanmar border. They advocate for a more tolerant and less stigmatising environment that can encourage open communication between adolescents and their families and support shared decision making in sexual relationships.

Abbreviations

ANC: Antenatal clinic; EGA: Estimated gestational age; FGD: Focus group discussion; HIV: Human immunodeficiency virus; MKT: Maw Ker Thai migrant clinic; MLA: Mae La refugee camp clinic; NGO: Non-governmental organisations; SDG: Sustainable development goals; SMRU: Shoklo Malaria Research Unit; SRH: sexual and reproductive health

Acknowledgements

We thank Dingo Keidar for translation and transcription, Daraporn Prakunwisit for quality checks and Myo Chit Min for creating the map for this study.We would further like to thank all colleagues and staff of SMRU for supporting this project and all study participants and their families for sharing their experiences and views.

Funding

This project was funded by the MSc Programme in International Health and Tropical Medicine, Centre for Tropical Medicine and Global Health, Nuffield Department of Medicine, University of Oxford.

Authors' contributions

CA participated in the design of the study, data acquisition, data analysis and interpretation and drafted the manuscript. GF participated in the design of the study and helped to draft the manuscript. EP participated in data analysis, data interpretation and helped to draft the manuscript. NSW, MP and MKP conducted data acquisition. PC helped to draft the manuscript. FN provided general supervision of the research. RM participated in the design of the study, data interpretation and drafting of the manuscript. All authors read and approved the final manuscript.

Competing interests

The authors declare that they have no competing interests.

Author details

[1]Centre for Tropical Medicine and Global Health, Nuffield Department of Medicine, University of Oxford, Oxford OX3 7FZ, UK. [2]Nuffield Department of Population Health, University of Oxford, Old Road Campus, Headington, Oxford OX3 7FZ, UK. [3]Shoklo Malaria Research Unit, Mahidol-Oxford Tropical Medicine Research Unit, Mahidol University, Mae Sot 63110, Thailand. [4]Mahidol-Oxford Tropical Medicine Research Unit, Mahidol University, Bangkok 10400, Thailand.

References

1. UNFPA. Sustainable development goals. New York: UNFPA; 2015. http://www.unfpa.org/sdg. Accessed 22 Aug 2017
2. World Health Organisation (WHO). Adolescent pregnancy: fact sheet number 364. Geneva: WHO; 2014. http://www.who.int/mediacentre/factsheets/fs364/en/. Accessed 22 Aug 2017
3. United Nations Population Fund (UNFPA). Adolescent pregnancy: a review of the evidence. New York: UNFPA; 2013. http://www.unfpa.org/sites/default/files/pub-pdf/ADOLESCENT%20PREGNANCY_UNFPA.pdf. Accessed 22 Aug 2017
4. Global Burden of Disease Pediatrics Collaboration. Global and national burden of diseases and injuries among children and adolescents between 1990 and 2013: findings from the global burden of disease 2013 study. JAMA Pediatr. 2015; https://doi.org/10.1001/jamapediatrics.2015.4276.
5. United Nations Population Fund (UNFPA). Girlhood, not motherhood. New York: UNFPA; 2015. http://www.unfpa.org/publications/girlhood-not-motherhood. Accessed 22 Aug 2017
6. Ruedinger E, Cox JE. Adolescent childbearing: consequences and interventions. Curr Opin Pediatr. 2012; https://doi.org/10.1097/MOP.0b013e3283557b89.
7. Malabarey OT, Balayla J, Klam SL, Shrim A, Abenhaim HA. Pregnancies in young adolescent mothers: a population-based study on 137 million births. J Pediatr Adolesc Gynecol. 2012; https://doi.org/10.1016/j.jpag.2011.09.004.
8. Santhya KG. Early marriage and sexual and reproductive health vulnerabilities of young women: a synthesis of recent evidence from developing countries. Curr Opin Obstet Gynecol. 2011; https://doi.org/10.1097/GCO.0b013e32834a93d2.
9. Siegel RS, Brandon AR. Adolescents, pregnancy, and mental health. J Pediatr Adolesc Gynecol. 2014; https://doi.org/10.1016/j.jpag.2013.09.008.
10. UNFPA. State of the world population report 2015. New York: UNFPA; 2015. https://www.unfpa.org/sites/default/files/sowp/downloads/State_of_World_Population_2015_EN.pdf. Accessed 22 Aug 2017
11. McMichael C, Gifford S. Narratives of sexual health risk and protection amongst young people from refugee backgrounds in Melbourne, Australia. Cult Health Sex. 2010; https://doi.org/10.1080/13691050903359265.
12. Wong LP. An exploration of knowledge, attitudes and behaviours of young multi-ethnic Muslim-majority society in Malaysia in relation to reproductive and premarital sexual practices. BMC Public Health. 2012; https://doi.org/10.1186/1471-2458-12-865.
13. Chandra-Mouli V, McCarraher DR, Phillips SJ, Williamson NE, Hainsworth G. Contraception for adolescents in low and middle income countries: needs, barriers, and access. Reprod Health. 2014; https://doi.org/10.1186/1742-4755-11-1.
14. Ochako R, et al. Barriers to modern contraceptive methods uptake among young women in Kenya: a qualitative study. BMC Public Health. 2015; https://doi.org/10.1186/s12889-015-1483-1.
15. Brenner D. Inside the Karen insurgency: explaining conflict and conciliation in Myanmar's changing borderlands. Asian Secur. 2017; https://doi.org/10.1080/14799855.2017.1293657.
16. The Border Consortium. Annual report Jan –Dec 2016. Thailand: TBC; 2016. http://www.theborderconsortium.org/media/80489/2016-annual-report-jan-dec.pdf. Accessed 22 Aug 2017
17. UNHCR. Strategic roadmap for voluntary repatriation: refugees from Myanmar in Thailand, 2015–2017. Thailand: UNHCR. March 2015. Downloaded fromhttps://reliefweb.int/report/thailand/unhcr-strategic-roadmap-voluntary-repatriation-refugees-myanmar-thailand-2015-2017 on 22 Aug 2017.
18. Human Rights Watch. From the tiger to the crocodile: abuse of migrant workers in Thailand. New York: Human Rights Watch; 2010. https://www.hrw.org/sites/default/files/reports/thailand0210_insert_low.pdf. Accessed 22 Aug 2017

19. Dunlop N. Invisible people: Stories of migrant labourers in Thailand. http://www.mekongmigration.org/wp-content/uploads/2012/10/f13438945381.pdf. Accessed 22 Aug 2017.

20. McMichael C. Unplanned but not unwanted? Teen pregnancy and parenthood among young people with refugee backgrounds. J Youth Stud. 2013; https://doi.org/10.1080/13676261.2012.744813.

21. Ngum Chi Watts MC, Liamputtong P, McMichael C. Early motherhood: a qualitative study exploring the experiences of African Australian teenage mothers in greater Melbourne, Australia. BMC Public Health. 2015; https://doi.org/10.1186/s12889-015-2215-2.

22. Benner MT, et al. Reproductive health and quality of life of young Burmese refugees in Thailand. Confl Heal. 2010; https://doi.org/10.1186/1752-1505-4-5

23. Website Shoklo Malaria Research Unit. http://www.shoklo-unit.com. Accessed 22 Aug 2017.

24. Silverman D. Doing qualitative research. London: SAGE Publications LTD; 2013.

25. Bailey J. First steps in qualitative data analysis: transcribing. Fam Pract. 2008; https://doi.org/10.1093/fampra/cmn003.

26. Braun V, Clarke V. Using thematic analysis in psychology. Qual Res Psychol. 2006; https://doi.org/10.1191/1478088706qp063oa.

27. Letourneau NL, Stewart MJ, Barnfather AK. Adolescent mothers: support needs, resources, and support-education interventions. J Adolesc Health. 2004; https://doi.org/10.1016/j.adohealth.2004.01.007.

28. Bunting L, McAuley C. Research review: teenage pregnancy and motherhood: the contribution of support. Child Fam Soc Work. 2004; https://doi.org/10.1111/j.1365-2206.2004.00328.

29. Fellmeth et al. Pregnant migrant and refugee women's perceptions of mental illness on the Thai-Myanmar border: a qualitative study. BMC Pregnancy Childbirth. 2015; https://doi.org/10.1186/s12884-015-0517-0.

30. Falb K, McCormick M, Hemenway D, Anfinson K, Silverman J. Violence against refugee women along the Thai–Burma border. Int J Gynaecol Obstet. 2013; https://doi.org/10.1016/j.ijgo.2012.10.015.

31. Srikanthan A, Reid RL. Religious and cultural influences on contraception. JOGC. 2008; https://doi.org/10.1016/S1701-2163(16)32736-0.

32. Brand G, Morrison P, Down B. How do health professionals support pregnant and young mothers in the community? A selective review of the research literature. Women Birth. 2014; https://doi.org/10.1016/j.wombi.2014.05.004.

33. LaMancuso K, Goldman RE, Nothnagle M. "Can I ask that?" perspectives on perinatal care after resettlement among Karen refugee women, medical providers and community-based doulas. J Immigr Minor Health. 2016; https://doi.org/10.1007/s10903-015-0172-6.

34. Patton GC, et al. Our future: a lancet commission on adolescent health and wellbeing. Lancet. 2016; https://doi.org/10.1016/S0140-6736(16)00579-1.

35. Bearinger LH, Sieving RE, Ferguson J, Sharma V. Global perspectives on the sexual and reproductive health of adolescents: patterns, prevention, and potential. Lancet. 2007; https://doi.org/10.1016/S0140-6736(07)60367-5.

36. Denno DM, Hoopes AJ, Chandra-Mouli V. Effective strategies to provide adolescent sexual and reproductive health services and to increase demand and community support. J Adolesc Health. 2015 Suppl 1; doi: https://doi.org/10.1016/j.jadohealth.2014.09.012.

15

Essential newborn care practices and associated factors among home delivered mothers in Damot pulasa Woreda, southern Ethiopia

Tesfaye Yitna Chichiabellu[1*], Baze Mekonnen[2], Feleke Hailemichael Astawesegn[3], Birhanu Wondimeneh Demissie[4] and Antehun Alemayehu Anjulo[5]

Abstract

Background: Globally 3.1 million children die each year in their neonatal period (first 28 days of life) according to World Health Organization (WHO) 2011 report. Half of these surprisingly occur within the first 24 h of delivery and 75% occur in the early neonatal period.

Methods: A community based cross-sectional study design was carried out from March 2016 to April, 2016 in Damot Pulasa district, Wolaita zone, Southern Ethiopia to assess selected essential newborn care practices and associated factors among home delivered mothers in Damot pulasa district. Data were entered into Epi Info version 3.5.1 and exported to SPSS version 20 software for analysis. Multiple logistic analyses were done to control possible confounding variable. A P-value less than 0.05 was taken as a significant association.

Result: The study showed that the prevalence of essential newborn care practice was 24%. Multivariate logistic regression analysis revealed that variables like ANC visit (AOR =0.213,P = 0.015,CI = 0.102–0.446),PNC visit (AOR = 0.209, P = 0.00,CI = 0.110–0.399), advice about essential newborn care practice (AOR =0.114,P = 0.0001, CI = 0.058–0.221),urban areas women (AOR =2,P = 0.042, CI = 1.024–3.693), planned pregnancy (AOR = 7, P = 0.00, CI =3.732–11.813), and knowledge about newborn danger signs (AOR = 0.277, P = 0.006, CI = 0.110–0.697) were the independent predictors of ENBC practices.

Conclusion: Generally, coverage of essential newborn care practices was low. ANC visit, advice about ENBC, PNC visit, residence, planned pregnancy and knowledge about newborn danger signs were predictors of essential newborn care practice in the study area. Therefore, Health facilities should enhance linkage with health posts to increase ANC and PNC service utilization. Health extension workers should also promote and give health education about pre-lacteal feeding, early bathing, planned pregnancy, newborn danger signs and application of materials on the newborn stump.

Keywords: Essential newborn care practice, Newborn

* Correspondence: yefaste2005@gmail.com
[1]Department of Nursing, College of Health Science and Medicine, Wolaita Sodo University, P.O.Box: 138, Wolaita Sodo, Ethiopia
Full list of author information is available at the end of the article

Plain English summary

Though many efforts had been made to overcome newborn mortality in Sub-Saharan Africa, it is continued to be great public health problems. Essential newborn care is a comprehensive strategy designed to improve the health of newborns through interventions before conception, during pregnancy, at and soon after birth, and in the postnatal period. Data associated with socio-demographic variables, maternal health services utilization, knowledge, counseling from a health worker, source of information, and traditional practices were collected. Even though majority of the women used boiled blade to cut the cord and tied with threads, application of butter on the umbilical stump practiced by most of the women. In addition to low coverage of initiation of breast feeding within one hour and giving colostrum, the majority, of the women in this study gave pre-lacteals. Bathing of the newborn after 24 h was practiced by the majority of the women. The level of coverage of essential newborn care practices in the district was generally low. The associated factors of essential newborn care practice were; ANC visit, advice about ENBC, PNC visit, residence, planned pregnancy and knowledge about newborn danger.

In conclusions; Health facilities should enhance linkage with health postse to increase antenatal and postnatal care service utilization. Health extension workers should also promote and give health education about pre-lacteal feeding, early bathing, planned pregnancy, newborn danger signs and application of materials on the newborn stump.

Background

Globally 3.1 million children die each year in their neonatal period (first 28 days of life) according to World Health Organization (WHO) 2011 report. Half of these surprisingly occur within the first 24 h of delivery and 75% occur in the early neonatal period (0 to 6 days after delivery) because of preterm births, severe infections and birth asphyxia [1]. Though many efforts had been made to overcome newborn mortality in Sub-Saharan Africa, it is continued to be great public health problems. Every year 2.9 million babies die during the neonatal period [2]; it is also the time of greatest risk for stillbirths and maternal deaths [3].

One of the targets of the MDG was a two-thirds reduction in infant and child mortality by 2015; it was intended to achieve by involving skilled birth attendants, increasing immunization coverage against six vaccine preventable diseases, improving the status of women through education, and enhancing women participation in the labor force [4].

Globally, around 40 million mothers give birth at home per year without any trained health worker. Factors like lack of good quality care during labor and birth;

socio-economic aspects of poverty; poor health status of women; lack of autonomy and decision making authority; and illiteracy to health system related factors like poor antenatal and obstetric care; absence of trained birth attendant; inadequate referral system; lack of transportation facilities; poor linkages between health centers and communities favored the morbidities and mortalities of pregnant women, perinatal and neonate [5]. In Ethiopia, according to Ethiopia Mini Demographic Health Survey 2014 report, only 15% of births take place at a health institution, 40% of women receive Antenatal Care (ANC) from a skilled provider, and 12% of women receive a postnatal care (PNC) within the first two days of birth [6]. This favors neonatal morbidity and mortality rates to be high in Ethiopia; around 122,000 newborns die every year and the neonatal mortality rate is 37 per 1000 live births [7, 8].

WHO recommended Essential Newborn Care (ENBC) practices to reduce the risk of the main causes of neonatal deaths in both community and facility deliveries [8]. ENBC is a comprehensive strategy designed to improve the health of newborns through interventions before conception, during pregnancy, at and soon after birth, and in the postnatal period [9].ENBC practices, as recommended by WHO, include drying (wiping) and wrapping the newborn immediately after birth, initiating skin-to-skin contact, dry cord care (not applying any potentially harmful substance to the umbilical cord), immediate initiation of breastfeeding and delayed bathing (for at least 6 h) [10].

Ethiopia government has been striving to achieve the 3rd Sustainable Development Goal (SDG3) which is to ensure healthy lives and promote well-being for all, at all ages [11]. However, the neonatal mortality rates in Damot pulasa is still remained higher than the national level; it is 38 per 1, 000 live births [12]. Thus, new innovative strategies must be developed for safe home deliveries including essential neonatal care in order to change the practice at the household level, besides devising means of proper care of the neonate in domestic settings and ensuring proper referral of those neonates who cannot be managed at home [13]. A study showed that home-based counseling strategy using volunteers and designed for scale-up can improve newborn care behaviors in rural communities [14].

Traditional Birth Attendants (TBAs), relatives, neighbors and other aged women from the community who lack the requisite knowledge of safe delivery and newborn care practices; Meanwhile, their intervention to support mothers who give birth at home is inevitable. This may increase maternal and newborn morbidity and mortality among home delivered mothers. Traditional practice like pre-lacteal feeding, avoiding of first milk and application of material on the newborn stump was practiced by the majority of study participant in the study area. Therefore, improving newborn survival is a major priority in child health today and the government sets universal sustainable development goals which state to end preventable deaths of newborns and under-five children by 2030. Therefore, this study aimed to assess selected essential newborn care practices and associated factors among home delivered mothers in Damot pulasa district.

Methods and materials

Study area

A community based cross-sectional study design was conducted from March 2016 to April 2016 in Damot Pulasa district, Wolaita zone, Southern Ethiopia. Damot Pulasa located at 365 Km from Addis Ababa, the capital city of Ethiopia. The population of the district was estimated to be 130,515 with an estimated number of women of reproductive age group 30,818 which is 23.6% of the total population. The town has an urban kebele and 22 rural kebeles, in terms of health facilities; there are 5 governmental health centers, 8 private clinics, 1 private pharmacy, 1 drug vender and 1urban and 22 rural health posts.

Populations

The study population was randomly selected women of reproductive age group who had given birth at home in the past one year in Damot Pulasa district which encompasses 450 women who participated in the study. Those mothers who had given live birth at home within one year preceding the data collection date included in the study. The source population was list of households who had women's in the reproductive age and who had given birth at home in Damot pulasa district.

Sample size determination

The required sample size was determined by using single population proportion formula by taking 23% of expected prevalence for essential newborn care practice [8], assuming 5% margin of error and 95% confidence level, design effect of 1.5 and 10% for non-response rate. The calculated sample size was 450.

Sampling technique and procedures

Cluster multi-stage sampling technique was employed for the Selection of the sampling units. In the district, there are 22 rural and an urban kebeles. From 22 rural kebeles10 were selected by simple random sampling. The total sample size was allocated for each selected kebeles proportionally to the number of households within each kebele. Then systematic sampling technique was used to select a household where participant exist. The index case was selected and interviewed using

lottery method when more than one eligible respondent present in a house.

Data collection tools and procedures

Data associated with socio-demographic variables, maternal health services utilization, knowledge, counseling from a health worker, source of information, and traditional practices were collected using interviewer administered questionnaire adapted from similar studies [8, 14, 18] (Additional file 1). The data were collected by B.Sc. nurses who are fluent speakers of the local languages.

Data processing and analysis

Data was checked visually for completeness, and then coded and entered in to Epi Info version 3.5.1 and exported in to Statistical Program Social Science (SPSS) version 20 software for analysis. Binary and multiple logistic regressions were run to assess the associations of various factors with essential newborn care practice. The results were presented in the form of tables, figures and summary statistics. A P-value less than 0.05 was taken as a significant association.

Results

Socio-demographiccharacterstics

In this study, a total of 450 women have participated and the response rate was 100%. In terms of religion, majority of the respondents were protestant, which accounts 238 (52.9%) and 434 (96.4%) were Wolaita in ethnicity. One hundred ninety-five (43.3%) were illiterate and 310 (68.9%) were housewife. With regard to marital status and place of residence, 444 (98.7%) were married and 393 (87.3%) were rural dweller (Table 1).

Maternal health services

A total of 364 (80.9%) of respondents belonged to the age group 19–41 years and the mean age of respondents was 30.8 ($\pm$ 4.05). Majority of the study subjects conceived their last baby unintentionally, which accounts 383 (85.1%). Thirty two (7.1%) received at least one ANC visit. From all mothers, 363 (80.7%) prepared themselves for birth. From the total study subjects, 120 (26.7%) utilized PNC service and from these mothers, 35 (29%) utilized the service within 7-41 days (Table 2).

Health service availability

Concerning health service availability, 318 (70.7%) mothers had health facilities (health post)in the nearby site. Home delivered mothers mentioned the following reasons why they gave birth at home; Two hundred eighty-three (62.9%) "Not seriously ill", 247 (54.9%) "Had TBAs", 126 (28%) "Unwelcoming of health workers approach" and 123 (27.3%) "An experience of safe home delivery before" Moreover, the majority of women

Table 1 Socio-demographic characteristics of the respondent in Damot pulasa district, Wolaita Zone, Southern Ethiopia, 2016

Variable	Frequency (n = 450)	Percentage (%)
Religion		
Protestant	238	52.9
Catholic	124	27.6
Orthodox	76	16.9
Muslim	12	2.7
Educational status		
No education	195	43.3
Primary level	175	38.9
Secondary level	67	14.9
Higher education	13	2.9
Ethnic group		
Wolaita	434	96.4
Gammo	8	1.8
Amhara	7	1.6
Gurage	1	.2
Occupation		
Housewife	310	68.9
Farmer	13	2.9
Merchant/Trade	100	22.2
Daily labor	27	6.0
Marital status		
Married	444	98.7
Widowed	6	1.3
Residence		
Urban	57	12.7
Rural	393	87.3
Age at current pregnancy		
< 20 years	2	0.4
20–34 years	364	80.9
34–49 years	84	18.7
Planned pregnancy		
Yes	67	14.9
No	383	85.1
Parity		
1	44	12.8
2–4	194	56.6
> = 5	105	30.6

Table 2 Maternal health services of respondents, in Damot pulasa district, Wolaita Zone, Southern, Ethiopia, 2016

Variable	Frequency (n = 450)	Percentage (%)
Receive ANC		
Yes	32	7.1
No	418	92.9
Number of ANC visit		
Once	13	40.6
Twice	10	31.25
Three times	6	18.75
Four times	3	9.4
Advice about ENBC		
Yes	32	7.1
No	418	92.9
Preparation for delivery		
Yes	363	80.7
No	87	19.3
Receive PNC		
Yes	120	26.7
No	330	73.3
Time for frequency of PNC		
Less than 4 h	12	10
4–23 h	20	16.7
1–2 days	27	22.5
3–6 days	26	21
7–41 days	35	29

(92.2%) women who had information about when to start breastfeeding, 141 (34%) mothers started breastfeeding within the first one hour of birth. From all mothers, 390 (86.7%) of them had knowledge about colostrum and 262 (67%) mothers mentioned the importance of colostrum. Four hundred six (90.2%) of women told that it is possible to expose the neonate for morning sunlight; In addition to this, 432 (96%) of women mentioned that, exposing the neonate for vaccination has no problem (Table 4) (Figs. 2 and 3).

Newborn care practice of the respondent

From all mothers, 408 (90.7%) remembered where they positioned the neonate immediately after delivery. Of all mothers, 259 (63.5%) put their newborn baby on their abdomen immediately after delivery (Table 5).

Safe cord cutting

Almost all mothers, 434 (96.4%) used boiled new razor blade in order to cut their newborn baby and 288 (64%) study subjects applied butter on the cord after the cord was cut.

participated in this study, 356 (79.1%) decided to deliver at home by themselves (Table 3) (Fig. 1).

Knowledge of the respondents

From the total study subjects, 417 (92.7%) of the women had information about newborn care. Among 415

Table 3 Health service utilization of respondents, in Damot pulasa district, Wolaita Zone, Southern Ethiopia, 2016

Variable	Frequency (n = 450)	Percentage (%)
Availability of HF		
Yes	450	100
Type of HF		
Health post	318	70.7
Health center	132	29.3
HF provide delivery		
Yes	227	50.4
No	179	39.8
I don't know	44	9.8
Decision for place of birth		
Self	356	79.1
Husband	77	17.1
Relatives	17	3.8

Initiation of early exclusive breastfeeding

From the total study subjects, 206 (45.8%) initiated breastfeeding within an hour of birth. From the total of 224 (49.8%) women who gave pre-lacteals, 218 (97.3%) gave water and 6 (2.7%) gave butter. Two hundred twenty three (49.6%) of the respondents gave first milk to the newborn and 247 (54.9%) mothers fed their breast greater than or equal to eight times.

Thermal care (bathing time)

From all mothers, 362 (80.4%) mothers dried/wrapped the newborn baby. Of whom 190 (52.2%) dried/wrapped the newborn before delivery of the placenta. One hundred sixty-six (45.6%) mothers used a pre-prepared towel to dry/wrap up the newborn. About 294 (65.3%) of them bathed the newborn after 24 h. The majority of study subjects, 249 (55.3%) mothers made skin to skin contact of mother and newborn.

The prevalence of essential newborn care practices

The prevalence of cord cutting, initiation of breastfeeding and thermal care practices were studied in this study. This study revealed that the prevalence of cord cutting, initiation of breastfeeding and thermal care practices were 434 (96.4%), 206 (45.8%) and 294 (65.3%) respectively (Fig. 4).

Associated factors of essential newborn care practices

In order to determine the association of independent variables with essential newborn care practices both bivariate and multivariate analysis were used. Variables that showed association with the outcome variables in the bivariate analysis were selected for multivariate analysis.

Crude analysis revealed that variables like ANC visit (COR 0.213, 95% CI: 0.102–0.446), advice about ENBC (COR 0.166, 95% CI: 0.078–0.354), PNC visit (COR0.135,95% CI:0.083–0.217), place of residence (COR2.244, 95% CI:1.251–4.025), planned pregnancy (COR 6.863, 95% CI: 3.943–11.943), birth preparedness (COR 3.511, 95% CI: 1.635–7.541), knowledge about newborn danger signs (COR 5.276, 95% CI: 2.232–12.471), and knowledge about newborn care (COR 1.892, 95% CI: 1.223–2.928) were felt to be the key predictors of essential

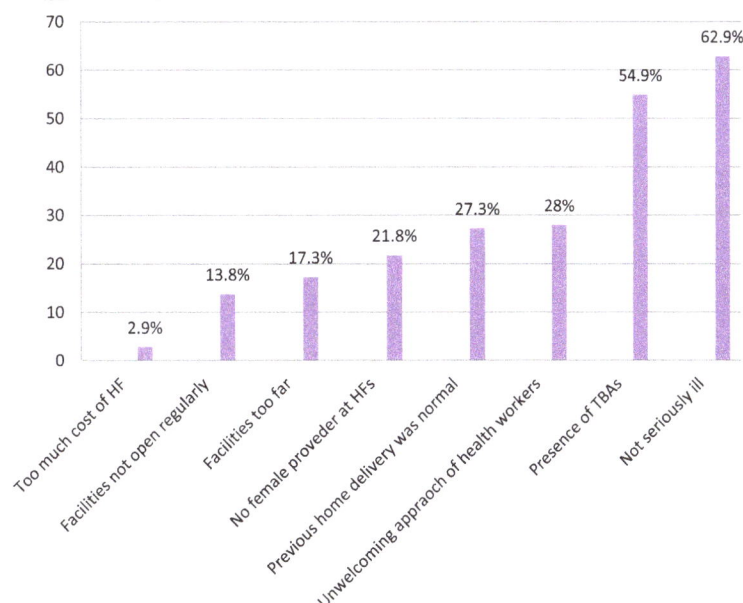

Fig. 1 Reasons of women not delivered at health facilities, in Damot pulasa district, Wolaita Zone, Southern Ethiopia, 2016

Table 4 Knowledge of the respondents, in Damot pulasa district, Wolaita Zone, Southern Ethiopia, 2016

Variable	Frequency (n = 450)	Percentage (%)
Information on newborn care		
Yes	417	92.7
No	33	7.3
Information to start breastfeeding		
Yes	415	92.2
No	35	7.8
Time to start breastfeeding		
First one hour	141	34.0
After one hour	274	66.0
Knowledge on first milk		
Yes	390	86.7
No	60	13.3
Advantage of first milk		
Advantageous	262	67.0
Disadvantageous	129	33.0
Expose neonate for morning sunlight		
Yes	406	90.2
No	44	9.8
Expose neonate for vaccination		
Yes	432	96.0
No	18	4.0
Information when to bath the neonate		
Yes	436	96.9
No	14	3.1
Time of bathing		
First 24 h	303	69.5
After 24 h	133	30.5
Knowledge about neonatal problems		
Good knowledge	87	19.3
Poor knowledge	363	80.7

newborn care practice and were used to form multivariable logistic regression analysis (Table 6).

Multivariate logistic regression was done for variables that had statistically significant association with essential newborn care practice in crude analysis. Multivariate logistic regression analysis revealed that variables like ANC visit (AOR 0.264, 95% CI:0.090–0.773), advice about essential newborn care practice (AOR 0.114, 95% CI:0.058–0.221), PNC visit (AOR 0.209, 95% CI:0.110–0.399), place of residence (AOR 2, 95% CI:1.024–3.693), planned pregnancy (AOR 7, 95% CI:3.732–11.813), and knowledge about newborn danger signs (AOR 0.277, 95% CI:0.110–0.697) were the independent predictors of essential newborn care practice after controlling the potential confounders (Table 6).

Discussion

Generally, in this study the coverage of essential newborn care practice was low. Even though majority of the women used boiled blade to cut the cord (96.4%) and tied with threads (98.2%), application of butter on the umbilical stump (64%) of the women practiced. I n addition to low coverage of initiation of breast feeding within one hour (45.8%) and giving colostrums (49.6%),the majority, (49.8%) of the women in this study gave pre-lacteals. Bathing of the newborn after 24 h was practiced by the majority (65.3%) of the women.

The prevalence of ENBC practice was 24% which was higher than the research done in Awebel district East Gojam Zone [8] which was 23.1% but which was much lower than the study conducted in Northwest Ethiopia, Mandura district [15] which was 41%. Cord cutting was practiced by the majority 96.4% of the women, using new blade, which was much higher than the study conducted in, Nawalparasi district of Nepal (48.31%) [16], Northern Ghana which revealed 90.8% [17], Sub urban areas of western Nigeria (90.3%) [18], study conducted in Northwest Ethiopia, Mandura district was (59.8%) [15],and the study conducted in four regions of Ethiopia which was 88.3% [6], the reason for this might be good awareness and custom followed in the study area but the finding was in line with the study conducted at Awebel district, East Gojam of Ethiopia (97.6%) [8]. Majority of the study participants (98.2%) the cord was tied with thread which was higher than the study conducted in the four regions of Ethiopia (48.5%) [6], this might be due to awareness in the study community. Even though majority of the women used boiled blade to cut the cord and tied with threads, application of butter on the umbilical stump (64%) of the women practiced in the study area which is higher than the study conducted in Northern Ghana (14.4%) and the study conducted in Northwest Ethiopia Mandura district was (18.18%) [15, 17] but which was lower than the study conducted in the four regions of Ethiopia (88.3%) [6].

Initiation of breastfeeding within one hour in the study area was 45.8% which was higher than the study conducted in rural Bangladesh (40%), East Gojam of Ethiopia (41.6%). This finding was not incongruent with the study conducted in India (65%), Nepal (51.3%), Northern Ghana (80%), Eastern Uganda (50%), Western Nigeria (65.3%), four regions of Ethiopia (52.1%), Northwest Ethiopia and Southwest Ethiopia (50%) [6, 15–21] respectively. The Majority, 49.8% of the women in this study gave pre-lacteals. The finding was higher as compared to study conducted in the four regions of Ethiopia (12.4%) gave pre-lacteals [6], but lower than the study conducted in East Gojam of Ethiopia Awebel district, 11.2% gave pre-lacteals [8]. The reason might be traditional beliefs of the community. Breastfeeding of the

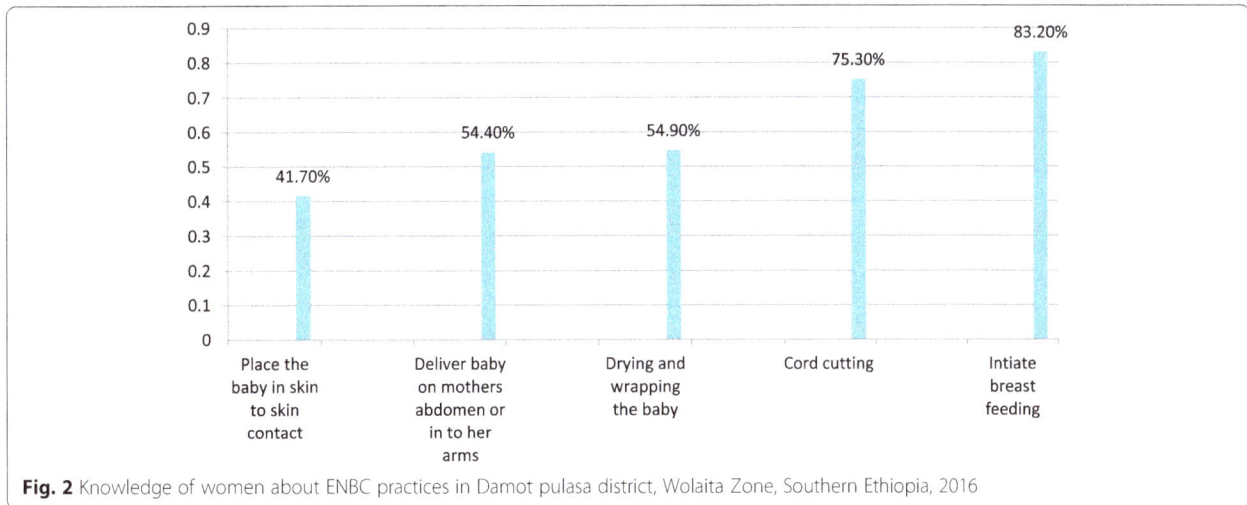

Fig. 2 Knowledge of women about ENBC practices in Damot pulasa district, Wolaita Zone, Southern Ethiopia, 2016

first milk (colostrum) was given (49.6%) of the women in the study area. This is lower than a case study of tribal women, Gujarat (63%) [22]. The reason for this was (33%) of the respondent believed that first milk was disadvantageous and from this (31%) believed that it would cause diarrhea,(60.5%) constipation and (58.9%) believed that it would decrease the growth of the newborn.

Bathing of the newborn after 24 h was practiced by the majority (65.3%) of the women in the study area which was in line with the study conducted in East Gojam of Ethiopia, Awebel district (65.6%) [8]. But this finding was lower than study conducted in Northern Ghana (93.6%), Rural Nepal (72.2%), South Sudan (99%), Easter Uganda (100%), Western Nigeria (98.2%), study conducted in four regions of Ethiopia (74.7%) [6, 16–18, 20, 23].

In this study women who didn't get ANC visit were 73.6% less likely to practiced essential newborn care practice as compared to those who initiated ANC visit (AOR = 0.213,P = 0.015,CI = 0.102–0.446), which is

supported by the study conducted in Northern Ghana which suggested that women who initiated ANC visit were two times more likely to practiced essential newborn care practice as compared to women who initiated ANC visit late [17]. This might be due to women who attended ANC have the chance of getting information about the components and the importance of newborn care practice from health care providers.

The finding of this study also showed that women who didn't get PNC visit early were 79% less likely practiced ENBC when compared to women who didn't get immediate PNC visit (AOR = 0.209, P = 0.00,CI = 0.110–0.399). This finding was supported by the study conducted in rural communities of Awebel district, East Gojam of Ethiopia, which stated that immediate PNC visit was statistically significant with ENBC practice of women and those women who had got immediate PNC visit after delivery were 3.2 times more likely to practice ENBC when compared with those who had not got immediate PNC after delivery [8]. This could be health extension workers

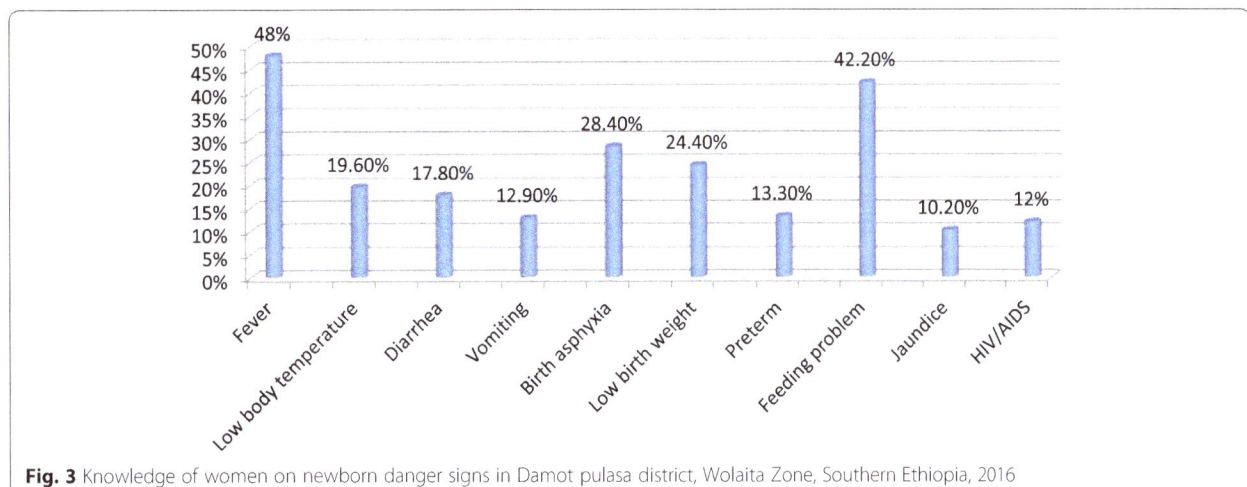

Fig. 3 Knowledge of women on newborn danger signs in Damot pulasa district, Wolaita Zone, Southern Ethiopia, 2016

Table 5 Newborn care practices of respondents, in Damot pulasa district, Wolaita Zone, Southern Ethiopia, 2016

Variable	Frequency (n = 450)	Percentage (%)
Position the neonate		
Yes	408	90.7
No	42	9.3
Place of positioning the neonate		
On the mother's abdomen	259	63.5
Near the delivery surface	86	21.1
On another bed separately	52	12.7
Transferred to father/relatives	9	2.2
I don't remember	2	.5
Dry/wrapping the neonate		
Yes	362	80.4
No	88	19.6
Time of dry/wrap the neonate		
Before delivery of placenta	190	52.2
Immediately after delivery of placenta	169	46.4
I did not remember	5	1.4
Material used for dry/wrap the neonate		
Pre-prepared towel	166	45.6
Piece of blanket/Gabi	72	19.8
Available material	126	34.6
Material used to cut the cord		
Boiled /un-boiled new razor blade	434	96.4
Used razor blade	16	3.6
Remember material used to tie the cord		
Yes	442	98.2
No	8	1.8
Material used to tie the cord		
Thread	442	100
Apply material after cord cutting		
Yes	288	64.0
No	162	36.0
Type of material applied on the cord		
Butter	288	100
Initiate exclusive breastfeeding		
Yes	226	50.2
No	224	49.8
Time of initiating exclusive breastfeeding		
First one hour	206	45.8
After one hour	244	54.2
Give pre lacteals		
Yes	224	49.8
No	226	50.2
Pre-lacteals given		

Table 5 Newborn care practices of respondents, in Damot pulasa district, Wolaita Zone, Southern Ethiopia, 2016 (Continued)

Variable	Frequency (n = 450)	Percentage (%)
Water	218	97.3
Butter	6	2.7
Give first milk		
Yes	223	49.6
No	227	50.4
Frequency of breastfeeding		
< 8 times	203	45.1
> = 8 times	247	54.9
Remember time of bathing		
Yes	442	98.2
No	8	1.8
Time of bathing		
First 24 h	156	34.7
After 24 h	294	65.3
Skin to skin contact		
Yes	249	55.3
No	201	44.7

and community health workers might gave proper advice about essential newborn care practice.

Those mothers who had got ENBC advice during ANC visit or other meetings were 83.4% more likely practiced ENBC practice as compared to women who did not got the advice (AOR =0.114, P = 0.0001, CI = 0.058–0.221). It was supported by study done, Awebel district which showed that women who had got advice about ENBC practices during monthly pregnant mothers' group meeting were 4.8 times more likely to practice ENBC as compared with those women who had not got advice about ENBC practices during monthly meeting [8]. The reason could be the health care providers could discuss about essential newborn care practice during ANC visit.

In this study, urban areas women were two times more likely practiced ENBC practice when compared to rural areas women (AOR =2, P = 0.042, CI = 1.024–3.693). The finding was supported by a study conducted in Mandura district which stated that women in urban areas were three times more likely to have good newborn care practices as compared to rural areas [15]. This might be due to accessibilities of health service and good knowledge secondary to better educational status of urban women when compared to rural areas women.

Those women who planned there pregnancy were seven times more likely practiced newborn care when compared to women who did not plan their pregnancy (AOR = 7, P = 0.00, CI =3.732–11.813). The reason for

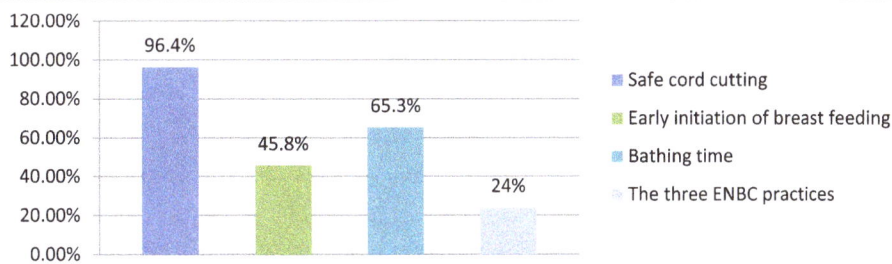

Fig. 4 Distribution of the three essential newborn care practices, in Damot pulasa district, Wolaita Zone, Southern Ethiopia, 2016

this could be women who had planned pregnancy might be more likely to use maternal and child health services.

The study showed that those women who were knowledge about newborn danger signs practiced ENBC 72% more likely when compared to women who had poor knowledge about newborn danger signs (AOR = 0.277, P = 0.006, CI = 0.110–0.697). This finding was supported by the study conducted in rural areas of Northern Ghana which states that women who could mention at least four danger signs of the neonates were four times more likely to give good neonatal feeding to their babies [17]. This could be most of the women in the sample may not have adequate knowledge about newborn care. This might be due to majority of the women did not get an adequate message about newborn care during antenatal care follow up. Findings in this study should be interpreted in the light of the inherent limitations of the study. Recall bias was a possibility since the women were

Table 6 Factors associated with the three essential newborn care practices by bivariate and multiple logistic analyses in Damot pulasa district, Wolaita Zone, Southern Ethiopia, 2016

Variable	ENBCP		COR	AOR
	Yes (%)	No (%)		
Receive ANC				
Yes	18	14	1	1
No	90	328	0.213(0.102–0.446)	0.264(0.090–0.773)*
Advice about ENBC				
Yes	19	13	1	1
No	61	252	0.166(0.078–0.354)	0.114(0.058–0.221)*
Receive PNC				
Yes	64	56	1	1
No	44	286	0.135(0.083–0.217)	0.209(0.110–0.399)*
Residence				
Urban	22	35	2.244(1.251–4.025)	2(1.024–3.693)*
Rural	86	307	1	1
Planned pregnancy				
Yes	40	27	6.863(3.943–11.943)	7(3.732–11.813)*
No	68	315	1	1
Birth preparedness				
Yes	8	75	3.511(1.635–7.541)	0.467(0.200–1.087)
No	100	267	1	1
Knowledge about newborn danger signs				
Good knowledge	6	102	5.276(2.232–12.471)	0.277(0.110–0.697)*
Poor knowledge	81	261	1	1
Knowledge about newborn care				
Good knowledge	49	209	1.892(1.223–2.928)	0.760(0.460–1.257)
Poor knowledge	59	133	1	1

inquired about events which occurred during a two year period. However, the questioning was focused on the most recent experiences of essential newborn care practices in order to minimize this possibility.

Conclusions

In this study, the level of coverage of essential newborn care practices in the district was generally low. Traditional practice like: pre-lacteal feeding, avoiding of first milk and application of material on the newborn stump were practiced by majority of study participant in the study area. This finding also revealed that most essential newborn interventions were not reaching the newborns. ANC visit, advice about ENBC, PNC visit, residence, planned pregnancy and knowledge about newborn danger signs were predictors of essential newborn care practice in the study area. Therefore Damot pulasa district health office should promote strong community based behavior change communication on the importance of ENBC practices to change the poor ENBC practices in the study area. Health facilities should enhance linkage with health posts to increase ANC and PNC service utilization. Health extension workers should promote and give health education about pre-lacteal feeding, early bathing, planned pregnancy, newborn dander signs and application of materials on the newborn stump.

Abbreviations

ANC: Anti Natal Care; EDHS: Ethiopian Demographic and Health Survey; ENBC: Essential Newborn Care; MDG: Millennium Development Goal; NMR: Neonatal Mortality Rate; PNC: Post Natal Care; SDG: Sustainable Development Goal; SPSS: Statistical Program Social Science

Acknowledgments

We would like to thank Addis Ababa University and Wolaita Sodo University. Our gratitude also extends to Wolaita zone health department and Damot pulasa district health office for their unreserved cooperation.

Funding

Addis Ababa University.

Authors' contributions

TY was involved in conception, designing the study, writing proposal, analysis interpretation of data and manuscript writing. BW, AA and FH were involved in designing the study, analysis, interpretation of data and manuscript writing. All authors agreed to be accountable for all aspects of the work.

Competing interest

We declared no financial, personal or professional competing interests influenced this paper.

Authors Information

[1]Lecturer in Department of Nursing, College of Health Science and Medicine, Wolaita Sodo University.
[2]Lecturer in Department of Nursing, School of nursing and midwifery, Addis Ababa University,
[3]Assistant Professor in School of Public Health, College of Medicine and Health Science, Hawassa University.
[4]Lecturer in Department of Nursing, College of Health Science and Medicine, Wolaita Sodo University.
[5]Lecturer in Department of Medical Laboratory, College of Health Science and Medicine, Wolaita Sodo University.

Author details

[1]Department of Nursing, College of Health Science and Medicine, Wolaita Sodo University, P.O.Box: 138, Wolaita Sodo, Ethiopia. [2]Department of Nursing, School of nursing and midwifery, Addis Ababa University, Addis Ababa, Ethiopia. [3]School of Public Health, College of Medicine and Health Science, Hawassa University, Hawassa, Ethiopia. [4]Department of Nursing, College of Health Science and Medicine, Wolaita Sodo University, Sodo, Ethiopia. [5]Department of Medical Laboratory, College of Health Science and Medicine, Wolaita Sodo University, Sodo, Ethiopia.

References

1. WHO, PMNCH. A Global Review of the Key Interventions Related to Reproductive, Maternal, Newborn and Child Health (RMNCH). Geneva: WHO and the Partnership for Maternal Newborn & child health (PMNCH); 2011.
2. UN Inter-agency Group for Child Mortality Estimations. Levels and trends in child mortality. In: Estimates developed by the UN inter-agency Group for Child Mortality Estimation. New York: UN IGME; 2013.
3. Pattinson R, Kerber K, Buchmann E, Friberg IK, Belizan M, Lansky S, et al. Stillbirths: how can health systems deliver for mothers and babies? Lancet. 2011;377:1610–23.
4. World Health Organization: Estimates.In State of the World's Newborns. Washington, DC: Saving Newborn Lives, Save the Children/ USA; 2001:1–49.
5. Save the Children 2014. Ending newborn deaths: Ensuring every baby survives. 2014. [https://www.savethechildren.net/sites/default/files/libraries/ENDING-NEWBORN-DEATHS.pdf]. Accessed 3 Mar 2014.
6. Callaghan-koru JA, Seifu A, Tholandi M, De G-j J, Daniel E, Rawlins B, et al. Newborn care practices at home and in health facilities in 4 regions of Ethiopia. BMC Pediatr. 2013;13(198).
7. Central Statistical Agency and ICF International. Ethiopia Demographic and Health Survey 2011. Addis Ababa, and Maryland. https://dhsprogram.com/pubs/pdf/fr255/fr255.pdf. Accessed Mar 2014.
8. Kokebie T, et al. Community Based Essential Newborn Care Practices and Associated Factors among Women in the Rural Community of Awabel District. Int J Adv Sci Res. 2015;01(01):17–27.
9. Narayanan I, Rose M, Cordero D, Faillace S, Sanghvi T. Perinatal / neonatal essential newborn care. Virginia: Basics Support Institutionalizing Child Surviv Proj (BASICS II) United States Agency Int Dev Arlington; 2004.
10. WHO. Pregnancy, Childbirth, Postpartum and Newborn Care: A Guide for Essential Practice. Geneva: WHO Press World Health Organization; 2006.
11. Shiff man J. Issue attention in global health: the case of newborn survival. Lancet. 2010;375:2045–9.
12. Liu L, et al. Global, regional, and national causes of child mortality: an updated systematic analysis for 2010 with time trends since 2000. Lancet. 2012;379(9832):2151–61.
13. Central Statistical Agency. Ethiopia Mini Demographic and Health Survey. Addis Ababa; 2014.

14. Penfold S, Manzi F, Mkumbo E, Temu S, Jaribu J, D Shamba D, Mshinda H, Cousens S, Marchant T, Tanner M, SchellenbergDandSchellenberg J. Effect of home-based counselling on newborn care practices in southern Tanzania one year after implementation: a cluster-randomised controlled trial. BMC Pediatr. 2014;14:187.

15. Tegene T, Andargie G, Nega A, Yimam K. Newborn care practice and associated factors among mothers who gave birth within one year in Mandura District, Northwest Ethiopia. Clinics Mother Child Health. 2015;12: 172. https://doi.org/10.4172/2090-7214.1000172.

16. Kaphle HP, Yadav DK, Neupane N, Sharma B. Newborn care practices in rural communities of Nawalparasi District , Nepal. JHAS. 2013;3(1):35–9.

17. Saaka M, Iddrisu M. Patterns and determinants of essential newborn care practices in rural areas of northern Ghana. Int J Popul Res. 2014;(5):1–10.

18. Adelaja LM. A survey of home delivery and newborn care practices among women in a suburban area of Western Nigeria. ISRN Obstet Gynecol. 2011; 2011:9.

19. Vijayalakshmi S, Patil R, Datta SS. Community-based study on newborn care practices and its determinants in rural Pondicherry,India. J Neonatal Biol. 2014;3:158. https://doi.org/10.4172/2167-0897.1000158.

20. Waiswa P, Peterson S, Tomson G, Pariyo GW. Poor newborn care practices - a population based survey in eastern Uganda. BMC Pregnancy Childbirth. 2010;10:9.

21. Debelew GT, Afework MF, Yalew AW. Determinants and causes of neonatal mortality in Jimma zone, Southwest Ethiopia: a multilevel analysis of prospective follow up study. PLoS One. 2014;9(9):e107184. https://doi.org/10.1371/journal.pone.0107184.

22. Shah BD, Dwivedi LK. Newborn care practices: a case study of tribal women, Gujarat. Health. 2013;05(08):29–40.

23. Rosales AC, Hedrick JA, Cherian DT, Moore EC, Brown KM, Walumbe E. Essential newborn care in rural settings: the case of Warrap state in South Sudan. African Evaluation Journal. 2014;2(1) Art. #80, 6 pages. https://doi.org/10.4102/ aej.v2i1.80.

16

The feasibility of task-sharing the identification, emergency treatment, and referral for women with pre-eclampsia by community health workers in India

Umesh Charanthimath[1], Marianne Vidler[2], Geetanjali Katageri[3*], Umesh Ramadurg[4], Chandrashekhar Karadiguddi[1], Avinash Kavi[1], Anjali Joshi[1], Geetanjali Mungarwadi[1], Sheshidhar Bannale[5], Sangamesh Rakaraddi[6], Diane Sawchuck[7], Rahat Qureshi[8], Sumedha Sharma[2], Beth A. Payne[2], Peter von Dadelszen[9], Richard Derman[10], Laura A. Magee[9], Shivaprasad Goudar[1], Ashalata Mallapur[3], Mrutyunjaya Bellad[1], and the Community Level Interventions for Pre-eclampsia (CLIP) India Feasibility Working Group, Zulfiqar Bhutta, Sheela Naik, Anis Mulla, Namdev Kamle, Vaibhav Dhamanekar, Sharla K. Drebit, Chirag Kariya, Tang Lee, Jing Li, Mansun Lui, Asif R. Khowaja, Domena K. Tu and Amit Revankar

From 2nd International Conference on Maternal and Newborn Health: Translating Research Evidence to Practice
Belagavi, India.

Abstract

Background: Hypertensive disorders are the second highest direct obstetric cause of maternal death after haemorrhage, accounting for 14% of maternal deaths globally. Pregnancy hypertension contributes to maternal deaths, particularly in low- and middle-income countries, due to a scarcity of doctors providing evidence-based emergency obstetric care. Task-sharing some obstetric responsibilities may help to reduce the mortality rates. This study was conducted to assess acceptability by the community and other healthcare providers, for task-sharing by community health workers (CHW) in the identification and initial care in hypertensive disorders in pregnancy.

Methods: This study was conducted in two districts of Karnataka state in south India. A total of 14 focus group discussions were convened with various community representatives: women of reproductive age ($N = 6$), male decision-makers ($N = 2$), female decision-makers ($N = 3$), and community leaders ($N = 3$). One-to-one interviews were held with medical officers ($N = 2$), private healthcare OBGYN specialists ($N = 2$), senior health administrators ($N = 2$), Taluka (county) health officers ($N = 2$), and obstetricians ($N = 4$). All data collection was facilitated by local researchers familiar with the setting and language. Data were subsequently transcribed, translated and analysed thematically using NVivo 10 software.

(Continued on next page)

* Correspondence: geetanjali_mk@yahoo.co.in
[3]Department of Obstetrics and Gynaecology, S Nijalingappa Medical College, Bagalkot, Karnataka, India
Full list of author information is available at the end of the article

(Continued from previous page)

Results: There was strong community support for home visits by CHW to measure the blood pressure of pregnant women; however, respondents were concerned about their knowledge, training and effectiveness. The treatment with oral antihypertensive agents and magnesium sulphate in emergencies was accepted by community representatives but medical practitioners and health administrators had reservations, and insisted on emergency transport to a higher facility. The most important barriers for task-sharing were concerns regarding insufficient training, limited availability of medications, the questionable validity of blood pressure devices, and the ability of CHW to correctly diagnose and intervene in cases of hypertensive disorders of pregnancy.

Conclusion: Task-sharing to community-based health workers has potential to facilitate early diagnosis of the hypertensive disorders of pregnancy and assist in the provision of emergency care. We identified some facilitators and barriers for successful task-sharing of emergency obstetric care aimed at reducing mortality and morbidity due to hypertensive disorders of pregnancy.

Keywords: Task-sharing, Community health workers, Pre-eclampsia, Blood pressure, Antihypertensives, Magnesium sulphate

Background

Globally, maternal mortality has fallen by 45% over the past two decades [1]. Since 1990, India has made significant progress in reducing the maternal mortality ratio by 68.7%. The latest estimate calculated by the World Bank was 174 per 100,000 live births. Furthermore, there has been a substantial increase in accessing antenatal care and delivery in hospital [2, 3]. Nevertheless, India accounts for 15% of global maternal deaths annually [4].

Hypertensive disorders of pregnancy (HDP) are some of the main causes of maternal death globally, and, in India, are estimated to cause 7.1% of maternal mortality. Symptomatic HDP, including pre-eclampsia, gestational hypertension and chronic hypertension, often occur late in pregnancy. Repeated blood pressure (BP) monitoring is advised in pregnancy for early detection of hypertension which would optimise outcomes [5]. Women with HDP require enhanced surveillance by appropriately trained healthcare professionals providing evidence-based care (including clinical, laboratory and ultrasound assessments) to guide timing of delivery along with initiation of life-saving therapies (use of oral antihypertensive and magnesium sulphate).

Targets for many health indicators are not met as expected and hence it is important to explore means of strengthening the health system. One of the barriers to providing universal coverage of health services is the inadequacies of health care professionals, especially in many low and middle Income countries (LMICs) [6]. In 2005, the World Health Organization (WHO) estimated that more than 90% percent of maternal deaths are avoidable with moderate levels of health care and task-sharing or shifting. Task-shifting, as defined by the WHO, is when "specific tasks are moved, where appropriate, from highly qualified health workers to health workers with shorter training and fewer qualifications in order to make more efficient use of available resources for health". Task-sharing is a strategy in which health care workers take on

additional duties with sufficient training and supervision [7]. Sharing of tasks from health professionals to community health workers (CHW) can improve access to care and optimize the use of limited human resources in many resource-poor settings [8]. "Task-sharing" the serial measurement of blood pressure, risk stratification, and initiation of both life-saving therapies and referral, may be effective in reducing HDP associated morbidity and mortality and serve to bridge the gap of health service delivery to women residing in rural India. This study aims to better understand the facilitators and barriers to implementation of this strategy in Karnataka, India.

Study area

This study was conducted in Belagavi and Bagalkote districts of rural Karnataka, in South India (Fig. 1). The healthcare infrastructures of Karnataka are inadequate for serving the rural and remote areas where there are health worker shortages and large distances from health facilities [3]. The National Rural Health Mission (NRHM) has instituted community health worker programmes throughout the region to increase service utilisation in the hope of improving health outcomes [3]. For study site characteristics, see Table 1.

Community health workers

Community health workers in India include Auxiliary Nurse Midwives (ANM) and Accredited Social Health Activists (ASHA). ANMs provide care at the sub-centre, covering a population of 3000 to 5000 [9]. ANMs are trained in various topics related to maternal and child health, such as the provision of antenatal care, skilled attendance at delivery, postpartum care, and the management of pregnancy complications. NRHM guidelines from 2012 are used to train and authorise ANMs to administer 50% magnesium sulphate for cases of severe pre-eclampsia and eclampsia [10]. In 2005, the Government of India launched the ASHA programme to bring door-to-door

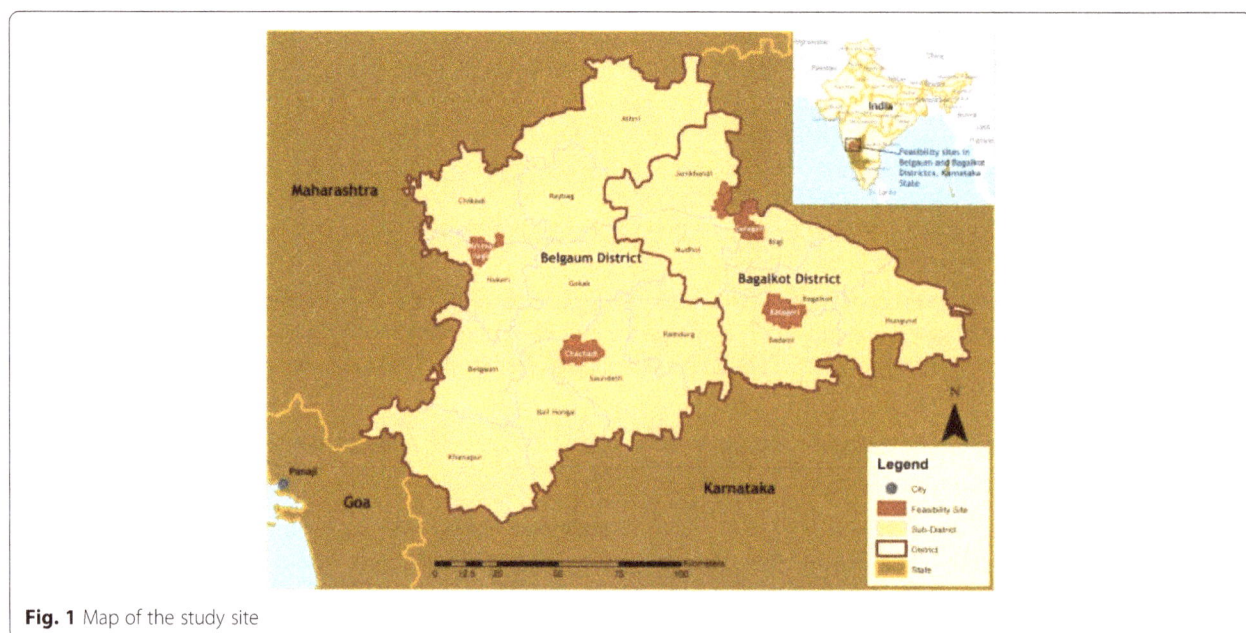

Fig. 1 Map of the study site

health services to rural areas. ASHAs are females between the ages of 25 to 45 years, with an education equivalent to grade eight or higher, who are selected by the local government to serve in their residential areas. Each ASHA extends her services to a population of about 1000 individuals. ASHAs are trained to provide health care advice in the homes (provision of basic maternity care, child care and nutrition counselling), create community health awareness, conducting social mobilisation, treatment of infections, maintenance of health records and increase utilization of existing health services. ASHAs are trained in district training centres for a period of 4 weeks with the upgrading of knowledge being done by the Lady Health Visitors and Medical Officers of the respective primary health centres. ASHAs have been deemed to bridge the gap between the community, ANMs, primary health centres, and referral facilities [11].

Table 1 Site characteristics

	India	South India	Karnataka
Site characteristics			
Population	1028,610,328[a]		61095297[d]
# States	35	5	(30 Districts)
Dominant religion	Hindu[c]	Hindu[c]	Hindu[c]
Women's literacy	55%[c]	68%[c]	58%[c]
Employment	36% currently employed[c]	41% currently employed[c]	40% currently employed[c]
Rural /Urban	32% urban[a]		39% urban[d]
Fertility rate	2.8[c]	1.9[c]	2.1[c]
Maternal mortality ratio	178 per 100,000 live births[b]	105 per 100,000 live births[a]	144 per 100,000 live births[a]
Maternal health care utilization			
ANY ANC	76.4%[c]	94%[c]	89%[c]
≥ 4 ANC	48%[c]	89%[c] (3+)	76%[c](3+)
Facility delivery (%)	39%[c]	79%[c]	65%[c]
Skilled attendant at delivery	47%[c]	84%[c]	70%[c]

[a]World Health Organization Country Profile: India 2012
[b]Office of the Registrar of India, 2013
[c]Demographic Health Survey 2013
[d]Rural Health Statistics in India 2012

Methods

This qualitative study was conducted as part of a larger country assessment in the preparation of a cluster randomized control trial, the Community Level Interventions for Pre-eclampsia (CLIP) Trial (NCT01911494).

This study consisted of focus group discussions (FGD) and in-depth interviews (IDI). FGDs were preferred to encourage group dialogue from all participants. Researchers selected various participant groups including community leaders, male and female decision-makers and women of reproductive age. The community leaders are representatives from the local government or other members who are held in high esteem by the community. They play an important role in decision-making, affecting their respective locality. The male and female decision-makers were the family members who took responsibility for healthcare related decisions for the family. In-depth interviews were conducted with medical officers, senior health administrators and obstetricians from both private and government institutions. These groups were chosen to represent the spectrum of the communities' and health care providers' views (Table 2). Fourteen FGDs and twelve IDIs were conducted between January and March 2013. Data saturation was noted after these interviews and FGDs.

Local clinicians and researchers with the knowledge of cultural nuances and dynamics, with no known association with the respondents, were chosen and trained for qualitative study methods to facilitate interviews and focus group discussions. Focus group and interview guides were developed for the study and were semi-structured to promote a natural discussion progression. The FGDs were conducted in the local language, *Kannada*, to best promote interaction with participants and obtain the richest data. All FGDs were facilitated by one researcher and assisted by a second researcher who recorded field notes including non-verbal communication. IDIs were conducted in English. All FGDs and IDIs were audio recorded. The first FGD incorporating 55 women of reproductive age was conducted as a pilot to sensitise the local research team regarding effective ways of data collection in qualitative research.

The remaining stakeholder groups were convened separately and comprised a varied number of participants (between seven and eighteen). Participants were identified through local health system networks of ASHA and ANMs. Male and female decision-makers in the family were approached for participation when they accompanied women of reproductive age to local health centres.

All audio recordings were later transcribed verbatim and translated into English for analysis, with the incorporation of field notes. Data were analysed using NVivo 10 software. Transcripts were coded by one rater (MV),

Table 2 Characteristics of focus group participants

#	Stakeholder Group	District	Education status				Total Participants
			A	B	C	D	
1	Community Leaders	Bagalkote	0	6	1	0	7
2	Community Leaders	Bagalkote	1	8	1	0	10
3	Community Leaders	Belagavi	–	–	–	10	10
4	Male Decision-Makers	Bagalkote	3	3	2	0	8
5	Male Decision-Makers	Belagavi	0	9	2	0	11
6	Female Decision-Makers	Bagalkote	8	2	0	0	10
7	Female Decision-Makers	Belagavi	12	4	2	0	18
8	Female Decision-Makers	Belagavi	11	2	0	0	13
9	Women of Reproductive Age	Belagavi	–	–	–	55	55
10	Women of Reproductive Age	Bagalkote	0	15	1	0	16
11	Women of Reproductive Age	Bagalkote	3	8	3	0	14
12	Women of Reproductive Age	Belagavi	0	15	2	0	17
13	Women of Reproductive Age	Belagavi	3	8	3	0	14
14	Women of Reproductive Age	Belagavi	0	10	6	0	16
			41 (18.7%)	90 (41.1%)	23 (10.5%)	65 (29.68%)	
TOTAL							219

A – Illiterate
B- Primary/Secondary Schooling
C – Pre university / University
D – Don't Know

after which all coded transcripts and themes were cross-checked by the local research team to resolve or clarify any misinterpretation. Using deductive reasoning, results were then grouped into predetermined key themes. During analysis, inductive reasoning was used to incorporate new and unexpected ideas. This produced a comprehensive analysis structure to reflect the richness and variety of responses.

Results

Participants in the community leaders FGD had diverse backgrounds: some were illiterate with no formal schooling while others had completed university education or college. They ranged in age between 24 and 51 years. Male decision-makers were aged between 18 to 57 years; 85% were illiterate, most identified themselves as labourers and farmers and were often the husband or father/father-in-law of the pregnant woman. Female decision-makers were 28 to 65 years of age, most had no formal schooling and could not read or write (71%), and the majority identified themselves as housewives and mothers-in-law. Women of reproductive age had an average age of 23 years, nearly all of them were housewives (91%), most were pregnant at the time of data collection (79%), and over half (66%) had at least one child under the age of five.

Two IDIs were conducted with medical officers, each responsible for one primary health centre which serves as the entry point to the health system. Senior district health system administrators ($N = 4$) were invited to participate, as they coordinate reproductive health services throughout the district and have a unique perspective. They are actively involved in the implementation of reproductive and child health services by local, state and central government. Three were obstetricians and gynaecologists; and one, a general surgeon.

Two obstetricians from secondary and four from tertiary facilities serving in the private and government sectors, with varying experience and training were interviewed. They provided specialist care to women coming from the study area. For more participant details, see Table 2 and Table 3.

Home blood pressure monitoring visits by ASHA workers

Most community leaders agreed that ASHAs could safely measure BP in the home; however, some had concerns regarding their knowledge, education, effectiveness, training, experience and supervision. Overall, there was an acceptance of ASHAs being tasked with the measurement of BP at home once they were appropriately trained.

"In the future, ASHAs might do if they are well educated and trained about BP measurement" (Community Leader)

"A life is dependent on appropriate BP measurement. How will you come to know that ASHAs have understood? It is not possible. Is there any exam?" (Community Leader)

Nearly all decision-makers agreed that a shift of this activity to ASHAs would be acceptable in their communities. In contrast, one group of male decision-makers strongly opposed this suggestion and argued that they would be unable to judge if an ASHA had not been properly trained and the possibility of a misdiagnosis was high.

"Because even a MBBS qualified person who has studied for 4-5 years cannot do it, then how can an SSLC graduate do...if training would suffice then everybody would have taken training" (Male Decision-Maker)

Table 3 Characteristics of In-depth Interview participants

#	Stakeholder	Training	Level of Care	Pregnancies/ Week
1	Medical Officer	MBBS	Primary	50–60
2	Medical Officer	MBBS	Primary	10–15
3	Private Practitioner	MBBS, MD in OBG	Tertiary	40–50
4	Private Practitioner	MBBS, MD in OBG	Tertiary	280–300
5	Senior Health Administrator	MS General Surgery	NA	NA
6	Senior Health Administrator	MBBS & Diploma in OBG	NA	NA
7	Taluka Health Officer	MBBS, Diploma in OBG	Secondary	200–250
8	Taluka Health Officer	MBBS & Diploma OBG	Secondary	50–60
9	Obstetrician	MBBS, MD in OBG	Tertiary	250
10	Obstetrician	MBBS, DGO, MD in OBG	Tertiary	200–300
11	Obstetrician	MBBS, Diploma in OBG	Tertiary	45
12	Obstetrician	MBBS, MD in OBG	Tertiary	–

Two Medical officers and three obstetricians expressed confidence in ASHAs measuring BP if they were provided with a reliable easy-to-use digital device. Some obstetricians who were already using a digital apparatus spoke about the problems associated with these devices, such as erroneous readings, battery life and expressed concern whether ASHAs would be able to overcome these challenges. These practitioners did not comment on the technique required to measure accurate BP. They appeared to feel strongly that this job requires experience and qualification; and less-educated or under-trained workers like ASHAs could not do it effectively.

Most Women of reproductive age were happy to accept ASHAs for recording blood pressure at home. Health administrators did not support BP measurement by ASHAs. Private practitioners were not familiar with the capabilities of the ASHA workers and had no opinion or suggestions to make.

Initiation of treatment with oral antihypertensive by ANMs

All community leaders and male decision maker supported treatment by ANMs except two, who strongly opposed treatment. The remaining participants supported this task-sharing by ANMs, but stressed the need for swift transport to the higher facility for further management. These respondents believed that ANMs had been adequately trained to provide oral emergency treatment but there should be someone who takes the responsibility for training and supervision.

"In my opinion, not all ANMs are experienced especially newly appointed ones. Some ANMs are experienced, such ANMs should be designated to give the medicines when the doctor is not there".
(Community Leader)

"No......No.... Who will do that? They cannot give treatment in an emergency"

(Male Decision-Maker)

The women of reproductive age were ready to accept medications from ANMs in emergency situations. Some obstetricians accepted the new role for the ANM; however, some voiced concerns regarding their ability to manage side-effects resulting from the use of the medication. All obstetricians emphasised the importance of proper training and urgent referral.

"I don't support this. Methyldopa causes sedation so before giving that drug we convince them, we counsel them. So the same thing is done by ANM they will

have to be well educated of everything" (OBGYN tertiary care hospital)

Administration of magnesium sulphate loading dose by ANMs

Community leaders accepted that with proper training, ANMs could be permitted to administer magnesium sulphate treatment in urgent cases. They expressed that such an emergency intervention might increase the likelihood of a woman's survival before she reaches a referral centre. Female decision-makers and women of reproductive age expressed strong acceptance for receiving treatment from ANMs and expressed faith in care by ANMs. Obstetricians supported the administration of a loading dose of magnesium sulphate as it is safe intervention, needs no extensive monitoring and believed that it would reduce the complications associated with preeclampsia and eclampsia. All groups were in favour of giving magnesium sulphate but stressed appropriate training. A few mentioned that ANMs should contact a medical officer before giving the treatment and arrange for transport. Health administrators emphasised the importance of ensuring uninterrupted availability of drugs and proper training prior to task-sharing.

Availability of transport and acceptability of referral

FGD and interview participants emphasized that treatment should not be continued at the community level and woman needed to be referred from the community to higher referral centre. With the availability of robust free ambulance services by the state government in this locality (free ambulance service on dialling 108), transport was not seen as much of a challenge. Women of reproductive age claimed that they would refuse emergency treatment and referral if a family member was unavailable to decide on her behalf or accompany her.

Discussion

The study aimed to identify facilitators and barriers for task-sharing in the identification and emergency treatment of pregnant women with HDP (Fig. 2). Enhanced antenatal and postnatal surveillance at home by the ASHA workers with measurement of BP and when indicated, administration of oral antihypertensives and intramuscular magnesium sulphate by the ANM prior to referral form the key components of the CLIP (NCT01911494) Trial.

There was strong community support for home visits by CHW to measure the blood pressure of pregnant women; however, respondents were concerned about their knowledge, training and effectiveness. The treatment with oral antihypertensive agents and magnesium sulphate in emergencies was accepted by community representatives but medical practitioners and health administrators had reservations, and insisted on emergency

| Lack of qualified manpower | Increased demand for services | Need for scale-up services | Reduction in adverse outcomes | Poor geographical accessibility | Cost effectiveness |

FACILITATORS

TASK SHARING

BARRIERS

| Effective training | Lack of administrative support | Monitoring and supervision | Career progression or scale up | Acceptability and safety | Incentive package |

Pictorial representation of Facilitators and barriers for task sharing

Fig. 2 Pictorial representations of facilitators and barriers for task-sharing

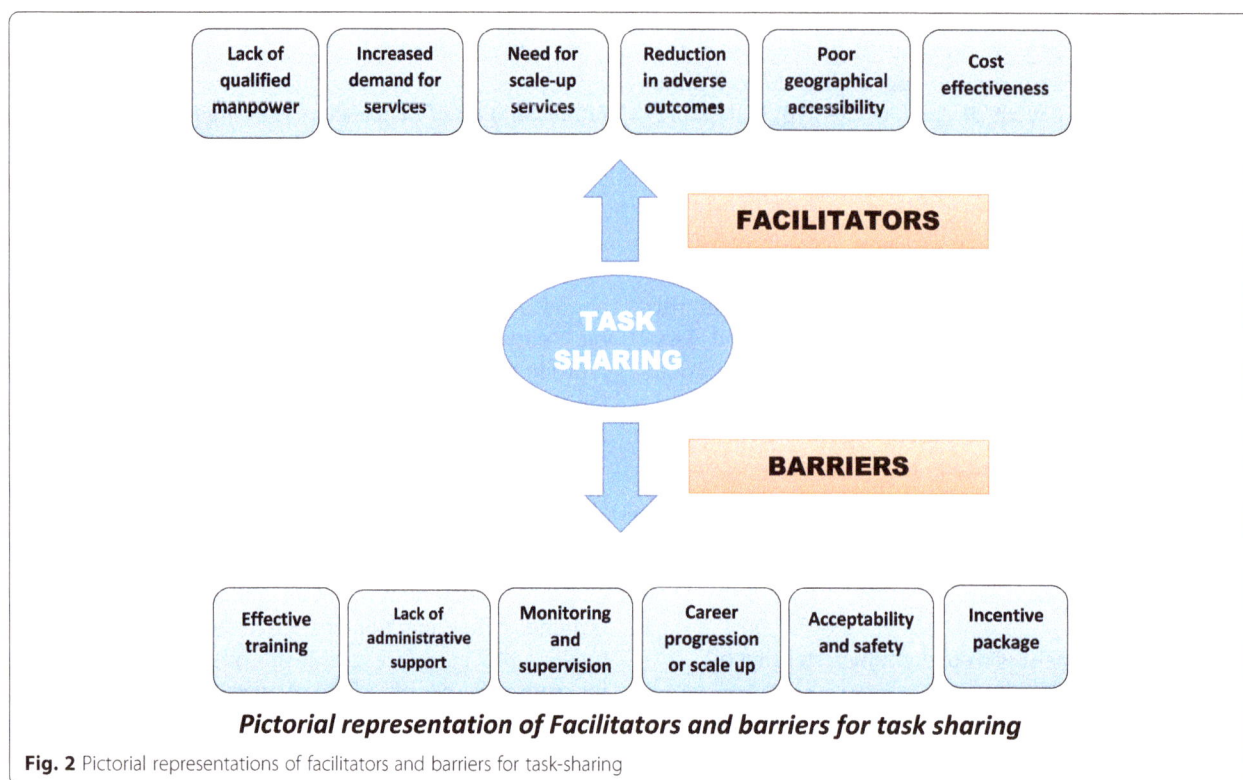

transport to a higher facility. The most important barriers for task-sharing were concerns regarding insufficient training, limited availability of medications, the questionable validity of blood pressure devices, and the ability of CHW to correctly diagnose and intervene in cases of hypertensive disorders of pregnancy.

Task-sharing is a process which has been proposed to overcome manpower shortages faced by the health care system. This shifts the tasks to "lay workers" or CHW who are not formally trained in the task assigned to them but can be expected to carry out the responsibilities after some training and with supervision [8]. This causes an improvement in early diagnosis and treatment of emergency conditions and is cost-effective [12, 13]. Task-sharing could improve access to health workers in resource-constrained settings and possibly have an impact on reducing mortality and morbidity [8].

More commonly, tasks expected from the "lay workers" are related to preventive and health promotional activities. The importance of "Community Embeddedness" of the lay worker has been stressed [14]. Women of reproductive age and decision makers in this study favoured home visits by the ASHA for BP monitoring. This has also been noted by other studies that found that this could be because it would reduce visits to the hospital for measurement of BP which were missed at times due to lack of knowledge, poor transportation facilities, competing responsibilities and commitments, loss of daily wages due to the visit and

financial constraints [15]. People tend to preferably seek health care if the facility is close by rather than at a great distance [16]. Pregnant women and female decision-makers also supported this as the ASHA belongs to their locality and lives in close proximity; and could be helpful during emergencies, as other studies have reported [12].

The ASHA workers are not trained in measuring BP or other clinical examinations but are capable of identifying the danger signs of HDP [11]. The use of CHW for the measurement of BP in chronic hypertension has been reported in several studies, with favourable outcomes in the participants [17, 18]. A study done in north India demonstrated that ASHA workers could be trained to measure BP and concluded that they could be used for monitoring hypertension antenatally [19].

Some obstetricians raised concern regarding the use of an oscillometric digital apparatus, as well as validation and errors in recording. It is however important that the BP devices be validated for the purpose they are intended. The Microlife 3AS 1–2 semi-automatic handheld BP device, used by the ASHAs in the CLIP Trial has been validated for use in pregnant women including those with pre-eclampsia. This handheld device can be used effectively by unskilled personnel after minimal training [20, 21]. The concerns about errors in the BP readings can be substantially reduced by proper ongoing training sessions, validation and calibration of the device [22, 23].

WHO recognises that lay workers are more likely to be motivated if their tasks include curative aspects along with the preventive [8]. The ANMs were expected to administer methyldopa orally if the woman was found to have severe hypertension, in addition to magnesium sulphate injection intramuscularly in certain clinical scenarios, prior to referral. The ANMs are familiar with many drugs, Intravenous fluids, and injectable medications and vaccines [10]. Women of reproductive age and decision makers voiced trust in the ANM for treating women with HDP using oral antihypertensives and referring them to higher centres for further management. Since the antihypertensive in question here is in tablet form, skill development is not needed for administration.

Task-sharing in the provision of healthcare is not a new concept and has been implemented widely for the management of various conditions such as malaria, HIV, and tuberculosis (TB) [24–28]. Lewin et al. found that the use of lay health workers improved the uptake of immunization and breastfeeding practices; and also decreased morbidity and mortality from common childhood illnesses and additionally led to improved TB treatment outcomes [29].

Some obstetricians expressed concern about the ANM giving methyldopa due to concerns of adverse effects; however, it is widely recommended for use in HDP [30]. Methyldopa is found to be safe in HDP when used to prevent maternal and foetal complications. Though it may sometimes cause sedation or drowsiness, there is no evidence of acute complications in HDP with a loading dose of methyldopa [31–33].

The other task expected of the ANMs was the administration of magnesium sulphate injection intramuscularly before referral. The Magpie trial revealed that administration of magnesium sulphate leads to a 58% reduction in the risk of convulsions and its safety is well established [34, 35]. Magnesium sulphate is on the WHO Essential Medicines List for the use in severe pre-eclampsia and eclampsia [36]. Obstetricians interviewed in this study were also supportive of the administration of magnesium sulphate before referral and perceived it be safe. According to the guidelines for skilled birth attendants in India, ANMs are authorised to use 10 g magnesium sulphate as a deep intramuscular injection (5 g on each buttock) prior to referral in severe pre-eclampsia and eclampsia. Although provision of magnesium sulphate is in the current ANM guidelines, it is rarely followed in practice. This could be overcome by administrative support and effective training [10].

An adjunctive study conducted in tandem with the present study found that ANMs perceived magnesium sulphate to be an antihypertensive and nifedipine to be an anticonvulsant. It is necessary to address these misconceptions. Nevertheless, ANMs expressed confidence in the administration of intramuscular injections and this self-assessed competence could be strengthened to enable them to use magnesium sulphate appropriately [37].

In evaluating the role of CHW for strengthening child health programmes in Mali, the authors found that provision of continuous training, transport means, adequate supervision and motivation through financial incentives and remuneration are important [38]. In a similar study done in Pakistan to evaluate task sharing with Lady Health Workers for the identification and management of pre-eclampsia, the authors concluded that appropriate training, equipment availability and supervision is a must for successful implementation [39]. In this study too, the need for training and adequate supervision were brought up during the discussions, to be important pre-requisites for the proposed task-sharing. Many studies have reported significant capacity for skill development if the trainees have refresher training in skills to which they were not previously exposed, this being one of the most important factors favouring task-sharing [15].

Recommendations and guidelines have been framed for task- sharing but it has been emphasized that the lower cadre of providers who may be entrusted with new responsibilities will have to fit into the existing health system framework. This is unique to each region, and hence national and local bodies should frame and adopt policies which are relevant to their communities. There must be strong support for these workers based on governance, financing, the supply of medicines and equipment and support from the rest of the formal health system for referral services [8, 40]. Mombo et al. state that task-sharing, if implemented properly, has the potential to play a major role in better access to and more equitable provision of basic health care. However, failure to follow appropriate methods and poor planning and implementation could be counterproductive, with compromised health care delivery [41]. This study found during discussions and interviews that most of the participants favoured task-sharing and emphasised the need for adequate training, supervision and logistical support for the CHW.

Conclusion

This qualitative study found strong support for task-sharing activities such as home based blood pressure monitoring by community health workers; initiation of emergency treatment and transfer of pregnant women identified as having hypertensive disorders of pregnancy to higher centers by health care providers for further management. The concerns raised were inadequate knowledge, training, experience, supervision and ability of lower cadre health workers to appropriately deliver these services in the community. These concerns could be addressed by community engagement, repeated training to bridge the knowledge gap and active monitoring of the newly assigned tasks by trained personnel. The future implication of this study is to help in implementing a larger trial to evaluate whether these task-sharing can help in reducing mortality and morbidity among pregnant women suffering from HDP and can strengthen existing healthcare infrastructure with constraint human resources.

Strengths of the study

This study was conducted in collaboration with Indian and multinational researchers who are experienced in developing qualitative protocols and analysis. Their experience has generated robust study design. The local site researchers are familiar with the local Kannada language, which helped participants express their opinions freely and contributed to a better understanding by the facilitators.

Limitations of the study

Primary health centre staff identified the participants from the local community and this may have resulted in selection bias. The participants who did not access primary care through the formal health care delivery system were unlikely to be contacted for participation. The participants who were never exposed to such FGDs could have been hesitant in expressing their thoughts freely or may have withheld their comments. Even though the researchers were well-trained to facilitate equal inputs from all the participants, group dynamics and cultural barriers may have enhanced or hindered the dialogues by some participants. Non–probabilistic sampling methods limit the ability to generalize results.

Abbreviation
ANM: Auxiliary nurse-midwives; ASHA: Accredited social health activists; CHW: Community health workers; DGO: Diploma in gynaecology and obstetrics; FGD: Focus group discussion; HDP: Hypertensive disorders of pregnancy; IDI: In-depth interview; MBBS: Batchelor of medicine/bachelor of surgery; MD: Medicine doctor; OBGYN: Obstetrician and gynaecologist; SBA: Skilled birth attendant; WHO: World Health Organisation; WRA: Women of reproductive age

Acknowledgements
This work is part of the University of British Columbia PRE-EMPT (Pre-eclampsia/Eclampsia, Monitoring, Prevention and Treatment) initiative supported by the Bill & Melinda Gates Foundation. We gratefully acknowledge contributions of the Community Level Interventions for Pre-eclampsia (CLIP) India Feasibility Working Group: Zulfiqar Bhutta, Sheela Naik, Anis Mulla, Namdev Kamle, Vaibhav Dhamanekar, Sharla K Drebit, Chirag Kariya, Tang Lee, Jing Li, Mansun Lui, Asif R Khowaja, Domena K. Tu and Amit Revankar. We also acknowledge the support of KLE University, JN Medical College, SN Medical College, University of British Columbia, Government of Karnataka, the district health administration of Belgaum and Bagalkote Districts. We also thank health centre staff and community leaders for their participation and their efforts in motivating community participation. We additionally acknowledge the research office staff for assisting in data translation and transcription. Finally, a special thanks to all the focus group and interview participants.

Funding
This study was undertaken as a part of the PRE-EMPT (Pre-eclampsia Eclampsia Monitoring Prevention and Treatment) grant awarded to the University of British Columbia, a grantee of the Bill & Melinda Gates Foundation. The funding body had no role in the design or conduct of the study or in the reporting of the results. Publication charges for this supplement were funded by the University of British Columbia PRE-EMPT (Pre-eclampsia/Eclampsia, Monitoring, Prevention and Treatment) initiative supported by the Bill & Melinda Gates Foundation.

Authors' contributions
UC, GK and UR were involved in the preparation of the study materials, data collection and prepared the manuscript. AJ, SB, SR, CK, GM, AK were involved in data collection. RD, SG, SS, MV, AM, MB, DS, BP, LAM were responsible for protocol preparation and overseeing the study. PVD and RQ were the Principal Investigators. All authors read and approved the final manuscript.

Competing interests
The authors declare that they have no competing interests.

Author details
[1]KLE Academy of Higher Education and Research's, J N Medical College, Belagavi, Karnataka, India. [2]Department of Obstetrics and Gynaecology, and the Child and Family Research Unit, University of British, Columbia, Vancouver, BC, Canada. [3]Department of Obstetrics and Gynaecology, S Nijalingappa Medical College, Bagalkot, Karnataka, India. [4]Department of Community Medicine, S Nijalingappa Medical College, Bagalkot, Karnataka, India. [5]Department of Pharmacology, S Nijalingappa Medical College, Bagalkot, Karnataka, India. [6]Department of Anatomy, S Nijalingappa Medical College, Bagalkot, Karnataka, India. [7]Department of Research, Vancouver Island Health Authority, Victoria, BC, Canada. [8]Division of Women and Child Health, Aga Khan University, Karachi, Sindh, Pakistan. [9]School of Life Course Sciences, Faculty of Life Sciences and Medicine, King's College London, London, England. [10]Department Kings of Obstetrics, Thomas Jefferson University, Philadelphia, PA, USA.

References
1. Ending Preventable Maternal Mortality: USAID Maternal Health Vision for Action Evidence for Strategic Approaches - January 2015. Available on URL - https://www.usaid.gov/sites/default/files/documents/1864/MH%20Strategy_web_red.pdf Accessed on 28th Dec at 10.00 am.
2. Trends in Maternal Mortality: 1990 to 2015 Estimates by WHO, UNICEF, UNFPA, World Bank Group and the United Nations Population Division. Available on URL - http://www.afro.who.int/sites/default/files/2017-05/trends-in-maternal-mortality-1990-to-2015.pdf Accessed on 12th Dec 2017 at 09.00 pm.
3. Adamson PC, Krupp K, Niranjankumar B, Freeman AH, Khan M, Madhivanan P. Are marginalized women being left behind? A population-based study of institutional deliveries in Karnataka, India. BMC Public Health. 2012;12(30):1–6.
4. Alkema L, Chou D, Hogan D, Zhang S, Moller AB, Gemmill A, et al. Global, regional, and national levels and trends in maternal mortality between 1990 and 2015, with scenario-based projections to 2030: a systematic analysis by the UN maternal mortality estimation inter-agency group. Lancet. 2016 Jan 30;387(10017):462–74. https://doi.org/10.1016/S0140-6736(15)003-7.Epub 2015 Nov13.

5. Montgomery AL, Ram U, Kumar R, Jha P The million death study collaborators. Maternal mortality in India: causes and healthcare service use based on a nationally representative survey: PLoS One, January 2014 | Volume 9 | Issue 1 | e83331.

6. Ritchie LMP, Khan S, Moore JE, Timmings C, Lettow M, Vogel JP, et al. Low- and middle-income countries face many common barriers to implementation of maternal health evidence products. J Clin Epidemiol Aug 2016; 76:229–237.

7. Combating Global Health Worker Shortages Task shifting and sharing may provide one solution, AJN report, Dec 2012, Vol 112 (12).

8. WHO recommendations, Optimizing health worker roles to improve access to key maternal and newborn health interventions through task shifting. Available on URL; http://apps.who.int/iris/bitstream/10665/77764/1/9789241504843_eng.pdf Accessed on 22nd Nov 2017 at 10.00pm.

9. Indian Public Health Standards (IPHS) Guidelines for Sub-Centres Revised 2012. Available on URL; http://health.bih.nic.in/Docs/Guidelines/Guidelines-Sub-Centers-(Revised)-2012.pdf Accessed on 25th June 2017 at 10.00 am.

10. Skilled birth attendance (SBA). A handbook for auxiliary nurse midwives lady health visitors & staff nurses, 2010. Available on URL; http://tripuranrhm.gov.in/Guidlines/Staff_Nurses.pdf. Accessed on 5th January 2018 at 11.00 pm.

11. Skills that Save Lives, ASHA Module 6: Available on URL; http://nhsrcindia.org/sites/default/files/Skills%20that%20Save%20Lives%20ASHA%20Module%206%20English.pdf Accessed on 10th January 2018 at 10.00pm.

12. Ochieng MB, Akunja EA, Edwards N, Mombo D, Marende L, Kaseje DC. Perceptions of health stakeholders on task shifting and motivation of community health workers in different socio demographic contexts in Kenya (nomadic, peri-urban and rural agrarian). BMC Health Serv Res. 2014; 14(Suppl 1):1–13.

13. Dawson AJ, Buchan J, Duffield C, Homer CSE, Wijewardena K. Task shifting and sharing in maternal and reproductive health in low-income countries: a narrative synthesis of current evidence. Health Policy Plan. 2014;29(3):396–408. https://doi.org/10.1093/heapol/czt026.

14. Campbell C, Scott K. Retreat from Alma Ata? The WHO's report on Task Shifting to community health workers for AIDS care in poor countries. Glob Public Health. 2011;6(2):125–38.

15. Ejembi CL, Norick P, Starrs A, Thapa K. New global guidance supports community and lay health workers in postpartum hemorrhage prevention. Int J Gynaecol Obstet. 2013;122(3):187–9.

16. Rao BV, Schellenberg D, Ghani AC; Overcoming health systems barriers to successful malaria treatment: Trends Parasitol, April 2013, Vol. 29, No 4; 164–180.

17. Sankaran S, Ravi PS, Wu YE, Shanabogue S, Ashok S, Agnew K, et al. An NGO-implemented community –clinic health WorkerApproach to providing long-term Care for Hypertension in a remote region of southern India. Glob Health. 2017;5(4):668–77.

18. He J, Irazola V, Mills KT. HCPIA investigators. Effect of a community health worker–led multicomponent intervention on bloodpressure control in low-income patients in Argentina: a randomizedclinical trial. JAMA. 2017;318(11):1016–25.

19. Amarchand R, Sharma H, Krishnan A. Community health workers can be trained to measure blood pressure: experience from India. Reg Health Forum. 2013;17(1):26–31.

20. Greeff A, Nathan H, Stafford N, Liu B, Shennan AH. Development of an accurate oscillometric blood pressure device for low resource settings. Blood Press Monit. 2008;13(6):342–8.

21. Nathan HN, Greeff A, Hezelgrave NL, Chappell NC, Shennan AH. An accurate semiautomated oscillometric blood pressure device for use in pregnancy (including pre-eclampsia) in a low-income and middle-income country population: the microlife 3AS1-2. Blood Press Monit. 2015;20:52–5.

22. Ramse M. BLOOD PRESSURE MONITORING: AUTOMATED OSCILLOMETRIC DEVICES, Knowing Your Monitoring Equipment; Copyright © 1991 by Little, Brown and Company. J Clin Monit. 1991;7;56–57.

23. Pickering TG, Hall JE, Appel LJ, Falkner BE, Graves J, et al. Recommendations for blood pressure measurement in humans and experimental animals part 1: blood pressure measurement in humans a statement for professionals from the Subcommittee of Professional and Public Education of the American Heart Association Council on high blood pressure research. Hypertension. 2005;45:142–61.

24. Zachariah R, Ford N, Philips M, Lynch S, Massaquoi M, Janssens V, et al. Task shifting in HIV/AIDS: opportunities, challenges and proposed actions for sub-Saharan Africa. Trans R Soc Trop Med Hyg. 2009;103(6):549–58. https://doi.org/10.1016/j.trstmh.2008.09.019.

25. Druetz T, Ridde V, Kouanda S, Ly A, Diabaté S, Haddad S. Utilization of community health workers for malaria treatment: results from a three-year panel study in the districts of Kaya and Zorgho, Burkina Faso. Malar J. 2015;14:71.

26. Delacollette C, Van der Stuyft P, Molima K. Using community health workers for malaria control: experience in Zaire. Bull World Health Organ. 1996;74(4):423–30.

27. Ong'ang'o JR, Mwachari C, Kipruto H, Karanja S. The effects on tuberculosis treatment adherence from Utilising community health workers: a comparison of selected rural and urban settings in Kenya. PLoS One. 2014;9(2):e88937.

28. Garg S, Nanda P, Dewangan M. Role of community health workers in improving TB detection on scale: a case study from the *Mitanin* programmein Chhattisgarh, India. BMJGH. 2016; DOI: 10.1136/bmjgh-2016-EPHPabstracts.21 Published 7 July 2016

29. Lewin SA, Dick J, Pond P, Zwarenstein M, Aja G, van Wyk B, et al. Lay health workers in primary and community health care. Cochrane Database Syst Rev. 2005 Jan 25;1:CD004015.

30. Magee LA, Pels A, Helewa M, Rey E, Dadelszen PV, et al. SOGC CLINICAL PRACTICE GUIDELINE; diagnosis, evaluation, and Management of the Hypertensive Disorders of pregnancy: executive summary: no. 307, May 2014.

31. JNC 7 Express, The Seventh Report of the Joint National Committee on Prevention, Detection, Evaluation, and Treatment of High Blood Pressure. National High Blood Pressure Education Program. Available on URL - https://www.nhlbi.nih.gov/files/docs/guidelines/express.pdf Accessed on 5th Jan 2018 at 11.00 am.

32. Cockburn J, Moar VA, Ounsted M, Redman CW. Final report of study on hypertension during pregnancy: the effects of specific treatment on the growth and development of the children. Lancet. 1982;1(8273):647–9.

33. Magee LA, Abalos E, Dadelszen PV, Sibai B, Easterling T, Walkinshaw S. For the CHIPS study group. How to manage hypertension in pregnancy effectively. Br J Clin Pharmacol. 72(3):394–401.

34. Magpie L D Trial Office, Nuffield Department of Medicine, Level 5, John Radcliffe Hospital, Headington, Oxford OX3 9DU, UK. Email lelia.duley@ndm.ox.ac.uk; The Magpie Trial: a randomised trial comparing magnesium sulphate with placebo for pre-eclampsia.Outcome for women at 2 years. RCOG 2006 BJOG An International Journal of Obstetrics and Gynaecology. 2007;114:300–9.

35. Bain ES, Middleton PF, Crother CA. Maternal adverse effects of different antenatal magnesium sulphate regimens for improving maternal and infant outcomes: a systematic review. BMC Pregnancy Childbirth. 2013;13:195.

36. WHO Model List of Essential Medicines for Children, 20th List (March 2017); Available on URL - http://www.who.int/medicines/publications/essentialmedicines/6th_EMLc2017.pdf Accessed on 25th Jan 2018 at 9.00 am.

37. Ramadurg U, Vidler M, Charanthimath U, Katageri G, Bellad M, Mallapur A, et al. Community health worker knowledge and management of pre-eclampsia in rural Karnataka state, India. Reprod Health. 2016 Sep 30; 13(Suppl 2):113.

38. Perez F, Ba H, Dastagire SG, Altmann M. The role of community health workers in improving child health programmes in Mali. BMC Int Health Hum Rights. 2009 Nov 10;9:28. https://doi.org/10.1186/1472-698X-9-28.

39. Salam RA, Qureshi RN, Sheikh S, Khowaja AR, Sawchuck D, Vidler M, et al. Potential for task-sharing to lady health workers for identification and emergency management of pre-eclampsia at community level in Pakistan. Reprod Health. 2016;13(Suppl 2):107.

40. Fulton BD, Scheffler RM, Sparkes SP, Auh EY, Vujicic M, Soucat A. Health workforce skill mix and task shifting in low income countries: a review of recent evidence. Hum Resourc Health [Electronic Resource]. 2011;9(1):1.

41. Mombo DS, Kaseje DCO. Health services consumers perceptions on task shifting of primary healthcare functions to community health Workers in Rural Butere sub County, western Kenya. Univ J Public Health. 2015;3(3):120–7.

17

Fertility preservation decision making amongst Australian transgender and non-binary adults

Damien W. Riggs[*] and Clare Bartholomaeus

Abstract

Background: Historically, transitioning gender was seen as precluding transgender people from having children in the future. However, there are now increased reproductive options available to transgender people, with such options also available to non-binary people (i.e., people whose gender is not exclusively male or female). These options include undertaking fertility preservation if genetic children may be desired in the future. Despite these increased options, there is still only a limited amount of international research exploring the views of transgender and non-binary people on fertility preservation.

Methods: This mixed-methods study draws on a convenience sample of Australian transgender and non-binary adults, focused on their decision making about fertility preservation. The questionnaire was constructed by the authors, drawing on previous research. Participants were recruited via Australian organisations and groups made up of and/or working with people who are transgender or non-binary. The questionnaire was open from January– February 2018. The final sample included 409 participants. Statistical analyses were conducted on the closed-ended responses. Open-ended responses were analysed via a conventional content analysis.

Results: Decisions about fertility preservation were influenced by views on the importance of genetic relatedness, willingness to delay transition, economic resources, already having children or desiring children in the future, and the views of significant others. Advice or counselling prior to decision making was received only by a minority of participants. Very few participants (7%) had undertaken fertility preservation, although 95% said that fertility preservation should be offered to all transgender and non-binary people. Participants who viewed genetic relatedness as important were more likely to have undertaken fertility preservation.

Conclusions: The findings indicate that fertility preservation should be made available as an option to all transgender or non-binary people prior to undertaking treatment which may impact on fertility. However, it should also be recognised that not all people who are transgender or non-binary will want to undertake fertility preservation, and that not all people may be able to afford to.

Keywords: Transgender, Non-binary gender, Decision making, Fertility preservation, Reproductive desires

* Correspondence: damien.riggs@flinders.edu.au
College of Education, Psychology and Social Work, Flinders University, GPO
Box 2100, Adelaide, SA 5001, Australia

Plain English summary

In the past, transgender people were seen as automatically excluded from having children. However, the reproductive rights of transgender people have been increasingly recognised, as too have those of non-binary people (i.e., people whose gender is not exclusively male or female). This may include preserving fertility should transgender or non-binary people wish to have children in the future. Yet there is little research which explores the views of transgender and non-binary people on fertility preservation.

To explore such views, a questionnaire was designed by the authors. The questionnaire was completed by 409 transgender and non-binary adults in Australia.

The findings from the questionnaire show that the people who completed the survey made decisions about fertility preservation depending on several reasons. The reasons included how important it was to be genetically related to a child, how willing they were to wait to transition gender, how much money they had, whether they had children already or if they wanted to have children in the future, and the views of people around them. Only a small number of people who completed the survey had preserved their fertility. Nearly all said that fertility preservation should be offered to all transgender and non-binary people.

The findings suggest that the option for preserving fertility should be available to all people who are transgender or non-binary. However, not all transgender or non-binary people will want to preserve their fertility, or will be able to afford it.

Background

Historically, transitioning gender was seen as precluding transgender people from having children in the future, with sterilisation often being mandatory, or treated as axiomatic in the context of gender affirming surgery. As such, whilst some transgender people may have had children prior to transitioning, the potential for future children was typically not considered. The World Professional Association for Transgender Health (WPATH) *Standards of Care for the Health of Transsexual, Transgender, and Gender Nonconforming People* (SOC), however, in their seventh version [1], introduced a focus on reproductive rights. The SOC recommend that fertility preservation should be offered to anyone considering undertaking medical treatment which may have a permanent impact on their fertility. Such treatment specifically relates to gender affirming surgeries undertaken by transgender women or men which lead to irreversible sterility, and hormone therapies that such women and men may undertake that can permanently impact on gamete quality [2]. People with a non-binary gender (i.e., people whose gender is not exclusively male or female) may undertake similar medical treatments, although research suggests that non-binary people may be less likely to do so than transgender people who have a binary gender. [3] Importantly, however, such research also suggests that the lower rates at which non-binary people access medical treatments may be a product of perceived or actual barriers to services arising from a lack of clinician awareness about non-binary genders. [3] Perhaps as a consequence of such a lack of awareness, the experiences of non-binary people in terms of reproduction have often been overlooked in previous research, or as will be seen below, are often collapsed in with the experiences of transgender people who have a binary gender. This is a problem given non-binary people are likely to have specific needs and experiences.

The country in which transgender or non-binary people live constitutes a formative context in terms of experiences of fertility preservation. Therefore, it is important to provide a brief background to the Australian context as it is the setting for the study reported in this paper. There are no specific laws or policies banning transgender or non-binary people from undertaking fertility preservation or assisted reproductive technology in Australia, although in some jurisdictions legislation enables providers to object on religious grounds. However, fertility preservation is expensive and is only covered by the Australian public healthcare system if it is classified as being medically necessary. Whilst for oncology patients fertility preservation is seen as medically necessary, for transgender and non-binary people it is not. Estimates from 2010 suggest that, depending on the clinic, sperm banking costs $300–$400 a year in storage fees, sperm aspiration costs $1000–$1500, egg banking or embryo storage costs $300–$500 a year in storage fees, and IVF may cost $15,000–$20,000 (all in Australian dollars) [4]. These costs must be located in the context of legislation, which in some Australian states mandates that in order for a person to change their gender marker on their birth certificate, they must have undergone some form of surgery, which for many people will result in sterility. As such, not only is fertility preservation costly in Australia, but for many transgender and non-binary people it is also necessary if they wish to preserve their fertility prior to undertaking surgeries that will allow for formal recognition of their gender.

In terms of the importance of fertility preservation, previous research suggests that whilst lower numbers of transgender (and in some research non-binary) people are already parents than would be expected from general population data, the numbers of transgender and non-binary people who wish to become parents in the future is not negligible [5–7]. These studies report that transgender and non-binary people become parents in multiple ways, including by giving birth, by a partner giving birth, by surrogacy, by foster care or adoption, or by step parenting. As the latter pathways to parenthood would suggest, existing research indicates that transgender or non-binary people may be less focused on being genetically-related to their children than the broader population [7–10]. Studies have also found that transgender women are more likely to already have children than transgender men [7, 11, 12].

Whilst there are increasing options available for transgender or non-binary people to undertake fertility preservation, there is still only a limited amount of international research exploring the views of transgender people on this topic, and even less with non-binary people. De Sutter et al.'s [11] groundbreaking study examined the views of 121 transgender women, most of whom lived in Europe. Their study found that over three quarters of respondents thought that sperm freezing should be offered to all transgender women before hormonal treatment, although only half would have seriously thought about doing this or would have done it themselves if it had been available. A similar study conducted more recently with 50 transgender men in Belgium found that 37.5% of respondents would have considered freezing germ cells if the technique had been available [12]. Similarly, literature drawing on case reviews highlights that the uptake of fertility preservation is low [13], particularly amongst transgender young people [14, 15]. Research has also found that to date few people have used their preserved gametes to conceive children [14]. In terms of gender, previous research and case reviews indicate that transgender women are more likely to undertake fertility preservation than transgender men [8, 14, 16].

In terms of decision making about fertility preservation, studies have found that this can be influenced by perceived psychological and physiological challenges associated with either ceasing hormone treatments in order to undergo fertility preservation [17], or delaying surgical and medical transition [8, 11, 17]. Decision making about fertility preservation may also be influenced by the associated financial costs [8, 9, 18], along with not being aware that fertility preservation is an option, not knowing that hormone treatments may make it difficult to have genetically-related children, travel time to the nearest fertility clinic, and the newness of technologies such as egg freezing [8, 19]. In terms of individual factors, research has found that for some people the idea of using stored gametes to conceive a child can be dysphoria inducing, and that some individuals express concerns about passing on poor genes [11].

Whilst previous research has included comment on decision making, as summarised above, this has occurred in the context of research on intentions, experiences and outcomes for transgender (and occasionally non-binary) people who plan to undertake, or who have

already undertaken, fertility preservation. The present study sought to focus specifically on decision making about fertility preservation amongst a convenience sample of transgender and non-binary people, and was guided by the following research questions:

1. Is genetic relatedness valued, does this relate to undertaking fertility preservation, and how is genetic relatedness accounted for?
2. How does gender-affirming medical treatment relate to fertility?
3. How prevalent is fertility preservation and who is most likely to undertake it?
4. What influences decision making about fertility preservation, and does decision making occur in the context of professional advice or counselling?

Methods

The mixed-methods study design was intended as a scoping study given the relative lack of previous research specifically on decision-making. Ethical approval for the research was granted by the Flinders University Social and Behavioural Research Ethics Committee (project number 7867).

Participant recruitment

Participants were recruited via emails to Australian organisations and groups made up of and/or working with people who are transgender or non-binary, including broader 'LGBT' organisations. Organisations and groups were asked to share information about the questionnaire via their social media (Facebook and/or Twitter) and via an email to their members. Thirty-five organisations and groups were contacted and approximately half shared the details of the questionnaire. The researchers did not have access to member names or email addresses. The questionnaire was open from January–February 2018. No financial incentive was offered to participants.

To be included in the final sample, at minimum participants needed to have answered socio-cultural demographic questions, and whether or not they had undertaken fertility preservation. In total 442 people commenced the questionnaire. Of those, 28 people started the questionnaire but did not respond to any items. An additional five people started the questionnaire but did not complete the minimum questions required. Of the final sample of 409 participants, participants on average spent 12 min completing the questionnaire.

Questionnaire

Participants were invited to complete an online questionnaire hosted on SurveyMonkey. No identifying information (i.e., names or email addresses) was collected as part of the questionnaire, and the IP addresses of participants were not tracked. SurveyMonkey servers use secure encryption, and access to the data collected is available only to the researchers (i.e., it is not available to SurveyMonkey staff). The first page of the questionnaire included background information to the research and links to a full information sheet and a list of support resources. Participants were asked whether they consented to participate in the questionnaire by selecting 'Yes' or 'No' after reading the information on the first page of the questionnaire. Participants selecting 'Yes' were directed to the start of the questionnaire. Those selecting 'No' were redirected to a page welcoming them to return and complete the questionnaire at another time.

The questionnaire, designed by the authors, drew upon previous research to focus on key variables which are likely to shape decision making around fertility preservation (e.g., [11]). The questionnaire first asked participants to provide demographic information, including gender, age, Australian State or Territory of residence, and sexual orientation. Participants were then asked to give information relating to their current relationship status, whether or not they had children (and/or planned to have children in the future), and if they already had children, whether they did so before or after transitioning gender. Participants were then asked 'is it important to you that you share a genetic relationship with your children?', 'have you undergone gender affirming treatment which may impact on fertility?' (and if so, what form this took), and 'have you previously undertaken fertility preservation?'. Depending on participant responses to the last question, they were then directed to one of two pages.

Participants who indicated they had undertaken fertility preservation were asked an open-ended question about how they had made this decision, whether or not they had received advice or counselling prior to their decision, whether they had delayed their gender transition in order to undertake fertility preservation, and how likely they were to use stored gametes in the future (1 = not very likely, 2 = somewhat likely, 3 = quite likely, 4 = very likely). Participants who indicated they had not undertaken fertility preservation were asked an open-ended question about how they made this decision, whether they had received any advice or counselling prior to making this decision, and whether they would have considered delaying their gender transition in order to undertake fertility preservation. Both of these pages concluded by asking whether participants thought that fertility preservation should be available to all transgender and non-binary people. In sum, participants who indicated they had undertaken fertility preservation were presented with a total of 15 questions to answer, and participants who indicated they had not undertaken fertility preservation were presented with 14 questions to answer.

Data analysis

Questionnaire data were exported from SurveyMonkey into SPSS 21.0. Descriptive statistics were generated for socio-cultural demographics (gender, Australian State or Territory, sexuality, and current relationship status, see Table 1 below), and for child-related demographics (have children or not, when they had children, and whether or not sharing a genetic relationship with children is important, see Table 2 below). Descriptive statistics were also generated for mean age at which fertility preservation was undertaken and likelihood of using stored gametes (see below), and treatments that may impact on fertility preservation and willingness to delay transition in order to undertake fertility preservation (see Table 4). Finally in terms of descriptive statistics, these were generated for whether or not participants had undertaken fertility preservation (and if so, what type), and whether or not they had received counselling or advice prior to their decision (see Table 5).

Drawing on previous research, inferential statistics were then performed on specific variables likely to be related to one another. These were: 1) having children already (or not) and gender, 2) views on the importance of genetic relatedness and fertility preservation, 3) age and gender-affirming treatments, 4) gender and having undertaken fertility preservation, 5) gender and

Table 1 Socio-cultural demographics (N = 409)

	Category	N (%)
Gender	Female	97 (23.7)
	Male	131 (32.0)
	Non-binary	149 (36.4)
	Agender	32 (7.8)
State or Territory	Australian Capital Territory	10 (2.4)
	New South Wales	92 (22.5)
	Northern Territory	6 (1.5)
	Queensland	102 (24.9)
	South Australia	50 (12.2)
	Tasmania	24 (5.9)
	Victoria	106 (25.9)
	Western Australia	19 (4.6)
Sexuality	Heterosexual	31 (7.6)
	Bisexual	65 (15.9)
	Gay	31 (7.6)
	Lesbian	37 (9.0)
	Pansexual	99 (24.2)
	Queer	109 (26.7)
	Asexual	37 (9.0)
Currently in Relationship	Yes	214 (52.3)
	No	195 (47.7)

Table 2 Child-related demographics

	Category	N (%)
Already have Children (n = 64)	Yes, and would like to have more	12 (18.8)
	Yes, and do not plan to have more	39 (60.9)
	Yes, and undecided about having more	13 (20.3)
When had Children	Before transitioning	48 (75.0)
	After transitioning	10 (15.62)
	Both before and after transitioning	6 (9.38)
Do not have Children (n = 345)	No, but would like to in the future	114 (33.0)
	No, and do not plan to have children	119 (34.5)
	No, and undecided about having children in the future	112 (32.5)

willingness to delay gender transition in order to undertake fertility preservation, and 6) gender and the wish that fertility preservation had been undertaken. Additional tests were run on any relationship between advice or counselling received about fertility preservation and gender. Log-likelihood ratio tests (LLR) were used for all of the inferential statistics involving two categorical variables, given the existence of small cell sizes. For each LLR percentages are reported for each category so as to provide the reader with a breakdown of differences between groups. For the analysis of variance, Levene's Test of Equality of Variance was used to test the assumption of equal variances, and to test the linearity of the data the Lack of Fit test was used. For each, results were non-significant, indicating that there were equal variances across groups examined, and that the data were linear.

Open-ended responses were analysed via a conventional content analysis, following the guidelines outlined by Hsieh and Shannon [20]. This involved 1) repeated readings of the data corpus, 2) developing codes by highlighting key words that capture frequently occurring concepts, 3) reducing codes in order to minimise overlaps, 4) examining codes for patterned responses, in order to group codes into categories, and 5) examining categories to determine whether or not they accurately reflect the data corpus. As noted by Hsieh and Shannon, a limitation of conventional content analysis is that it does not utilise member checking or inter-rater reliability. Given the questionnaire was anonymous, member checking was moot for the present study. In terms of inter-rater reliability, Hsieh and Shannon note that all analyses are subjective, and thus should be viewed as offering one interpretation derived by the researcher. Nonetheless, the content analysis undertaken by the first author was reviewed and confirmed by the second author.

Results

Participant demographics

Participants ranged in age from 18 to 72 years ($M = 28.54$, $SD = 11.25$). Other socio-cultural demographics are outlined in Table 1.

In terms of having children, 64 of the participants were already parents, and 345 participants were not (see Table 2). Of the parent participants, 64% became parents via their partner giving birth, 28% gave birth to their child, 5% were step parents, and 3% were foster parents. Further in terms of parent participants, 48% were female, 28% were non-binary, 18% were male, and 6% were agender, LLR (2, 64) = 53.97, $P < 0.001$. For participants who were not parents, 33% desired to have children in the future, of whom 44% were non-binary 36% were male, 12% were female, and 8% were agender, LLR (20, 397) = 47.87, $P < 0.001$.

Importance of genetic relatedness

In terms of views on the importance of sharing a genetic relationship with children, 244 participants responded to this question, of whom 82 (33.6%) thought that genetic relatedness was important, and 162 (66.4%) thought it was not important. Focusing specifically on fertility preservation, of those who had undertaken fertility preservation 71% thought that genetic relatedness was important, and for those who had not undertaken fertility preservation 31% thought that genetic relatedness was important, LLR (1, 244) = 15.574, $P = 0.008$.

With regard to the open-ended question about the importance of genetic relatedness, a content analysis of the 91 responses to this question identified six key categories, as outlined in Table 3. Three categories pertained to participants who responded that genetic relatedness was *not* important to them. The most common response of these three categories was that participants were planning to adopt or foster, and thus had no interest in genetic relatedness. The other three categories pertained to participants who responded that genetic relatedness *was* important to them. The most common response of these three categories was a pragmatic acceptance that genetic relatedness was not possible, even if desired.

Gender-related medical treatment and its relationship to fertility

Participants were asked about any gender-affirming medical treatment they had undertaken which may impact on fertility. Responses are outlined in Table 4. A one-way between groups ANOVA was conducted to determine whether type of treatment undertaken differed by age. A statistically significant difference emerged, F (3, 237) = 14.49, $P < 0.001$. Post hoc comparisons using the Bonferroni test indicated that the mean age for participants who had undertaken gender affirming surgery

Table 3 Content analysis of importance of genetic relatedness

Viewed genetic relatedness as important	Category	N	Examples
No	Plan to adopt or foster children	21	"It doesn't matter, I'm hoping to adopt". "I feel it is selfish to prioritise a genetic relationship when there are so many children in the world without families"
No	A genetic relationship is not important	14	"Never saw why it made any difference". "It's not necessary for a child to be genetically related to their parents to have a normal and loving home environment".
No	Perception of having 'bad genes'	10	"I don't want to pass on genetic mental illness". "I have terrible genes and do not want them to continue".
Yes	Pragmatic acceptance that genetic relatedness is not possible	19	"It is important to me, but ultimately not likely to be possible so I'm working on letting that go". "I understood as I came to terms with my gender that I'd never bear my own children".
Yes	Would like the option of having a genetic relationship	13	"I would like the option to have biological children". "I want at least one other biological child for personal reasons, but it's not actually important to me otherwise".
Yes	Fine either way	14	"Ideally I would like to have another genetic child but I would also be happy to help raise a non genetic child". "Both me and my partner would like children to share our genetics but if that's not possible we want to adopt".

was higher ($M = 42.38$, $SD = 14.27$) than the mean ages for puberty blockers ($M = 20.50$, $SD = 3.20$), current use of hormones ($M = 29.43$, $SD = 10.93$), and past use of hormones ($M = 33.91$, $SD = 8.74$). Also outlined in Table 4 are responses to questions about whether participants considered, or would have considered, delaying transition in order to preserve fertility. 'Not applicable' responses pertained primarily to non-binary people, who did not plan to undertake any medical treatments that would impact upon their fertility.

Fertility preservation decision making

Table 5 outlines rates at which fertility preservation was undertaken, the form this took, whether advice or counselling was given prior to decision making, and whether participants who had not undertaken fertility preservation now wished otherwise (and whether they had received advice or counselling prior to their decision not

Table 4 Treatment and transition impact on fertility

	Category	N (%)
Treatment that may impact on fertility (n = 242)	Puberty blockers	6 (2.5)
	Hormones (current)	190 (78.5)
	Hormones (previously)	11 (4.5)
	Surgery related to reproductive organs	35 (14.5)
Delayed transition to preserve fertility (n = 26)	Yes	15 (57.7)
	No	11 (42.3)
Would have considered delaying transition to preserve fertility (n = 315)	Yes	64 (20.3)
	No	174 (55.2)
	Not applicable	77 (24.4)

to undertake fertility preservation). The mean age at which participants had undertaken fertility preservation was 25.24 years ($SD = 8.29$). The mean for likelihood of using stored gametes was 2.28 ($SD = 1.24$), meaning that participants reported that they were only somewhat likely to use their stored gametes in the future. Of the 335 participants who responded to the question about whether or not fertility preservation should be offered to all transgender and non-binary people, 317 (94.6%) answered yes.

Of those who had undertaken fertility preservation, 53% were female, 21% were non-binary, 18% were male, and 8% were agender, LLR (2, 28) = 13.910, $P < 0.001$. In terms of delaying gender transition in order to have undertaken fertility preservation, of those who answered yes 66% were female, 20% were male, and 14% were non-binary, LLR (6, 26) = 14.806, $P = 0.006$. With regard to advice or counselling received prior to undertaking fertility preservation, there were no statistically significant differences in terms of gender. For those who had not undertaken fertility preservation, a majority (68%) indicated that they had not received any advice or counselling about fertility preservation. Of those who had not received advice or counselling, 39% were non-binary people, 30% were male, 20% were female, and 11% were agender, LLR (16, 318) = 77.625, $P = 0.005$.

In terms of decision making for the 28 participants who had undertaken fertility preservation, a content analysis of the 22 open ended responses indicated that participants primarily focused on who helped them make the decision, rather than why they made the decision per se. As reported in Table 6, the most common response was that participants made the decision to undertake

Table 5 Fertility preservation decision making

	Category	N (%)
Previously undertaken fertility preservation (n = 398)	Yes	28 (7.0)
	No	370 (93.0)
What form of fertility preservation (n = 28)	Stored gametes after beginning puberty but before starting hormones	19 (67.9)
	Stored gametes after commencing hormones	8 (28.6)
	Stored fertilized embryos	1 (3.6)
Given advice or counselling prior to fertility preservation (n = 28)	Yes	16 (57.1)
	No	12 (42.9)
Wish had undertaken fertility preservation (n = 318)	Yes	27 (8.5)
	No	120 (37.7)
	Unsure	44 (13.8)
	Was not available/offered	35 (11.0)
	Still an option	92 (28.9)
Given advice or counselling about future fertility preservation options (n = 308)	Yes	70 (22.7)
	No (and I am fine with that)	161 (52.3)
	No (and I wish I had)	49 (15.9)
	Not applicable	28 (9.1)

fertility preservation due to their desire to have the option to have children in the future. Of the participants who had not undertaken fertility preservation, 155 responded to an open-ended question asking about how they had made this decision. A content analysis of these responses indicated six categories, as outlined in Table 6. The most common response was that cost was prohibitive to undertaking fertility preservation. Both having no interest in genetic relationships or having children, and the thought of children as inducing dysphoria, were also common responses.

Discussion

Drawing on a convenience sample of Australian transgender and non-binary people, this mixed-methods study found that only a minority of participants viewed being genetically related to children as important, though participants who had undertaken fertility preservation were more likely to hold this view. The relative lack of importance placed upon genetic relatedness amongst the sample echoes previous research with transgender (and in some studies non-binary) people in regards to fertility preservation and parenting [7–10], though differs significantly from research with cisgender populations, who have been found to strongly emphasise the importance of genetic relatedness [21].

Only a small number of participants had undertaken fertility preservation, and a majority of these participants had delayed their gender transition in order to preserve their fertility. For the majority who had not undertaken fertility preservation, delaying gender transition in order to preserve fertility was not considered. The relatively small number of participants who had undertaken fertility preservation also echoes previous research [13–15], as is the relative lack of willingness to consider delaying gender transition in order to preserve fertility [8, 11, 17]. Factors shaping the decision to undertake fertility preservation identified in the present research represent a novel contribution to the literature, whilst factors related to the decision not to undertake fertility preservation echo previous research [8, 9, 11, 17–19].

In terms of receiving advice or counselling about fertility preservation, over half of those who decided to preserve their fertility had received advice or counselling. For those who had not undertaken fertility preservation, less than a quarter had received advice or counselling. Previous research has paid little attention to whether advice or counselling is offered in the context of fertility preservation, despite the recommendations of the WPATH SOC that health care professionals discuss reproductive options prior to medical treatment. This finding is thus a novel contribution of the research reported in this paper.

Study strengths and limitations

The strength of the present study is that it represents the largest study to date of fertility preservation decision making undertaken with a non-clinical sample of transgender and non-binary people. The mixed-methods approach allows for an understanding of both the rates at which fertility preservation occurred amongst the sample and aspects of decision making related to this, as well as something of the meaning that participants attributed to decision making. The inclusion of non-binary people in the present study adds an important dimension to previous studies that have focused primarily on transgender people. In terms of limitations, the participants were all Australian and were comprised of a convenience sample, meaning that the findings may not be generalizable to other contexts. Additionally, responses to the open-ended questions around decision-making were on average relatively brief, meaning that more in-depth analyses of this qualitative data were not possible.

Directions for future research

Future research, including that planned as part of the present study, will benefit from focusing on experiences with fertility preservation. Whilst there are a small number of publications focused on this topic [8, 17, 22], a broader understanding is needed with regard to how

Table 6 Content analysis of decision making about fertility preservation

Question	Theme	N	Examples
How did you make a decision to undertake fertility preservation?	Individual's desire to have the option	11	"I decided to undertaken fertility preservation in case I still want to have children in the future" "I wanted to have children one day. I knew that soon my window would close and that my only option was to store sperm"
	Encouraged by medical professionals	4	"Recommended by health carers prior to starting HRT" "I started seeing an endocrinologist at a children's hospital who brought up the prospect of fertility preservation"
	Encouraged by partner	3	"Wife wanted kids" "I was neutral on the issue and my partner felt strongly about having the option"
	Encouraged by family members	4	"My parents thought the procedure would be a good idea" "My mother is insistent on having grandchildren"
How did you make the decision not to undertake fertility preservation?	Cost was prohibitive	44	"It was not available to me due to the sheer cost of it" "I was not going to be able to afford it"
	Not interested in genetic relationships and/or children	35	"Don't want genetic children, therefore fertility preservation is a non issue to me" "Never wanted children"
	Thought of children as dysphoria inducing	34	"I do not want children that are made through my genes. I do not want to bear children myself. The idea of childbirth adds to my dysphoria" "Conceiving and birthing a child sickens me and would humiliate me as a man"
	Have enough children already	20	"Nine children is enough" "I already have two children"
	Did not want to delay transition	11	"I wanted to begin my transition immediately as my priority was to treat the dysphoria. Future children were not a consideration" "Postponing hormones for possibly years until I was at the stage of my life to consider children was never an option"
	No genetic material available	11	"I can't have children anymore due to a genetic disorder" "I had cancer and chemo early which meant that I had no material to store regardless of transition"

diverse cohorts of transgender and non-binary people experience fertility preservation, as well as their thoughts on fertility and its relationship to gender more broadly. This may include research that explores in detail why many transgender and non-binary do not intend to have children, and how this relates to normative understandings of adulthood [23]. In other words, whilst it is important that researchers continue to investigate how transgender and non-binary people make decisions about fertility preservation, it is also important that researchers investigate how transgender and non-binary people choose to be child-free in the face of social norms about reproduction. In addition, future research could consider the experiences of transgender and non-binary people who undertake fertility preservation, including in terms of their desires to have children, and how they are impacted on by cisgenderism and norms around families and parenthood. Genetic reproduction and parenting, then, are but one part of the broader picture related to the decisions that transgender and non-binary people make about their lives.

Conclusions

Given that the WPATH SOC [1] are currently under revision, the findings reported in this paper offer important insights. The current SOC include the suggestion that fertility preservation should be encouraged. The findings reported in this paper suggest a more cautious approach, one that most certainly involves raising the topic of fertility preservation and exploring all options, but which acknowledges that potentially for a majority of transgender people fertility preservation will not be of interest, and that for many non-binary people fertility preservation remains an option, depending on any medical treatments undertaken (and the barriers to these that may exist, as noted in the introduction to this paper). Importantly, however, for those in the present study who had not undertaken fertility preservation, the greatest number who had *not* received advice or counselling about this were non-binary people. This suggests the need for greater awareness about the importance of discussing fertility preservation options with non-binary people, both amongst clinicians who work with non-binary people, and non-binary people themselves.

Finally, and given that the average age of participants in the present study who had undertaken fertility preservation was relatively young, this suggests that whether or not encouraging fertility preservation is useful will likely depend on the age of the person.

In terms of the wider clinical relevance of the findings, it is suggested that a focus on the meaning or importance of genetic relatedness may be a useful heuristic through which to provide counselling to transgender and non-binary people considering fertility preservation. This point may be especially salient given that those who had undertaken fertility preservation reported that they were on average only somewhat likely to use stored gametes in the future. Considering the high costs of fertility preservation including ongoing storage fees (alongside future costs of using the stored gametes), encouraging all transgender and non-binary people to undertake fertility preservation may not necessarily indicate best outcomes. Given the many pathways to parenthood available to transgender and non-binary people, other options besides genetic relatedness may be explored in order to mitigate the costs of fertility preservation if genetic relatedness is not viewed as important.

Abbreviations
LGBT: Lesbian, gay, bisexual and transgender; SOC: Standards of Care; SPSS: Statistical Package for the Social Sciences; WPATH: World Professional Association for Transgender Health

Acknowledgements
The authors wish to thank the organisations and groups who shared the questionnaire, as well as the participants who shared their experiences and views. They would also like to thank the members of TransMasc SA who provided feedback on the questionnaire.

Funding
This work was in part supported by the Australian Research Council under a Future Fellowship (FT130100087) awarded to the first author.

Authors' contributions
DR conceptualised the initial idea for the study and questionnaire. DR drafted the questionnaire and ethics application, and CB provided feedback on these. CB identified relevant organisations and groups to recruit participants and made contact with them. CB wrote the literature review. DR and CB wrote the methods section. DR analysed the questionnaire data and wrote the analysis and discussion sections. The full paper was reviewed by DR and CB prior to submission. DR and CB undertook all revisions. Both authors read and approved the final manuscript.

Authors' information
DR is an Associate Professor in social work at Flinders University, and an Australian Research Council Future Fellow. He is the author of over 200 publications, including the co-author of the book (with Clemence Due) *A critical approach to surrogacy: Reproductive desires and demands* (Routledge, 2018). CB is a Research Associate in the College of Education, Psychology and Social Work at Flinders University. She is the co-author of the book *Transgender people and education* with Damien Riggs (Palgrave Macmillan, 2017).

Competing interests
The authors declare that they have no competing interests.

References
1. World Professional Association for Transgender Health. Standards of care for the health of transsexual, transgender, and gender nonconforming people, 7th version; 2011.
2. De Roo C, Tilleman K, T'Sjoen G, De Sutter P. Fertility options in transgender people. Int Rev Psychiatr. 2016;28:112–9.
3. Clark BA, Veale JF, Townsend M, Frohard-Dourlent H, Saewyc E. Non-binary youth: access to gender-affirming primary health care. Int J Transgend. 2018;19:158–69.
4. Smith M. The baby game: how to make babies in a transgender relationship. Polare. 2010;2010:84.
5. James SE, Herman JL, Rankin S, Keisling M, Mottet L, Anafi M. The report of the 2015 U.S. transgender survey. Washington, DC: National Center for Transgender Equality; 2016. https://transequality.org/sites/default/files/docs/usts/USTS-Full-Report-Dec17.pdf. Accessed 20 Mar 2018
6. Pyne J, Bauer G, Bradley K. Transphobia and other stressors impacting trans parents. J GLBT Fam Stud. 2015;11:107–26.
7. Riggs DW, Power J, von Doussa H. Parenting and Australian trans and gender diverse people: an exploratory survey. Int J Transgend. 2016;17:59–65.
8. Mitu K. Fertility preservation: Technologies in search of users: Unpublished doctoral thesis. New York: Rensselaer Polytechnic Institute; 2016.
9. Tornello SL, Bos H. Parenting intentions among transgender individuals. LGBT Health. 2017;4:115–20.
10. von Doussa H, Power J, Riggs DW. Imagining parenthood: the possibilities and experiences of parenthood among transgender people. Cult Health Sex. 2015;17:1119–31.
11. De Sutter P, Kira K, Verschoor A, Hotimsky A. The desire to have children and the preservation of fertility in transsexual women: a survey. Int J Transgend. 2002;6.
12. Wierckx K, Van Caenegem E, Pennings G, Elaut E, Dedecker D, Van de Peer F, Weyers S, De Sutter P, T'Sjoen G. Reproductive wish in transsexual men. Hum Reprod. 2012;27:483–7.
13. Wierckx K, Stuyver I, Weyers S, Hamada A, Agarwal A, De Sutter P, T'Sjoen G. Sperm freezing in transsexual women. Arch Sex Behav. 2012;41:1069–71.
14. Chen D, Simons L, Johnson EK, Lockart BA, Finlay C. Fertility preservation for transgender adolescents. J Adolescent Health. 2017;61:120–3.
15. Nahata L, Tishelman AC, Caltabellotta NM, Quinn GP. Low fertility preservation utilization among transgender youth. J Adolescent Health. 2017;61:40–4.
16. Jones CA, Reiter L, Greenblatt E. Fertility preservation in transgender patients. Int J Transgend. 2016;17:76–82.
17. Armuand G, Dhejne C, Olofsson J, Rodriguez-Wallberg K. Transgender men's experiences of fertility preservation – a qualitative study. Hum Reprod. 2017;32:383–90.
18. Millar A, Kim BHK, Livne-Segev D, Fung R, Jarvi K, Millar AC. Attitudes, knowledge and beliefs regarding fertility preservation among people of transgendered experience: preliminary results. Can J Diabetes. 2015;39:536.
19. Strang JF, Jarin J, Call D, Clark B, Wallace GL, Anthony LG, Kenworthy L, Gomez-Lobo V. Transgender youth fertility attitudes questionnaire: measure development in nonautistic and autistic transgender youth and their parents. J Adolescent Health. 2018;62:128–35.
20. Hsieh HF. Shannon SE (2005). Three approaches to qualitative content analysis. Qual Hlth Res. 2005;15:1277–88.
21. Riggs DW, Due C. Support for family diversity: a three-country study. J Reprod Infant Psych. 2018;36:192–206.
22. James-Abra S, Tarasoff LA, green d, Epstein R, Anderson S, Marvel S, Steele LS, Ross LE. Trans people's experiences with assisted reproduction services: a qualitative study. Hum Reprod. 2015;30:1365–74.
23. Riggs DW, Bartholomaeus C. 'It's just what you do': Australian middle class heterosexual couples negotiating compulsory parenthood. Fem Psychol. 2017;28:373–89.

Permissions

List of Contributors

Prasanna Raj Supramaniam, Monica Mittal and Lee Nai Lim
Oxford University Hospitals NHS Foundation Trust, John Radcliffe Hospital, Headley Way, Headington, Oxford OX3 9DU, UK

Enda McVeigh
Nuffield Department of Women's and Reproductive Health, University of Oxford, Level 3, Women's Centre, John Radcliffe Hospital, Oxford OX3 9DU, UK

Jane Cover and Jeanette Lim
PATH, Seattle, WA 98109, USA

Allen Namagembe and Justine Tumusiime
PATH, Kampala, Uganda

Carie Muntifering Cox
St Catherine University, St. Paul Campus, 2004 Randolph Ave, St. Paul, MN 55105, USA

Heba H. Hijazi and Mohammad S. Alyahya
Department of Health Management and Policy, Faculty of Medicine, Jordan University of Science and Technology, Irbid 22110, Jordan

Amer M. Sindiani
Department of Obstetrics and Gynecology, Faculty of Medicine, Jordan University of Science and Technology, Irbid 22110, Jordan

Rola S. Saqan
Department of Pediatrics and Neonatology, Faculty of Medicine, Jordan University of Science and Technology, Irbid 22110, Jordan

Abdulhakeem M. Okour
Department of Public Health and Community Medicine, Faculty of Medicine, Jordan University of Science and Technology, Irbid 22110, Jordan

Hashini Nilushika Galappaththi-Arachchige
Norwegian Centre for Imported and Tropical Diseases, Department of Infectious Diseases Ullevaal, Oslo University Hospital, Postboks 4956 Nydalen, 0424 Oslo, Norway
Institute of Clinical Medicine, University of Oslo, Oslo, Norway

Siphosenkosi G. Zulu
Department of Infection Prevention and Control, Nelson R Mandela School of Medicine, College of Health Sciences, University of KwaZulu-Natal, Durban, South Africa

Elisabeth Kleppa and Kristine Lillebo
Norwegian Centre for Imported and Tropical Diseases, Department of Infectious Diseases Ullevaal, Oslo University Hospital, Postboks 4956 Nydalen, 0424 Oslo, Norway

Erik Qvigstad
Institute of Clinical Medicine, University of Oslo, Oslo, Norway
Department of Gynaecology, Women and Children's Division, Ullevaal University Hospital, Oslo, Norway

Patricia Ndhlovu
Imperial College London, Hammersmith Campus, London, UK

Birgitte Jyding Vennervald
Section for Parasitology and Aquatic Pathobiology, Faculty of Health and Medical Sciences, University of Copenhagen, Copenhagen, Denmark

Svein Gunnar Gundersen
Research Unit, Sorlandet Hospital, Kristiansand, Norway
Department of Global Development and Planning, University of Agder, Kristiansand, Norway

Eyrun Floerecke Kjetland
Norwegian Centre for Imported and Tropical Diseases, Department of Infectious Diseases Ullevaal, Oslo University Hospital, Postboks 4956 Nydalen, 0424 Oslo, Norway
Discipline of Public Health Medicine, Nelson R Mandela School of Medicine, College of Health Sciences, University of KwaZulu-Natal, Durban, South Africa

Myra Taylor
Discipline of Public Health Medicine, Nelson R Mandela School of Medicine, College of Health Sciences, University of KwaZulu-Natal, Durban, South Africa

Lilian T. Mselle
Department of Clinical Nursing, Muhimbili University of Health and Allied Sciences, Dar es Salaam, Tanzania

Thecla W. Kohi
Department of Nursing Management, Muhimbili University of Health and Allied Sciences, Dar es Salaam, Tanzania

Justine Dol
Faculty of Health, Dalhousie University, Halifax, Canada

Fidèle Mbadu Muanda
Programme National de Santé de la Reproduction (National Program for Reproductive Health) and Programme National de Santé de l'Adolescent (National Program for Adolescent Health), Ministry of Health, Avenue des Cliniques n 43/cliniques kinoises, Commune de la Gombe, Kinshasa, Democratic Republic of Congo

Ndongo Parfait Gahungu
L'Institut Supérieur de Développement Rural, Avenue des Cliniques n 43/cliniques kinoises, Commune de la Gombe, Kinshasa, Democratic Republic of Congo

Francine Wood
Department of Global Community Health and Behavioral Sciences, Tulane University School Public Health and Tropical Medicine, 1440 Canal Street, New Orleans, LA 70112, USA

Jane T. Bertrand
Department of Global Health Management and Policy, Tulane University School Public Health and Tropical Medicine, 1440 Canal Street, New Orleans, LA 70112, USA

Ulrika Rehnström Loi, Matilda Lindgren and Elisabeth Faxelid
Department of Public Health Sciences/IHCAR, Karolinska Institutet, SE-171 77 Stockholm, Sweden

Monica Oguttu
College of Health Sciences, School of Nursing Sciences, University of Nairobi, Nairobi, Kenya
Kisumu Medical Education Trust (KMET), Kisumu, Kenya

Marie Klingberg-Allvin
Department of Women's and Children's Health, Karolinska Institutet, SE-171 77 Stockholm, Sweden
School of Education, Health and Social Studies, Dalarna University, Högskolegatan 2, 791 31 Falun, Sweden

Anna Maria van Eijk, Linda Mason, Kelly Alexander and Penelope A. Phillips-Howard
Department of Clinical Sciences, Liverpool School of Tropical Medicine (LSTM) Pembroke Place, Liverpool L3 5AQ, UK

Kayla F. Laserson
Centre for Global Health Research, Kenya Medical Research Institute (KEMRI), Kisumu, Kenya

Division of Global Health Protection, Center for Global Health, Centers for Disease Control and Prevention (CDC), Atlanta, USA

Elizabeth Nyothach, Kelvin Oruko, David Obor, John Vulule and Clifford Oduor
Centre for Global Health Research, Kenya Medical Research Institute (KEMRI), Kisumu, Kenya

Jackton Omoto
Department of Obstetrics and Gynaecology, Siaya District Hospital, Ministry of Health, Siaya, Kenya

Aisha Mohammed
Division of Reproductive Health, Ministry of Health, Nairobi, Kenya

Alie Eleveld
Safe Water and AIDS Project, Kisumu, Kenya

Isaac Ngere
Ministry of Health, Siaya County, Kenya.

Godfrey Mbaruku, Robert Tillya, Selemani Mbuyita, Zacharia Mtema, Iddajovana Kinyonge, Ritha Godfrey and Silas Temu
Ifakara Health Institute, Dar es Salaam, Tanzania

Michelle Skaer Therrien and Suellen Miller
University of California, San Francisco, School of Medicine, Department of Obstetrics, Gynecology, and Reproductive Sciences, Safe Motherhood Program, California, USA

Philip Teg-Nefaah Tabong and Philip Baba Adongo
Department of Social and Behavioural Sciences, School of Public Health, University of Ghana, Accra, Ghana

Ernest Tei Maya
Department of Population, Family and Reproductive Health, School of Public Health, University of Ghana, Accra, Ghana

Terence Adda-Balinia, Dela Kusi-Appouh and Placide Tabsoba
Population Council, Accra, Ghana

Harriet Birungi
Population Council, City, Nairobi, Kenya

Gro Møller Christoffersen
University of Copenhagen, Faculty of Health and Medical Sciences, Blegdamsvej 3, 2200 Copenhagen N, Denmark

Peter James Bruhn
Department of Surgical Gastroenterology, Copenhagen University Hospital North Zealand, Dyrehavevej 29, 3400 Hillerød, Denmark

Rosanna de Neergaard
Department of Emergency Medicine, Zealand University Hospital Slagelse, Ingemannsvej 50, 4200 Slagelse, Denmark

Susanne Engel
Department of Culture, Municipality of Sermersooq, Kuussuaq 2, 3900 Nuuk, Greenland

Vibeke Naeser
Department of Obstetrics and Gynecology, Zealand University Hospital Næstved, Ringstedgade 61, 4700 Næstved, Denmark

Karen Hobday and Suzanne Belton
Menzies School of Health Research, Charles Darwin University, Darwin, Australia

Jennifer Hulme
Department of Emergency Medicine, University Health Network, University of Toronto, Toronto, Canada
Department of Family and Community Medicine, University of Toronto, Toronto, Canada

Caroline Homer
Centre for Midwifery, Child and Family Health, Faculty of Health, University of Technology Sydney, Sydney, Australia
Honorary Fellow, Menzies School of Health Research, Charles Darwin University, Darwin, Australia
Maternal and Child Health Program, Burnet Institute, Melbourne, Australia

Páscoa Zualo Wate
Centre for Midwifery, Child and Family Health, Faculty of Health, University of Technology Sydney, Sydney, Australia

Ndola Prata
Bixby Center for Population, Health and Sustainability, School of Public Health, University of California, Berkeley, USA

Precious Madula
School of Journalism and Information Communication, Huazhong University of Science and Technology, 1037 Luoyu, Road, Wuhan 430074, People's Republic of China
Mzuzu University, Private Bag 201, Luwinga, Mzuzu 2, Malawi

Fatch Welcome Kalembo and Atipatsa Chiwanda Kaminga
Mzuzu University, Private Bag 201, Luwinga, Mzuzu 2, Malawi

Hong Yu
School of Journalism and Information Communication, Huazhong University of Science and Technology, 1037 Luoyu, Road, Wuhan 430074, People's Republic of China

Carine Asnong and Emma Plugge
Centre for Tropical Medicine and Global Health, Nuffield Department of Medicine, University of Oxford, Oxford OX3 7FZ, UK

Gracia Fellmeth
Nuffield Department of Population Health, University of Oxford, Old Road Campus, Headington, Oxford OX3 7FZ, UK

Nan San Wai, Mupawjay Pimanpanarak and Moo Kho Paw
Shoklo Malaria Research Unit, Mahidol-Oxford Tropical Medicine Research Unit, Mahidol University, Mae Sot 63110, Thailand

Prakaykaew Charunwatthana
Mahidol-Oxford Tropical Medicine Research Unit, Mahidol University, Bangkok 10400, Thailand

François Nosten and Rose McGready
Centre for Tropical Medicine and Global Health, Nuffield Department of Medicine, University of Oxford, Oxford OX3 7FZ, UK
Shoklo Malaria Research Unit, Mahidol-Oxford Tropical Medicine Research Unit, Mahidol University, Mae Sot 63110, Thailand

Tesfaye Yitna Chichiabellu
Department of Nursing, College of Health Science and Medicine, Wolaita Sodo University, Wolaita Sodo, Ethiopia

Baze Mekonnen
Department of Nursing, School of nursing and midwifery, Addis Ababa University, Addis Ababa, Ethiopia

Feleke Hailemichael Astawesegn
School of Public Health, College of Medicine and Health Science, Hawassa University, Hawassa, Ethiopia

Birhanu Wondimeneh Demissie
Department of Nursing, College of Health Science and Medicine, Wolaita Sodo University, Sodo, Ethiopia

Antehun Alemayehu Anjulo
Department of Medical Laboratory, College of Health Science and Medicine, Wolaita Sodo University, Sodo, Ethiopia

Umesh Charanthimath, Chandrashekhar Karadiguddi, Avinash Kavi, Anjali Joshi and Geetanjali Mungarwadi
KLE Academy of Higher Education and Research's, J N Medical College, Belagavi, Karnataka, India

Marianne Vidler, Sumedha Sharma and Beth A. Payne
Department of Obstetrics and Gynaecology, and the Child and Family Research Unit, University of British, Columbia, Vancouver, BC, Canada

Geetanjali Katageri
Department of Obstetrics and Gynaecology, S Nijalingappa Medical College, Bagalkot, Karnataka, India

Umesh Ramadurg
Department of Community Medicine, S Nijalingappa Medical College, Bagalkot, Karnataka, India

Sheshidhar Bannale
Department of Pharmacology, S Nijalingappa Medical College, Bagalkot, Karnataka, India

Sangamesh Rakaraddi
Department of Anatomy, S Nijalingappa Medical College, Bagalkot, Karnataka, India

Diane Sawchuck
Department of Research, Vancouver Island Health Authority, Victoria, BC, Canada

Rahat Qureshi
Division of Women and Child Health, Aga Khan University, Karachi, Sindh, Pakistan

Peter von Dadelszen
School of Life Course Sciences, Faculty of Life Sciences and Medicine, King's College London, London, England

Richard Derman
Department Kings of Obstetrics, Thomas Jefferson University, Philadelphia, PA, USA

Damien W. Riggs and Clare Bartholomaeus
College of Education, Psychology and Social Work, Flinders University, Adelaide, SA 5001, Australia

Index

* 9 7 8 1 6 3 2 4 1 7 6 1 9 *